SARS Stories

SINOTHEORY

A series edited by Carlos Rojas and Eileen Cheng-yin Chow

BELINDA KONG

SARS Stories

AFFECT AND ARCHIVE
OF THE 2003 PANDEMIC

DUKE UNIVERSITY PRESS
Durham and London
2024

© 2024 DUKE UNIVERSITY PRESS
All rights reserved
Printed in the United States of America on acid-free paper ∞
Project Editor: Bird Williams
Designed by A. Mattson Gallagher
Typeset in Adobe Text Pro, Avenir LT Std, and Moonglow
by Westchester Publishing Services

Library of Congress Cataloging-in-Publication Data
Names: Kong, Belinda, [date] author.
Title: Sars stories : affect and archive of the 2003 Pandemic /
Belinda Kong.
Other titles: Sinotheory.
Description: Durham : Duke University Press, 2024. | Series:
Sinotheory | Includes bibliographical references and index.
Identifiers: LCCN 2023015275 (print)
LCCN 2023015276 (ebook)
ISBN 9781478025665 (paperback)
ISBN 9781478020929 (hardcover)
ISBN 9781478027812 (ebook)
Subjects: LCSH: SARS (Disease)—Social aspects—China. |
Epidemics in literature. | Pandemics—Social aspects—China—
History. | Pandemics—China—History. | SARS (Disease)—
China—History. | Racism—Health aspects. | Health and race. |
BISAC: HEALTH & FITNESS / Diseases & Conditions /
Contagious (incl. Pandemics) | SOCIAL SCIENCE / Ethnic
Studies / Asian Studies
Classification: LCC RA644.S17 K664 2024 (print)
LCC RA644.S17 (ebook)
DDC 362.1962--dc23/eng/20231024
LC record available at https://lccn.loc.gov/2023015275
LC ebook record available at https://lccn.loc.gov/2023015276

Cover art: Fong So 方蘇, *School Closed* (停課), 2003. Ink and
color on paper, 153 × 97 cm. From the series *Hong Kong 2003*
(香港 2003). Courtesy of the artist.

CONTENTS

vii Acknowledgments

1 **Introduction**

33 **1** **Pandemic Ordinariness**
Epidemic Romances and Female Sentiments

77 **2** **Pandemic Humor**
Digital Prosociality for the Epidemic Socius

112 **3** **Pandemic Resilience**
Deextinction and the Hong Kong Cantophone

180 **4** **Pandemic First Patients**
Deperilizing the Anglophone SARS Archive

238 **Afterword**

241 Notes
267 Bibliography
285 Index

ACKNOWLEDGMENTS

Though the origins of this book predate COVID-19, the current pandemic has given me a deeper appreciation for professional collegiality and connectivity. Especially when one is writing about Chinese experiences and sinophone cultures in as remote a place as Maine, and for a decade at a time, an invitation to present one's ongoing work and share still ripening ideas can seem a gift of community, something few of us now take for granted. Looking back over the time since the beginnings of this project, I want to express my gratitude to the many colleagues both near and far who have sustained faith in the value of this work. First and foremost, I thank Carlos Rojas, who has provided so many opportunities for my writing over the years, and whose superhuman ability to curate a million projects and "workshops" at any given time never ceases to amaze me. Thanks, too, to Andrea Bachner, who, along with Carlos, welcomed me to Duke University in 2014 for the Modern Chinese Literatures Workshop, and also to Angelina Chin, who invited me to my first Association for Asian Studies panel that year, back when I still thought my book was about biocapitalism! More locally, I thank David Hecht for organizing the Health Studies Workshop at Bowdoin College in 2018, Nancy Riley for budding up with me to present, and Priscilla Wald for her encouragement on the project at the time. Thanks to Kuei-fen Chiu and Yingjin Zhang, whose theme issue in *Modern Chinese Literature and Culture* gave me my first public forum for thinking through ideas of ordinariness. In March 2020, when everything moved online, Shiqi Lin and Kaiyang Xu were the first to introduce me to the notion of a "cloud panel," and theirs remains one of the earliest and most memorable of what has become a pandemic norm. Thanks to John Corso-Esquivel for inviting me to the Center for Public Humanities at Oakland University and giving me the chance to present part of this project when it took the reparative turn for good. Thanks to Jack Chen, for inviting me to present at the University of Virginia Asian Cosmopolitanisms Lab a portion of the book's final chapter as it was coming together. I am also grateful to Karen Kingsbury and Jie Zhang, who welcomed me onto their centennial panel on Eileen Chang at the 2021 ASIANetwork conference and fulfilled one of my lifelong dreams of being counted among Eileen Chang scholars. The camaraderie and intellectuality of this panel, which included Sherry Mou, Hsiu-Chuang Deppman, and Jiwei Xiao, makes me proud to do Asian Studies in the liberal arts. Thanks as well to Jing Zhang for allowing me to bring my research and teaching together in an activist forum for the powerful conversation at the New College of Florida on race, gender, and class-based violence soon after the tragic Atlanta spa shootings in 2021. Finally, thanks again to Carlos Rojas and to Keren He, for their 2022 Modern Language Association and Association for Asian Studies panels, respectively, and the inspiring conversations there with Michael Berry, Shiqi Lin, Haiyan Lee, Chris Berry, Roy Chan, and Ari Heinrich.

At various stages and in ways big and small, this project has also benefited from the support of innumerable people. I am grateful to the National Endowment for the Humanities for funding this book at its inception, and to Bowdoin College for funding two crucial sabbaticals during which I began and then completed the manuscript. Thanks also to Lynne Anderson at *The Conversation* for keen editorial instincts that gave me my first affirmation of the reparative approach to COVID material. To Jaeyeon Yoo for editorial perspicacity on through lines when I couldn't see them myself. To Eina Zhang for extraordinary advocacy and for pitching my piece to *b2o*—I am ever so grateful! To Shaohua Guo for brilliant and incisive feedback as much as C-drama tips for self-care. To Rachel Sturman for constant friendship and trusted counsel and Aquarian sisterhood, and for saying "Fly free, Belinda!" And to the countless students, colleagues, and friends at Bowdoin College who have nurtured and uplifted, mentored and affirmed, encouraged and inspired me through the years, especially Jeanne Bamforth, Rachel Beane, Nadia Celis, Connie Chiang, Paul Hoffman, Nancy Riley, Jayanthi Selinger, Jeff Selinger, Shu-chin Tsui, Dharni Vasudevan, Anthony Walton, Leah Zuo, and my colleagues in the Asian Studies Program and the English Department—I am grateful for your light. Finally, to the editorial team at Duke University Press: to Bird Williams, Chad Royal, James Moore, and Karen Carroll for shepherding the manuscript through the production stages; to Ryan Kendall for tirelessly and always cheerfully fielding my plethora of micro questions; and to Ken Wissoker for helping me distill the heart of this project and expertly guiding its writing to closure, in what has felt like an epic journey.

To my family, Jim and Yong Wilshire: from you I learn loyalty and heart, fierceness and compassion, dignity and humaneness, the values that I hope most animate this book; thank you for being my second parents. To Miu Ling Kong: thank you for safekeeping memories of our Hong Kong childhood and for sending masks that put a smile (and Little Twin Stars) on my face in those early COVID days. To Gail and Evan Thompson: thank you for opening your homes and hearts to me and for sharing seafood and dim sum (and so many enticing food photos). And to Hilary Thompson: you are the guiding spirit and grounding force who reminds me every day what it means to stay true to creative life. May the vegetables we muse among have the greatest longevity in the world.

After going through this nightmare summer together,
Will you and I face each other with greater humaneness?

Leung Ping-kwan (Ye Si),
"Love Poem in the Time of SARS"

Introduction

Prosociality in the Time of Pandemics

To not just survive the nightmare of disease but to feel greater humaneness toward each other as people—that is what matters in our experience of pandemics, so reflects the Hong Kong poet Leung Ping-kwan soon after the end of the 2003 SARS (severe acute respiratory syndrome) outbreak.[1] Yet reading the news during COVID-19 can wear down anyone's desire to feel embedded in a common world. To scrutinize constantly changing disease data and public health guidelines while wading through layers of partisan spin and georacial bias is often an exercise in selective attention, emotional calculation rather than social connectivity. Amid the protracted banalities of crisis, one has to turn to more mundane sources for comfort and strength, for meanings that arise from and abide within everyday life, and for an affirmative sense of peopleness to offset "affects of disaffection."[2] This book tells precisely these stories by looking back at the SARS pandemic, arguing for this archive's crucial significance especially in light of COVID-19. But we can also find a more recent example, a complex and revealing one, in the unexpected figure of a seventy-five-year-old Chinese grandmother reputedly turned onetime woman warrior.

On March 17, 2021—the morning after the Atlanta spa shootings that left eight people dead, six of them Asian women—Xie Xiao Zhen was punched in the face by a white male assailant while standing by a light pole at a San Francisco street intersection. In the ensuing days, her story went viral across both anglophone and sinophone media worldwide, not as yet another tragic example of anti-Asian violence and victimhood during COVID but as a tale of unexpected liveliness in dark times. Early news footage showed Xie at the scene afterward, left hand holding an ice pack to her swollen face and right hand brandishing a wooden board as she animatedly cursed her assailant in Taishanese, while he lay dazed and bloody-mouthed on a stretcher surrounded by police officers.[3] "Elderly Asian Woman Attacked in San Francisco Fights Back, Sends Alleged Attacker to Hospital," headlined multiple American news outlets appreciatively that week, citing eyewitness accounts of Xie "pummeling" her attacker.[4] Mainland Chinese news soon followed with features on "Overseas Chinese Grandma Suffers Attack but Forcefully Strikes Back" and "Granny Attacked in US Counterstrikes with All Her Might!"[5] Xie's grandson launched a GoFundMe campaign to help raise money for her medical expenses, and, within a week, the fund accrued almost one million dollars. Xie then decided to donate the money back toward fighting anti-Asian racism, insisting that the "issue is bigger than her," thereby prompting another round of international coverage. "Asian Grandmother Who Smacked Her Attacker with a Board Donates Nearly $1 Million," reported NPR.[6] "Valiantly Fighting Back against Hoodlum, Overseas Chinese Grandma in San Francisco to Donate Crowdfunding Proceeds," proclaimed the North American Chinese-language newspaper *World Journal*.[7] Xie's family finally set up a nonprofit, diverting over 80 percent of the proceeds toward "protecting the AAPI community, promoting safety, and preventing any further increase in Asian hate crimes."[8] When the family offered to refund those who do not support this charity, numerous donors left messages that they were donating again to offset any refund requests.

Within three months, the YouTube video of Xie's post-attack tirade, uploaded by the local KPIX television station, had garnered over a million views.[9] In the comments section, thousands of netizens across different racial and ethnic groups and from various countries applauded Xie's courage and spirit while expressing their heartache for her suffering. "[She] deserves a medal," remarked more than one poster, while others enthusiastically proclaimed "Good job, Grandma!" and "Respect to grandma!" Racial care as well as racial anger and racial grief emerged as prominent themes among self-identifying Asians, even as other netizens of color conveyed solidarity with their "Asian brothers and sisters."[10] The incident also incited much fury and pride among Xie's fellow Taishanese in her hometown and in the diaspora. The Guangdong-based cartoon journalist Chen Chunming, himself from Taishan, was inspired to sketch Xie in the pose of a fierce martial artist wielding her wooden board like a sword and barking out "daa nei puk gaai"—a colloquial Cantonese vulgarism that can be doubly translated, Chen explained, as either "beat you bastard" or "beat you till you go to hell," as Xie had been filmed swearing at her assailant as a "sei puk gaai" ("goddamn bastard"). This droll cartoon, along with a short video Chen created of it with the theme song from the Wong Fei Hong movie franchise as background music, also went viral in the sinophone media, further elevating Xie to the status of transnational ethnic folk hero. When this meme reached back to Xie's San Francisco family and they conveyed their gratitude to Chen, the latter responded that he wished not only to pay tribute to the granny but also to communicate a spirit of ethnic solidarity, for "the overseas Chinese to unite together and not be afraid of bullying."[11]

From one perspective, Xie's story epitomizes a generative hub of pandemic prosociality. As different components of her story spread globally, prosocial words and deeds, sentiments and connections proliferated, at first revolving around Xie as an individual but rapidly fanning out to encompass a much wider socius. Admiration for her transformed into positive group identifications within and across identity lines, cohering around common feelings of concern and care. At a time when the coronavirus has resurrected vehement orientalist and sinophobic attitudes across the Western world—a topic I will address more fully in chapter 4—the many instances of altruistic rallying around Xie testify to a strong countercurrent of social affects and attachments that are not reducible to disease fear and xenophobia. Indeed, against the backdrop of the pandemic's negative social effects, her story stands out as all the more extraordinary, with her fire and generosity moving others to speak and behave in kind. It is as if the global socius has been hungry precisely for an affirmative model to replicate and reciprocate amid its sense of collective crisis—especially given that this attack occurred during not only a spike in anti-Asian hate crimes in the United States since the start of the pandemic but also an ancillary wave of violence targeting specifically Asian seniors since the start of 2021. In the Bay Area alone, the eighty-four-year-old Thai immigrant Vicha Ratanapakdee was fatally shoved to the ground while taking his daily constitutional around his San Francisco neighborhood in January, and just a week before Xie's assault, the seventy-five-year-old Hong Kong immigrant Pak Ho was punched in the face while taking his usual morning walk around Oakland's Chinatown; both men died of their brain injuries.[12] According to the nonprofit organization Stop AAPI Hate, the 3,795 anti-Asian hate incidents reported to their center during the pandemic period from March 2020 to February 2021 "represent only a fraction of the number of hate incidents that actually occur," but this fraction already showcases "how vulnerable Asian Americans are to discrimination." Physical assault constitutes over 11 percent of the total reports, with Chinese Americans making up over 42 percent of targeted subjects, the largest reporting ethnic group.[13] Within this distressing context, Xie's story readily takes on an aura of myth.

As it happens, though, two key elements of this myth—Xie's ferocious thrashing of her attacker and the attacker's racial motivation—have been destabilized by new evidence. Steven Jenkins, Xie's assailant, turns out to be a homeless man with a history of mental illness who himself was the target of an unprovoked group assault just five minutes before encountering Xie. A seven-minute surveillance video released by the San Francisco Public Defender's Office shows Jenkins being punched and kicked forty times by four different people a few blocks away, and, when he walked off, he was followed by one of his attackers, who struck him five more times in the head before he escaped again. The second beating took place about ten yards from where Xie stood by her light pole, apparently hawking goods on the sidewalk like many street vendors in the city. Even as Jenkins ran from his attacker, the latter continued to tail him threateningly, prompting Jenkins to punch into the empty air in self-defense. As he reeled and flailed, in the seconds before he hit nearby Xie, his attacker was mere feet away on the other side of the pole. Security cameras also captured how, contrary to prevailing versions of the incident, Xie did not "pummel" Jenkins until he was down and immobilized. Instead, a security guard tackled Jenkins to the ground seconds after he struck Xie, at which point she picked up a wooden stick and slapped Jenkins's feet with it several times, as a crowd gathered and the police arrived.[14] According to Jenkins's lawyer, even before Jenkins approached Xie, he was already "bloodied ... disoriented and possibly concussed."[15]

This narrative approximates what Xie herself recounted to her local Chinese television station the day after. In this phone interview, Xie protested: "I'm seventy-some years old and he's only thirty-something, how on earth could I fight him? Some people are saying I bullied him, but when did I do that? The police pushed him and he fell into the concrete. Only then did I pick up a wooden stick from the street and hit the bottom of his feet a few times. That's all! I didn't beat him up!"[16] Even by Xie's own account, her fighting back was belated and negligible, not the phenomenal smackdown of viral lore. As Jenkins's defense attorney, Eric McBurney, writes in a press statement: "This situation is a tragedy on many fronts," with Jenkins as much a "victim" as Xie. Recognizing the larger context of escalated racial violence against Asian Americans during COVID but rejecting racism as a motivation for Xie's assault, McBurney highlights instead social apathy toward those experiencing homelessness and mental illness as contributing factors to this multilateral tragedy.[17] As he points out, the attacks on Jenkins happened "in broad daylight while pedestrians went about their business near the Farmers' Market" and "in the busy UN Plaza," with "not one person com[ing] to his aid."[18] McBurney himself is Asian American, born in Taiwan and adopted by a white family; having grown up "in small towns across the South" where he, as he puts it, was "the entire Asian population," he too understands unbelonging, he says, only too well.[19]

Additional details may continue to emerge around this case to complicate easy narratives and conclusions, but, for now, we can draw out a few themes. Most prominently, Xie's story has catalyzed a wave of surprising prosociality amid the tensions and divisions wrought by COVID. This pandemic prosociality takes forms both big and minute—as headline news and microaffirmations, crowdsourcing campaigns and small donations, social media activism and digital humor, cross-racial empathy and diasporic camaraderie. Many of these elements will reappear throughout this book in my examination of the 2003 SARS outbreak and its cultures of epidemic life. Furthermore, the prosociality precipitated by Xie's incident is transnational and translingual, and, while neither revolutionary nor permanent, it has been serially generative, activating innumerable instances of dispositions and emotions geared

INTRODUCTION　5

toward the well-being of others, including remote strangers and overseas communities. Recently, a group of evolutionary biologists and social scientists has theorized this concept of prosociality as not just a loose set of ideal principles but a "broad evolutionary worldview." In their book *Prosocial*, Paul Atkins, David Sloan Wilson, and Steven Hayes advance prosociality as an alternative framework to neoliberal paradigms of competition and self-interest, one that has the potential, they argue, to transform the lived human world by fostering multilevel relations of cooperation and care and creating "prosocial ecosystems" on a global scale.[20] Their book's opening example also involves an infectious disease outbreak: they describe how volunteer aid workers in Sierra Leone during the 2014–16 West African Ebola epidemic collaborated with local villagers rather than "imposing solutions from the outside" and how the two groups worked in concert to find strategies for viral containment while "respecting local customs and values."[21] So, for theorists of the concept, epidemic epicenters can be prime sites for engendering global prosocial practices. Likewise, my giving pride of place to Xie's tale constitutes one small attempt at reshaping pandemic discourse away from reflexive tropes of planetary calamity toward underrated modes of micro prosociality, retextualizing the psychic and affective environment in which we think and feel global disease across lines of difference. That is the guiding spirit of this book.

At the same time, people's eagerness to latch onto Xie as an icon of heroism amid pandemic racism—a paragon of what we might call crisis extraordinariness—risks reproducing empirical falsehoods and social erasures. First and foremost, Xie's own voice and narration of events, already multiply subalternized within a global hierarchy of languages and their respective power in epidemic knowledge production, have been mostly overridden, even by her champions and admirers. (This thematic nexus of language, power, and pandemic knowledge will reappear in chapters 3 and 4.) Moreover, the pervasive attention to high-profile pandemic-related issues has worked to sideline other endemic problems that turn out to be directly relevant to Xie's case, such as housing and mental health insecurity among precarious populations. Indeed, the prosociality radiating out from Xie has very pointedly excluded both Jenkins, who is swiftly branded the racist villain by a transnational public with little regard for his circumstances, and McBurney, who has received not only hate mail from other Asian Americans but also disapproval from his Taiwanese family for defending Jenkins.[22] In an ironic manner, this overshadowing of entrenched conditions through a selective spotlighting of top headlines of the moment parallels what many Asian Americanist scholars have underscored about anti-Asian racism, that it is not new with COVID but a persistent problem dating back to nineteenth-century yellow peril ideologies. Exclusively highlighting Xie's singular resilience may obscure the resilience of systemic racism itself. From a more minor perspective, though, we can see McBurney's commitment to affording Jenkins legal justice and a fair trial, despite the opposing tide of public and familial opinion, as a secondary order of prosocial ethics, as he foregrounds the long-standing plight of those who are homeless and pleads for greater compassion toward them. What McBurney advocates is not a dismissal of the assault charges against Jenkins but the weighing of these charges alongside a sympathetic and justice-based recognition of the latter's everyday reality and experiential world. Jenkins deserves a fair hearing, he insists, especially in the face of collective outrage born from a crisis milieu.

Against Pandemic Crisis Epistemologies

In "Against Crisis Epistemology," Kyle Whyte makes a key distinction between crisis and what he calls epistemologies of crisis. While real crises such as climate change do exist, crisis epistemologies, he argues, are those "practices of knowing the world that ... use crisis to mask colonial power." Focusing on the history of settler colonialism and the oppression of Indigenous populations in North America, Whyte writes: "Colonisation is typically pitched as being about crisis. People who perpetrate colonialism often imagine that their wrongful actions are defensible because they are responding to some crisis. They assume that to respond to a crisis, it is possible to suspend certain concerns about justice and morality."[23] Moreover, crisis rhetoric often entails a "presentist unfolding of time," whereby "a certain present is experienced as new" rather than as a repetition of historically sedimented modes of power, and this "structure of newness ... permits the validation of oppression." Whyte isolates in particular two tenets within this crisis temporality: unprecedentedness and urgency. Crisis epistemologies, he notes, tend to construct each current crisis as unprecedented, with "few usable lessons from the past" and "the novelty of being complex beyond anything previously encountered." Furthermore, every crisis is cast as urgent and imminent, in need of rapid response and possibly severe sacrifices, regardless of "harmful consequences" that may be "unfortunate, but acceptable."[24]

This presentist mindset then operates to "mask numerous forms of power, including colonialism, imperialism, capitalism, patriarchy, and industrialization."[25] In effect, crisis epistemologies perpetuate historical violences in the name of new crises.

Whyte's framework is all too resonant in the time of COVID. Across almost all arenas, this pandemic has been labeled an unprecedented global crisis necessitating urgent action, whether in terms of its health, economic, political, or social impact. This language is adopted by the World Health Organization, United Nations, World Bank, US Department of Homeland Security, and countless governments and media outlets worldwide.[26] One Dictionary.com poll finds *unprecedented* to be one of the most overused words during COVID, but even the website's editorial team feels obliged to concede that, while the word is "on everyone's lips . . . they aren't wrong; this is an unprecedented situation."[27] The presumed truth of this cliché seems irrefutable even to its satirists. Although many of these authorities also espouse coordination and cooperation, hence departing from an explicit script of colonial rationality, their crisis rhetoric reflects the presentist temporality Whyte outlines—as if this coronavirus outbreak has no pertinent history and no comparable precursors, not even the widely cited 1918 influenza pandemic, thus paving the way to validate extraordinary emergency measures that are then used to retroactively normalize an oppressive status quo. In this context, even though Giorgio Agamben has been criticized for pushing his biopolitical thesis about the "invention of an epidemic" in COVID's early months, a position that eerily aligned with right-wing science denialism at the time, he was not wrong to worry about state deployments of power during a public health emergency, as a disease outbreak can serve as an "ideal pretext for scaling . . . up beyond any limitation" "exceptional measures" that suspend basic rights and freedoms, thereby normalizing an "authentic state of exception."[28] Indeed, these apprehensions are especially warranted if we excavate the history of power behind pre-COVID pandemic discourse.

When I began this book around 2014, I, too, was centrally preoccupied with the subject of pandemic biopower and its potential for global expansion and entrenchment. For it was precisely during and after the 2003 SARS outbreak that these same tropes of pandemic crisis came to be articulated and cemented and the same assertions of urgency and unprecedentedness were used to justify exceptional governance procedures. Back then too, SARS was cast as an unprecedented crisis via an idiom of "firsts," billed by health authorities and infectious disease experts as much as international news media as the twenty-first century's "first new virus," "first emerging disease," "first new disease threat," "first dangerous pathogen," "first new global epidemic," and "first pandemic."[29] The international law scholar David Fidler in his 2004 book on SARS dubbed it "an epidemic of firsts" and argued that SARS was "the world's first post-Westphalian pathogen," rendering obsolete the older global health paradigm of state sovereignty and nonintervention and inaugurating a new model whereby nonstate entities become "legitimate governance actors in their own right."[30] In fact, it was apropos of SARS that the World Health Organization (WHO), for the first time in its then fifty-five-year history, issued a region-specific infectious disease–related travel advisory, warning against all nonessential travel to Guangdong and Hong Kong.[31] The various travel restrictions during COVID are therefore not new but have a direct precedent in SARS and its effects on global health response strategies. It was also on the heels of SARS that the World Health Assembly, WHO's decision-making body, revised the International Health Regulations in 2005 to hold member states directly accountable to WHO oversight, thereby formalizing powers that WHO had exercised only extrajuridically during the outbreak period, such as collecting and disseminating disease information derived from nonstate sources and without state consent.[32]

Across international news outlets back then too, SARS was ubiquitously portrayed as the global health crisis that demanded urgent and drastic action. According to one front-page *New York Times* article that May, it was only through "aggressive steps" and "sheer luck" that the United States "escaped the full fury" of the virus.[33] This emphasis on toughness to avert worse luck was echoed, after the pandemic's end, by an international group of scientists who concluded that "the world community was very lucky this time round" partly because "fairly draconian public health measures could be put in place with great efficiency in Asian regions where the epidemic originated." Had SARS broken out in North America or Western Europe, they speculated, containment would have been much more challenging "given the litigious nature" of people in Western democracies.[34] Exceptional biopolitics in the interest of global health was thus outsourced to Asia, which was posited as less concerned with human and civil rights to begin with and hence less prone to be hurt by their infringement and suspension. If Sara Ahmed sheds light on the white supremacist and jingoist rationales behind the rhetoric of Britain as a "soft touch nation" vis-à-vis asylum seekers, the idiom of biopolitical toughness around SARS trod a finer line, allotting just enough "softness" to the West to validate its liberal humanist superiority

INTRODUCTION   9

and just enough "hardness" to Asia to justify its fortunate otherness but ultimate moral inferiority.[35] I will unravel this colonialist projection vis-à-vis China in chapter 1.

This neocolonial orientalist facet of contemporary pandemic crisis discourse formed my other core concern at the book's inception. When I first delved into the cultural archive on SARS representations in Western popular media, I was shocked by how frequently the doomsday imagery and lexicon about an impending disease apocalypse recycled age-old sinophobic associations of Chinese bodies with pollution, filth, and pestilence. Numerous magazines at the time resorted to orientalist tactics without hesitation or embarrassment—as if to flaunt, in accord with the logic Whyte pinpoints, how the present crisis of pandemic disease obviates the immorality and harm of parading old racist stereotypes. If anything, a current of nationalist bravado ran through exaggerated performances of sinophobia that deliberately conflated anti-Chinese racism with anticommunist geopolitics. An April 2003 issue of the *Economist*, for example, featured on its cover a manipulated image of Mao Zedong in a face mask and the caption "The SARS virus: Could it become China's Chernobyl?" Similarly, the cover of a May 2003 issue of *Time* displayed a red chest x-ray and the caption "SARS Nation" with China's national flag superimposed. These images played a double signifying game. On the one hand, they functioned to metaphorically contain the pandemic as a strictly national—China's—problem rather than a truly planetary or human one. On the other, they yoked biological and racial signifiers to a specifically Chinese geopolitical iconography, anachronistically revitalizing potent symbols from the past (Mao, the red flag) and resituating them within contemporary crisis contexts (face masks, respiratory viruses, global pandemics) to intimate an ever-present communist threat now newly biologized and globalized.

Elsewhere, I have analyzed this discourse as pandemic bio-orientalism.[36] The component strands of this discourse are long-standing, but they coalesced uniquely around China and pandemic outbreaks during SARS. Media coverage at the time frequently insinuated that China's entry into a modern capitalist world system brings with it new types of danger to global life, as the country's and its people's entrenched cultural, social, and political practices prove to be a fertile breeding ground for deadly emergent pathogens. As Mei Zhan has argued, international debates surrounding the "zoonotic origin" of SARS at the time ultimately blamed the virus not on environmental factors but on "Chinese people's uncanny affinity with the nonhuman and the

10 INTRODUCTION

wild ... and the deadly filthiness of such entanglements." These "accusatory ambivalences," she notes, reflected not just familiar schemata of orientalist othering but also contemporary neoliberal anxieties about China's rising middle class and its "visceral practices of consumption."[37] In multiple ways, post-SARS pandemic discourse came to exceptionalize China as the planet's disease "ground zero"—a presumption that has become all too commonplace again during COVID, especially with the initial branding of the coronavirus as a "China virus" or "Wuhan virus." I will return to these perilizing motifs in the anglophone SARS archive in chapter 4.

Pandemic discourse, then, exemplifies an epistemology of crisis. By framing each epidemic as new while erasing the trail of prior outbreaks—and, by extension, the history of previous power deployments as well as the fact of our repeated mass survival—pandemic discourse mediates a way of knowing the world that uses disease crises to mask and perpetuate racial and geopolitical power. This discourse aligns with what Lauren Berlant calls a "genre of crisis," insofar as our long-standing and ongoing human reality of living with microorganisms and experiencing periodic epidemics now gets narrativized as a novel crisis condition of our unprecedentedly globalized world, "rhetorically turning an ongoing condition into an intensified situation in which extensive threats to survival are said to dominate the reproduction of life."[38] Even a dozen years after SARS, the trope of imminent species doom persisted without the need for an actual successor pandemic, though international media fanned trepidation by putting the West African Ebola epidemic at the forefront of global health news in the mid-2010s. As a May 2015 *New Scientist* issue captioned on its cover—above a colorful image of a giant viral particle that, upon closer inspection, turns out be ringed at its outer edge with skulls and crossbones: "THE NEW PLAGUE, we're one mutation away from the end of the world as we know it."[39] Then as now, the language of newness underscores that our current era is not just a repetition of the old, that we are in unknown territory with alien and constantly mutating microbial menaces. The visual aestheticization of disease terror and suspicion further suggests that what appears at first to be an innocent and pleasing art image can have death lurking at the periphery, almost invisible and blended into the background, hence all the more in need of constant vigilance.

This representation of illegible surfaces and hidden dangers also reverberates back to SARS iconography. In international media coverage at the time, prevalent images of masked Asian faces and crowds likewise summoned a sense of potentially fatal inscrutability and urban density. As Priscilla Wald

INTRODUCTION　11

observes, Western cultural narratives of disease outbreaks typically follow formulaic conventions, one of which is a "geography of disease" where "timeless, brooding Africa or Asia" is imagined as "the birthplace of humanity, civilization, and deadly microbes." Infectious diseases are constructed as third-world problems "leaking" into the Global North, in a one-way traffic of emergence and contagion.[40] Exactly so, post-SARS pandemic discourse frequently envisages planetary destruction and human extinction via Asia and Asian-originating germs and carriers. A prime example is a February 2004 issue of *Time*, the cover of which showed a giant egg about to be hatched and a baby bird beak poking through a crack in its shell, with the headline posing the ominous question: "Bird Flu: Is Asia hatching the next human pandemic?" The article then turned to avian flu as the "latest scourge to emerge from Asia," "spreading with alarming speed through Asia's poultry farms." According to the article, "the great fear of health officials around the world is that the virus could, like SARS, jump the species barrier, mutate into a deadly and highly contagious form and set off a worldwide pandemic"; this "next deadly global epidemic" would be "a slate wiper," but what endangers the world is not just the virus itself but "dissembling and stalling by local governments [that] have already allowed the pathogen to spread in Asia— not only in birds but also among the men and women who raise them for a living and the kids who gather eggs or simply kick up infected dust in their villages."[41] Given the combination of Asia's corrupt governments, the poor hygiene and general level of medical ignorance of its rural residents, and the rapidity of international travel enabled by globalization, Asia, the article warned, stands to jeopardize not just public health the world over but our very species survival, so that even the experts are afraid. The underlying message was that, while we may ethically lament the loss of Asian lives to lethal microbes, we should not slacken our vigilance toward Asian bodies because they host those microbes—if not every single body in actuality, then the collective Asian body in potentiality.

This bio-orientalist crisis epistemology underpinning pandemic discourse did not originate with SARS. As Ari Heinrich points out, the "intensity of [the] eruption of popular anti-Asian racism in the US, Europe and Australia [during COVID-19] draws on deeply entrenched stereotypes that date back more than 200 years."[42] Heinrich traces how eighteenth-century European travelers to China distorted the Qing court's relatively advanced system of smallpox management and inoculation into a more politically advantageous narrative of a special Chinese vulnerability to the disease. This misrepresentation later evolved into a "broader and more insidious stereotype linking Chinese identity to pathology: the notion that China was the 'sick man of Asia' . . . uniquely susceptible to ailments," from the plague to cholera, and this "pathological racism" went hand in hand with ideologies of empire as a civilizing mission, stretching into modernity with Chinese communism "portrayed as a contagious and potentially fatal disease of the spirit" requiring Western salvation.[43] As several Asian Americanist scholars have further shown, in nineteenth- and early twentieth-century America, Chinese immigrants and ethnic spaces were often demonized by health officials and the white public as sources of pestilence, with Chinese bodies represented and treated as a crisis of pollution within the national body.[44] The rise of public health as an institution and of public hygiene as a discourse of modernity served to reify preexisting yellow peril ideologies, providing a biomedical basis to white economic disgruntlement about labor competition and political anxieties about foreign infiltration. California emerged as the hub of this matrix. In San Francisco, successive outbreaks of tuberculosis, smallpox, syphilis, leprosy, and plague were blamed by local officials on Chinatown as the "plague spot," "cesspool," and "laboratory of infection" that poisoned the rest of the city, while in Los Angeles, health officials and citizens targeted Chinatown as "that rotten spot" of "filth and stench," with Chinese launderers and vegetable peddlers singled out as disease carriers and germ spreaders.[45]

It was in discerning the repetition of these historical patterns in the SARS archive that I realized how germane this scholarship on bio-orientalist histories of public health remains. It was also through this realization that I began to investigate the process by which the racialization and Asianization of infectious disease became increasingly tied to the geopolitics of US biosecurity after World War II. This research culminated in my article "Pandemic as Method," which, in the retrospective light of COVID, may seem prescient.[46] There I argue that, if we probe the concept of pandemic not as a neutral description of a natural phenomenon but as a set of discursive relations, we can see how our contemporary mode of thinking about pandemics is a product of layered histories of power, an assemblage of US geopower and biopower that can be traced from the post-9/11 War on Terror back to the Cold War period. Within this genealogy, Asia both near and far has been repeatedly targeted by American paradigms of biosecurity and infection control as the frontiers of bioterrorism and the diseased other, and, hence, as the rationale for establishing, consolidating, and augmenting biosecurity and biodefense programs. What a critical geopolitical archaeology further discloses about this history, which is not merely discursive but stretches over multiple fields of policymaking and finance in the name of human health, is its persistent ideological construction of Asia as the site of malicious biopolitical agents requiring special vigilance and response. This infectious disease paradigm's entrenchment by the new millennium illuminates why, even though SARS caused no fatalities in the United States, it prompted the National Intelligence Council to issue a report in August 2003 entitled *SARS: Down but Still a Threat*. This report's lexicon of national security was supplemented with maps prepared by the Central Intelligence Agency spotlighting China and Hong Kong as global pandemic hot spots.[47] If Kuan-Hsing Chen exhorts "critical intellectuals in countries that were or are imperialist to undertake a deimperialization movement by reexamining their own imperialist histories and the harmful impacts those histories have had on the world," my archaeology of pandemic discourse is one attempt at deimperializing US-centric infectious disease thinking.[48]

COVID Reappraisals

As noted above, this book began around 2014, about a decade after SARS's global end but still half a decade before COVID's onset. Back then, I believed that enough time had lapsed for pertinent materials around SARS to emerge, establishing a sufficiently stable empirical foundation from which I could then investigate pandemic discourses and fictions. No doubt, this assumption reflected a methodological bias on my part, one that clung to a version of Whyte's crisis temporality. On some level that remained tacit even to myself, I imagined pandemic time as decisively past and the SARS archive as comprising relatively inert objects awaiting retrieval and appraisal in a postcrisis scholarly time. This book, moreover, was originally conceived as half biopolitical critique and half literary and cultural analysis. Along the way, however, the proportion shifted. The former half came to recede in importance, condensed into a few paragraphs in this introduction, while the latter swelled into the bulk of the book. Chief in compelling this restructuring was COVID-19.

Throughout the early months of 2020, as the new coronavirus prompted Wuhan's lockdown and then spread from Italy to the United States as the pandemic's new epicenter, two sets of observations and questions progressively troubled me. The first was the utter predictive failure of biopolitical and biosecurity critiques regarding epidemic disease surveillance. By that point, I had already researched and written about these critical models and their chronic worry about the contemporary expansions of biosovereignty regimes. Because the primary focus of these macro critiques is on power and its unceasingly adaptive techniques, their vocabularies tend to be shaped by corresponding themes of permanent warfare and preemptive strikes, total surveillance and distributive control, with the specter of Agamben's planetary state of exception seeming ever more fully realized in the amplification and normalization of disease emergency politics.[49] Yet when Wuhan's COVID case counts rapidly mounted and the coronavirus swept across Western countries into the United States—the supposed center of global biopower and biosurveillance—a slow disillusionment sank in for me, as the limits of these critiques became ever more evident. For all the robust theorizing and ominous warnings about global consolidation of biosecurity strategies and surveillance networks around emerging pathogens, why did these same power structures fail so spectacularly to register, much less predict or prevent, what in retrospect seems to be the entirely foreseeable transmission of a respiratory virus across well-known routes of international travel? Then, when Agamben's first public reaction to Italy's outbreak was to proclaim the epidemic a hoax "invented" by the Italian government, effectively using the occasion to bolster his erstwhile thesis on states of exception rather than revising his own tenets in light of an unfolding global event, it was difficult not to detect a note of philosophical panic in his theoretical foreclosure and determined refusal to grapple with empirical counterevidence. Even more perturbing was how quickly he broadcasted his assessment—despite the by then confirmed death toll of over 2,700 in China—as though the imperative to fret about loss of Western freedoms rendered extraneous for contemplation reports of Chinese deaths.[50]

Later, as the US outbreak took on clearly racial contours and disproportionately impacted low-income minority communities, these same biopower critiques accrued additional gaps. Why are considerations of social inequality not central to any biopolitical articulation? In all the big-picture evaluations of global biosecurity, where is the concern with common people's lack of access to health security, even domestically here in America? Indeed, where are all the people in these biopolitical visions—not just people as abstracted subjects of governance, interchangeable bodies and data points within panoptic surveillance grids, or figures of bare life stripped of meaning except as evidentiary exhibits exposing a totalizing biopower but people as social citizens

INTRODUCTION   **15**

seeking basic access to healthcare and health resources, equitable treatment within medical systems, and safety from disease-driven racial stigma and violence? In retrospect, it struck me that biopolitical and biosecurity critics projected the wrong nightmares. They were not mistaken about the operations and augmentations of biosovereign regimes on a macro scale, but their accounts felt, in the face of an actual pandemic, ethically truncated and socially impoverished. In lieu of their absencing and flattening of people as persons, I began in those early months of COVID to seek out cultural platforms such as Chinese social media, where actual people materialized as actors and sources of agency in their own lives as they coped with an epidemic. If the category of agency presents a classic conundrum for biopolitical theory, this blind spot now appeared particularly glaring. How do we reconceive people as social agents and reorient our attention to their cultures of epidemic agency? How do we rethink epidemic agency beyond the top-down binary of compliance versus noncompliance, measured as these usually are by the yardstick of fluctuating guidelines and policies set by the very institutions that are supposed to have safeguarded public health and monitored epidemic emergence in the first place? In short, how do we move beyond critique-for-itself, beyond crisis biopolitics, beyond even critical deimperializing archaeologies?

While COVID shook the biosecurity footing of my project, its bioorientalist pillars, by contrast, were repeatedly reinforced. In the pandemic's early months, aside from the upsurge in anti-Asian hate incidents, Asian Americans were reportedly dying of the coronavirus at higher rates than any other racial group in urban areas such as San Francisco, due to systemic racial inequities that directly impacted their healthcare access, but this trend was underreported given the entrenched perception of Asian Americans as a successful and assimilated model minority.[51] Moreover, subtler modes of georacial chauvinism saturated both expert and lay attitudes, possibly exacerbating the pandemic's global toll. One index of this chauvinism was the early debate around face mask usage. Before Western authorities normalized the stance that face masks are an essential lifesaving public health measure, the WHO and US CDC as well as numerous Western governments vehemently advised against their use by the general public. Up until April 3, 2020, five weeks into the coronavirus's community spread in the United States, multiple top health officials at national and international levels issued unequivocal statements about the ineffectiveness of masks as a mitigation strategy.[52] Then-US Surgeon General Jerome Adams tweeted in impatient admonishment in late February: "Seriously people—STOP BUYING MASKS! They are NOT effective in preventing general public from catching #Coronavirus, but if health care providers can't get them to care for sick patients, it puts them and our communities at risk!"[53] While officials may have crafted their messages to combat panicked hoarding of supplies by the public and to conserve personal protective equipment for frontline healthcare workers, they simultaneously created a contradictory and unreliable information environment, especially when they later reversed their own policies and guidelines and then erased the trail of these reversals on their websites.[54] Ironically, as I will discuss in chapter 2, these health governance mistakes around public communication also characterized China's initial handling of SARS in 2003, but Western critics attributed them not to honest fumbles but authoritarian power.

What additionally stood out to me, as a second set of disturbing observations in COVID's early months, was the casual disregard and even implicit ridicule of Asian health practices among most Western authorities. By March 2020, China, Hong Kong, Taiwan, South Korea, and Singapore had all widely adopted the use of cloth masks and other face coverings.[55] Indeed, several scientific studies in the wake of SARS had established the effectiveness of face masks as a public health measure against coronaviruses and other respiratory illnesses.[56] These studies validated Asian "societal and cultural paradigms of mask usage" as a "rational" hygienic practice rather than simply a cultural quirk.[57] That Western agencies for months ignored this science-based practice and its track record of efficacy highlights how an unspoken georacial hierarchy of biomedical authority runs deep within global health epistemologies. Nonwestern societies, even those with greater experience in containing coronavirus outbreaks, are not viewed as sources of usable pandemic knowledge, much less purveyors of global pandemic education. This missed opportunity reveals another effect of imperialist pandemic knowledge formations. Yunpeng Zhang and Fang Xu have analyzed this dynamic in terms of what they call a "transpacific and transatlantic production of ignorance" surrounding COVID. In the pandemic's early months, even as Western countries eagerly sought out knowledge about the coronavirus, they simultaneously reproduced their own ignorance because "knowledge accumulated by experts from China as well as other Asian countries about the virus and mitigation strategies are [sic] marginalized, discredited, distrusted, if not dismissed altogether."[58] Zhang and Xu ultimately see these ignorance practices as rooted in "a conflation of orientalism, sinophobia and statephobia in the West," based on "cultural prejudice and racist bigotry" as well as "struggles for and the fear of losing power and authority" to China and other Asian countries.[59]

Writing in Germany in March 2020 and similarly pondering the delay in Western responses to COVID during the European outbreak, Marius Meinhof asked: "After seeing what the virus did in China, how could Europeans have underestimated it? Why did Chinese experiences not matter to them? Why did they not respond fiercely the moment when the first cases without known infection routes emerged?" This failure, he underscores, was not due to lack of information, as "terrifying news from China was available since late January: High death rates, permanent damage from the disease, people dying in their homes or in the street in front of overloaded hospitals, entire families dying." Meinhof's questions parallel my own regarding the failure of timely intervention by global surveillance networks and health institutions, but he probes a later moment in the timeline and raises the additional question of why "western observers did not see an urgent need to act." The problem, as he casts it, was not so much the triggering of a crisis epistemology as the astonishing deactivation of a crisis consciousness. He goes on to identify three types of orientalism at work: (1) an age-old "sinophobic racism" that faulted the Chinese for their dirty cultural habits, such as drinking "bat soup"; (2) a "colonial temporality" that partitioned the world into "backward" regions of disease calamities and "modern" nations that would remain largely untouched; and (3) a "new orientalism" that further otherized China as "the authoritarian 'other'" whose failure to contain the virus was taken as a sign of its political effeteness and, by extension, of Western liberalism's superiority. As Meinhof concludes, "what failed in Europe is not liberal democracy but postcolonial arrogance," which failed in "relating Chinese disasters to 'us.'"[60] Undoubtedly, this postcolonial arrogance also characterized America's initial passivity toward COVID.

Framed in terms of affect theory, these early dynamics bred a pandemic nonchalance in the West that led to a failure in what Ahmed calls the "sociality of pain" as well as a perpetuation of an unequal "politics of pain."[61] Under Western eyes, Chinese subjects with disease and sickness continue to channel historically sedimented emotions of dread and disgust, scorn and mockery, overriding empathetic identification with them as human subjects in pain and appropriate objects of grief. As Ahmed suggests, the cultural politics of emotion works to "differentiate between others precisely by identifying those that *can be* loved, those that *can be* grieved," and thereby "to secure a distinction between legitimate and illegitimate lives."[62] There exists "an intimate relation between lives that are imagined as 'grievable' . . . and those that are imagined as loveable and liveable in the first place."[63] Vis-à-vis COVID, entwined with the georacial politics of Western hubris toward Chinese knowledge was this cultural politics of emotional indifference toward Chinese lives and Chinese suffering and a sundered racial politics of grief. This matrix is the complementary inverse of Eric Hayot's argument that the imagination of Chinese pain has historically paired with tropes of Chinese cruelty to secure Western self-definitions of the sympathetic modern subject. It would seem the "ecliptic" relation Hayot theorizes, whereby China functions as a "horizon of horizons" for Western thought and "the exceptional object" guaranteeing the West's projections of its own universal virtuous norms, breaks down now precisely because this originary othering of sympathy toward Chinese pain lies at the core of Western philosophical humanism.[64] So, while the gloomy prophecies of biopolitical and biosecurity critics have failed to materialize, bio-orientalist formations have by contrast exploded. Indeed, in light of the current pandemic, I have come to wonder whether global biosovereignty can ever be a truly viable threat so long as huge swaths of the planet's human populations and their pain matter so little to those inhabiting Western centers of power and privilege. The more fundamental task, it now seems to me, is not to keep hammering home the same self-assured critiques of power but to lay down, multiply, and deepen aesthetic tactics and emotional pathways for affirming and deexceptionalizing Chinese humanity—if by human we mean simply people deserving of care, with their own practices of love, without the reflexive need to measure their lives' legitimacy against white Western standards of worth.

Toward Epistemologies of Pandemic Microagency, Sociality, and Care

As I meditated on these dilemmas and started to turn away from frameworks of crisis biopolitics, two alternative intellectual traditions surfaced as inspiration and resource: affect theory from queer feminist, critical race, and postcolonial perspectives; and various schools of social justice thought for which critique does not constitute an end-in-itself but serves to launch collective action and coalition. Amid COVID, these have been the hope-oriented and sociality-affirming intellectual practices I drew on to reenvision my project and finish the manuscript.

One of my early and most significant readerly epiphanies was Lauren Berlant's *Cruel Optimism*, particularly its fusing of affect and politics with sustained attention to and respect for the quotidian aspects of life at the social margins. Grappling with the deep-seated social precarity underlying the neoliberal West, Berlant zeroes in on structures of "crisis ordinariness"—where crisis is understood as "not exceptional to history or consciousness but a process embedded in the ordinary that unfolds in stories about navigating what's overwhelming." Similar to Whyte, they emphasize "systemic crisis" and "unfolding change" as commonplace realities confronting vulnerable subjects in late capitalism.[65] For many in the West today, they argue, the democratic promise of "the good life"—circumscribed for generations by fantasies of "upward mobility, job security, political and social equality, and lively, durable intimacy"—has dissolved as an actually achievable outcome. Instead, "the ordinary becomes a landfill for overwhelming and impending crises of life-building," but because people remain attached to "the good-life fantasy," they persevere in living, caught in an affective structure of "cruel optimism" where the very things they desire and work toward become obstacles to their well-being and sources of continual suffering.[66] This condition is not some extraordinary event arising from a radical rupture from the past; it does not single out "the historical present as the scene of an exception that has just shattered some ongoing, uneventful ordinary life that was supposed just to keep going on and with respect to which people felt solid and confident."[67] In terms kindred to Whyte's, Berlant notes: "Crisis rhetoric itself can assume a . . . kind of inflation. Often when scholars and activists apprehend the phenomenon of slow death in long-term conditions of privation, they choose to misrepresent the duration and scale of the situation by calling a *crisis* that which is a fact of life and has been a defining fact of life for a given population that lives that crisis in ordinary time."[68] Crisis ordinariness is lived in unexceptional ordinary time; it marks something constant, to be endured and lived with rather than overcome or lived past. On their conception, "being treads water; mainly, it does not drown."[69]

What moves me above all in Berlant's work is their insistence on recognizing the value of people's everyday practices of living, what they term "lateral agency" or "lateral politics" and what I call microagency. While crisis ordinariness produces an "impasse," this is not an existential paralysis à la Herman Melville's Bartleby, that favorite tableau of stunned and curled-up life so frequently conjured by political theorists. Instead, "people find themselves developing skills for adjusting to newly proliferating pressures to scramble for modes of living on."[70] Refusing to fall back on established political categories such as revolution and protest, transformation or some other exalted type of "heroic agency" as the de facto benchmark for what counts as agency at all—ideas of wholesale and colossal change that often privilege elite actors already endowed with an inordinate amount of social power and centrality, that naturalize a sovereign autonomous subject as the universal pregiven—Berlant urges us instead "to reinvent, from the scene of survival, new idioms of the political, and of belonging itself."[71] In particular: "We need better ways to talk about a more capacious range of activity oriented toward the reproduction of ordinary life," and "we need to think about agency and personhood not only in inflated terms but also as an activity exercised within spaces of ordinariness that does not always or even usually follow the literalizing logic of visible effectuality, bourgeois dramatics, and lifelong accumulation or self-fashioning," activities that engage in "self-continuity," "life maintenance," "ongoingness, getting by, and living on."[72] In effect, Berlant displaces exterior legibility and macro results as criteria for politics and prioritizes instead the lived meaning of micro actions. This model of lateral agency as the "life-affirming" creative energy of "subordinated peoples" amid crisis ordinariness will be pivotal for all the chapters in this book.[73] Throughout, I follow the spirit of Berlant's example by highlighting and recovering the stories and microagencies of those at the textual and contextual fringes of SARS, reconstructing worlds of pandemic meaning and value where the experiences and perspectives of globally marginalized epidemic subjects can take center stage.

In fact, a focus on small stories has been widely taken up during COVID. In their March 2020 "Theses for Theory in a Time of Crisis," for instance, Benjamin Davis and Jonathan Catlin urge readers to "share small stories, and tell your own," noting that "there is more to a crisis than the headlines. Possibilities for alternative futures are hidden in the granularities of day-to-day life."[74] Around the world, many pandemic archiving projects sprang up in COVID's early months, including at many colleges and universities. Collecting materials that chronicle people's daily experiences such as journal entries, photographs, artworks, emails, tweets, and blog posts, these humanistic projects put renewed emphasis on microstorytelling as comprising the core meanings of our communal present. These meanings do not have to await the recovery efforts of future archivists, however. As Shiqi Lin suggests, the "documentary impulse" that has flourished during COVID needs to be understood as collective attempts at building a "participatory digital archive" about pandemic life, not just by scholars and professionals but by common people. Lin ties these digital practices to a politics of everyday meaning-making and justice: "When our current language is still inadequate to capture the fears and uncertainties of living in this form of political injustice, to jot down traces of the present is not only a makeshift to process the gap between everyday experience, official discourse and media representation, but also an effort to reconstruct a lexicon from the everyday and of the everyday."[75] As global pandemic epicenters multiply, people have naturally intuited their capacity for lateral agency amid crisis injustice. Each small story told and shared testifies to this resourceful energy, whereby individuals create not just personal records for elite future memorialists but active and living communal meanings now, from the ground up and out of the minutiae of their own lives, bringing into being the contours of an actually shared global socius.

This critical spotlighting of pandemic sociality and microagency is particularly important for global knowledge production about China. As Xiaobing Tang argues, Cold War epistemologies continue to dominate Western perceptions of China today. He identifies a "dissidence hypothesis" that "presupposes any expression of criticism voiced in China to amount to an act of political dissidence subversive, and therefore intolerable, to the repressive regime," and this attitude "determines the relevance and value of a Chinese cultural product solely from a political calculation" and ultimately "draws on the demonization, with ... unmistakable racial undertones, of a menacing 'Red China' during the Cold War."[76] Similarly, Jenny Lau points to a narrow handover paradigm underpinning global discourses of Hong Kong, whereby every cultural product from the city is interpreted as obsessed with the politics of 1997 and the specter of communist rule. Such an "elitist historiography," she notes, "erases the concrete details of cultural experiences and ... complex social and psychological realities of life in Hong Kong," so that the city takes on significance for global commentators only if it fits into Western constructions of anticommunist resistance.[77] Lau made this argument in 2000, and it is perhaps even more pertinent today, on the heels of the globally high-profile 2014 Umbrella Movement and 2019 prodemocracy protests. In these at once aggrandizing but reductive hermeneutical frameworks, common people's micro practices of everyday living are often seen as irrelevant, mere dross in the grand dramas of power, rather than agentive acts in their own right. Tang's and Lau's critiques will play a key role in framing my analyses of SARS works in chapters 1 and 3, respectively.

For some time now, I have been seeking out scholars whose work helps decolonize elitist and persistently imperialist critical habits, who formulate ground-up epistemologies of contemporary Chinese agency and provide conceptual alternatives to the gridlock generated by the valorized categories of rebellion and dissent. These categories not only carry a tremendous amount of cachet in intellectual history and political discourse but often imply a moral cowardice surrounding their absence. Even vis-à-vis post-revolutionary China, these paradigms retain an implicit dominance. As Charles Laughlin observes in the controversy over Mo Yan's 2012 Nobel Prize in Literature, Western expectations for "Nobel laureates, especially those who were born in repressive societies, to be heroes," notwithstanding the patent "horrors of revolution" in modern Chinese history, ironically erase the "creative agency" of cultural producers who continue to live and labor within conditions of state repression.[78] A similar plea for acknowledging non-Western styles of agency and sociality motivates Erika Evasdottir's concept of "obedient autonomy." Writing on the discipline of archaeology in China, Evasdottir contends that Western templates of "uncompromising autonomy," whereby the world is "divided a priori into oppressors and oppressed," are inadequate for understanding identity and agency as a set of self-governing strategies within postsocialist China. She proposes obedient autonomy as an alternative framework that prioritizes "cooperative behaviors of mutual benefit rather than acts of 'dog eat dog' competition": in this system of "mutual interdependence," a person "becomes more involved in society, not less; becomes more connected, not separated; becomes someone who acts and effects change by participation, not destruction."[79]

Consonant arguments appear in several recent studies of Chinese visual culture. For instance, Margaret Hillenbrand argues against amnesia and censorship as normative explanations for how politically sensitive episodes in modern Chinese history get disavowed, noting that these frameworks "favor . . . top-to-bottom relations that locate agency in the state and treat the people as coercible herds." Analyzing a disparate archive of what she calls "photo-forms," she proposes public secrecy as a better model for grasping how collective silence under repressive governance is often "shared work," as people exercise "lateral sociality" in producing a complex culture of national public secrecy.[80] The "hushing of history," she writes, "is a densely collective endeavor in China . . . a highly agential process whose actors choose to obey the law of *omertà* for shifting, mindful reasons."[81] Myriad actors can choose to

INTRODUCTION **23**

maintain, skirt, play with, subvert, or satirize public secrets, and these acts mediate social agency without the flashiness of overt dissidence. In the global art field, Hentyle Yapp similarly contests "major narratives around resistance and romanticized notions of liberal free speech," whereby Chinese artists hailed as heroic dissidents garner value in the international art market when they "reify" Western images of "China as authoritarian." Yapp calls this dominant discourse "major and proper China," against which he poses "minor China" as a method to "rethink the terms, conditions, and operations that define not only whom or what we value but also *how we value*."[82] Likewise, in her study of the Chinese internet, Shaohua Guo challenges the narrow terms steering much Western commentary on digital developments in China, split as these are between "narratives of revolution" and "narratives of closure": the former pin high hopes on the potential of digital technologies to democratize authoritarian regimes, while the latter "foreground the omnipotence of the Chinese state in its power to enforce strict control over media and society, thereby closing the space for free expression." Both narratives, she points out, erect a "binary opposition between the state and its citizens [that] not only ignores the reality of a more sophisticated interplay between the two, but also results in a narrowly defined, politicized study of the Chinese Internet that neglects the daily experiences of netizens."[83] For Guo, the Chinese internet is at heart a manifestation of people's quotidian agency, "a product of the ways in which Chinese-language users navigate digital spaces and make sense of their everyday lives."[84] I will return to this conception of Chinese digital media as a space of social agency, already evident in the folk humor cultures during SARS, in chapter 2.

In various ways, these scholars all model the location of politics and culture, articulating what Eve Sedgwick calls "local theories and nonce taxonomies"—the tactical, localized, and contingent categories that subordinated subjects are continually "making and unmaking and *re*making" to navigate their social worlds within power relations of the moment.[85] Indeed, the dissidence hypothesis and handover paradigm mirror Sedgwick's conception of "paranoid reading"—whereby every act coming out of China or Hong Kong, regardless of temporal or local circumstance, is read suspiciously, as freighted with either tyranny or oppression, resistance or compromise.[86] In their excessive emphasis on macropolitical struggle, these critical habits effectively freeze China and Hong Kong as totalizing spaces of exception, as if to project onto them in reality what biopolitical theorists such as Agamben fear as only potentiality for the West, replicating anew the logic Edward Said identified long ago as orientalism's geopsychic partitioning of the world into self and other. But beyond the political register, these models are woefully incomplete, as they render insignificant and altogether invisible people's everyday survival practices, even when these have enduring meaning for the actors themselves. A pandemic event such as COVID or SARS can bring this insight home with sharpness and intensity, but the validity of people's self-organizing of life and life-meaning does not apply only in global emergencies. It is in this context, too, that a focus on affect gains magnified import, as it allows us to imagine the opposite of dissent not as acquiescence, capitulation, or complicity but as simply living and enduring, even creating and finding pleasure, with a whole range of ordinary emotions that saturate everyday life. Given the persistence of Western colonialist hermeneutics, tracing mundane feelings and attachments of, by, and toward Chinese subjects can itself constitute a praxis for recognizing non-Western forms of agency and sociality and for decolonizing hegemonic habits of interpreting non-Western others.

At its core, this book is concerned with not the polis but the socius—with redeeming and centering social practices and prosocial affects without burdening them with an obligatory politics. Hence, the artists and works I choose for analysis will not subscribe to a common political stance, such as pro- or anti-China or pro- or antidemocracy movement. Instead, I select for attention minor styles and minor genres, or minor moments within major texts, as key sites for understanding Chinese people's diverse microagencies and reparative desires, during and beyond SARS.[87] Domestic routines and ephemeral romances, female friendships and sentimental bonds, defunct small presses' untranslated novellas and digital bad jokes, televised award ceremonies and Cantopop songs, low-budget flicks and raunchy sex comedies, hospital records and epidemiological documents, spiritual documentaries and crowdsourced ghost tales—these are the archival materials out of which I curate noncrisis epistemologies of SARS. If Yoon Sun Lee looks to the "day-to-day routine" and "little things" as a means for uncovering the unsettled status of Asian Americans within racialized capitalist modernity, whereby "the everyday" is lived in terms of "muted recognition and constrained action" as well as "a minimal sociality," my study looks more optimistically to the ordinary and the minor for *maximal* sociality and care, of both self and others, beyond the organized exigencies of whatever polis.[88]

In this regard, beyond Berlant, several affect theorists are also influential here. Sianne Ngai's theory of "ugly feelings" productively gives critical due to those "minor and generally unprestigious feelings," such as irritation and envy, that have historically been relegated to the interpretive sidelines through congealed racial, gender, and class biases. For Ngai, these feelings are "explicitly *a*moral and *non*cathartic" and "have a remarkable capacity for duration," especially for marginal subjects in late capitalism.[89] I will extend her concept of ugly feelings to argue for Chinese women's affective sovereignty and to lay the groundwork for Chinese epidemic subjects' experiential sovereignty more generally in chapter 1. Carrying affect studies into the realm of justice, Ahmed's proposal of "just emotions" further teaches me that the "emotional struggles against injustice are not about finding good or bad feelings, and then expressing them" but "how we are moved by feelings into a different relation to the norms that we wish to contest, or the wounds we wish to heal . . . which opens up different kinds of attachments to others, in part through the recognition of this work *as* work."[90] If, as Ahmed remarks, "emotions are the very 'flesh' of time" and "show us how histories stay alive" while also "open[ing] up the possibility of restoration, repair, healing and recovery," my hope is that this book's recuperations and rescriptings of Chinese epidemic subjectivities, beyond the distortions and antipathies wrought by racist and imperialist histories, will help reshape my readers' affective relations to them and perform some restorative justice work.[91] Finally, against the "paranoid hermeneutics" of the dissidence hypothesis and handover paradigm, I assiduously follow Sedgwick's turn toward "reparative reading" for my SARS archive.[92] My desire, too, is to "assemble and confer plenitude" on my subjects—by showcasing Chinese practices of self- and prosocial care as "the many ways selves and communities succeed in extracting sustenance" that we can learn from, even derive hope and nourishment from, despite all prevailing prejudices.[93]

Concurrent with this affective turn has been my growing engagement with intellectual traditions around social justice work in North American contexts that couple political criticism with the theorizing of praxis. Whyte, for one, does not halt at the critique of crisis epistemologies but outlines what he calls "epistemologies of coordination," which "emphasize coming to know the world through kin relationships . . . moral bonds that are often expressed as mutual responsibilities" such as "care, consent, and reciprocity."[94] Epistemologies of coordination "do not tradeoff kinship relationships to satisfy desires for imminent action," operating instead in slower time to repair and rebuild frayed kinships, with a clear eye on "ethics and justice."[95] For Whyte, this knowledge paradigm has long shaped and sustained Indigenous peoples' responses to colonial violence and damaged ecologies, and its wider adoption "would go a long way to transform unjust and immoral responses to real or perceived crisis."[96] This coupling of justice with reparation has become more visible in recent health humanities scholarship, such as Karen Thornber's *Global Healing*, which leverages global narratives of illness to destigmatize disease and "create communities of care that promote healing and enable wellbeing."[97] Less recognized, perhaps, is the work of disability activists of color who have long given voice to the interlocking nexus of social justice, group survival, communal storytelling, and what Leah Lakshmi Piepzna-Samarasinha calls "care work." As Piepzna-Samarasinha narrates of her own journey, "Disability justice allowed me to understand that me writing from my sickbed wasn't me being weak or uncool or not a real writer but a time-honored crip creative practice. And that understanding allowed me to finally write from a disabled space, for and about sick and disabled people, including myself, without feeling like I was writing about boring, private things that no one would understand."[98] As she points out, lateral politics in the disability justice movement has long taken seemingly trivial forms, from zines, blogs, and social media to routine acts of "getting together at a kitchen table or a group Skype call to hesitantly talk about our lives, organize a meal train, share pills and tips, or post the thoughts about activism and survival we have at two in the morning." All this is "undocumented, private work—work often seen as not 'real activism.' But it is the realest activism there is," a kind of "care work in the apocalypse," "a story of collective struggle, community building, love and luck and skills."[99]

These paradigms of care and reciprocity, community and justice shape my approach to SARS's archives and affects in this book. If one consequence of pandemic crisis discourse has been an intensification of fear and animosity—of and toward otherness and difference, hardening around race hostility and xenophobia and spiraling into ever-greater disintegration of social kinship feelings, on both domestic and global scales—to reconstruct sentimental attachments, however small or trifling, between minor epidemic subjects is not just a retrieval of subaltern experience for its own sake but one critical path toward collective healing. It is within this cross-temporal pandemic zone that the SARS archive can yield profoundly reparative affects during COVID. Again and again in the ensuing pages, we will encounter pandemic reparations: even in the face of panoptic state power, the protagonist of China's first major SARS novel ends with an affirmation of her ordinary home life and its simple joys, such as walking the dog; even amid a fluctuating disease

INTRODUCTION **27**

information environment, a robust culture of digital SARS humor, including a plethora of nonpolitical bad jokes, flourished on the Chinese internet; even for a city as experienced in extinction threats as ex-colonial Hong Kong, a resilient happy-go-lucky sex worker would become the iconic figure of its SARS films; and even amid serial disease tragedies in Singapore, what may appear to be the trappings of techno-orientalism emerged as survival technologies of connectivity for the nation's index patient. These are only a few examples of the stories tracked here. By book's end, rather than doom and debility, the affects that linger, hopefully, will be hope and love.

An Array of SARS Scenes

The following chapters lay out an array of rhetorical styles and affective scenarios at some of SARS's epicenters. The materials span literary fiction (chapter 1), digital and social media (chapter 2), visual and sonic cultures (chapter 3), and science journalism and medical reports and records (chapter 4). My focus is on the sinophone broadly understood, inclusive of mainland Chinese literature, diasporic Chinese-language fiction, the Chinese digital mediascape, as well as Cantonese film, television, and music. In the last chapter, I probe the anglophone archive as a dominant linguistic switchboard for global pandemic meanings. My aim is not to present a comprehensive record of SARS articulations within any specific region, culture, or language; rather, I have selected for attention an assortment of epidemic scenes, mostly emerging from the outbreak's epicenters in 2003 China and Hong Kong, that can help undo pandemic crisis epistemologies. These scenes orchestrate alternative knowledges about how people lived with, and sometimes through, SARS without their epidemic experience being consumed by the tyrannical terms of disease catastrophe, mass death, and human extinction. Dystopian and apocalyptic narratives of biohorror or biothriller—such as Steven Soderbergh's *Contagion* (2011) or Max Brooks's *World War Z* (2006)—are thus not included here.[100] To summon Berlant again: this book tracks not so much conventional epidemic genres via "foreclosures of form" as "the ways the activity of being historical *finds* its genre." Rather than the usual suite of crisis tropes propagated by pandemic emergency discourse and what Priscilla Wald calls the outbreak narrative, SARS materializes here as a constellation of stories about people's "active habits, styles, and modes of responsivity"— with surprising turns into romance, comedy, farce, and spirituality.[101] As in

28   INTRODUCTION

the case of Xie Xiao Zhen, the genres we expect or crave may not tell the whole story, and it is in their cracks that we discover other microepistemes.

Chapter 1 concatenates three sinophone texts that foreground sentimental plotlines of female sexuality, domesticity, or friendship amid SARS: Joan Chen's 2012 short film *Shanghai Strangers* (*Feidian qingren*); Hu Fayun's 2004 internet novel *Such Is This World@sars.come* (*Ruyan@sars.come*); and Chen Baozhen's 2003 novella *SARS Bride* (*SARS xinniang*). Set respectively in Shanghai, Wuhan, and Guangzhou, all three works center on female feelings and relationships during SARS, mobilizing conventions of sentimental fiction to give shape to everyday epidemic experiences at Chinese urban sites. While they each link the 2003 outbreak to previous episodes of national or global crisis such as World War II, the Cultural Revolution, or the 1989 Tiananmen massacre, they nonetheless maintain the primacy of ordinary life's continuance rather than the ruptures of mass contagion and death. In this respect, they not only exemplify pandemic ordinariness but compel us to read with close attention those textual moments and motifs that bespeak commonplace microagencies of globally peripheralized epidemic subjects. The three authors' positions on gender and national politics may differ, but their texts all present a challenge to bio-orientalist projections of SARS China as a homogeneous space of filthy consumption, disease calamity, and exceptional biopower. This chapter also stays the longest with questions of gender, especially regarding what kinds of affective and ethical responses to a pandemic event get recognized as proper or properly political.

Chapter 2 turns to epidemic humor as another matrix of pandemic ordinariness and microagency during SARS, produced via the then fledgling sphere of Chinese digital media. Throughout the 2003 outbreak, epidemic humor was pervasive across both personal digitized networks and public internet forums, as people used new communication technologies not only to disseminate unofficial news about the virus but also to tell and share jokes about epidemic life. This digital humor culture constructed the sense of a mass socius yoked together by a common crisis yet collectively enduring it with ingenuity and wit. The bulk of these jokes were not political or even parapolitical but nonpartisan, insofar as they did not have critiques of the communist party-state at their core. Assuming such trivial, ephemeral, and bathetic forms as holiday greetings and love confessions, silly ditties and shoddy mimic poems, pseudomedical prescriptions and hodgepodge myth parodies, these cultural tidbits were widely circulated as amateur comic texts, presenting a rich spectrum of social expressions around SARS and compelling

INTRODUCTION 29

an expansive understanding of what counted as humor within the epidemic milieu. In contrast to satire's critical impetus and the carnivalesque's subversive energy, these SARS pieces mediated what I call small humor—the humor of deliberately bad jokes, forced puns, ridiculous buffooneries, and mock-inflated displays of emotion that invite the laughter of chuckles and giggles, smiles and grins, groans and eye rolls, channeling a gentle and generous laughing alongside rather than a spiteful or angry laughing at. Small humor is full of heart, animated at heart by a concern with the socius rather than the polis. It is fundamentally prosocial, aimed at shoring up a quick sense of shared bonds and the shared world within and despite everyday strife. During SARS, this small humor culture maintained an affective economy of communal care by spreading and reproducing feelings of sympathy, recognition, and solidarity, materializing an epidemic mass socius via micro digital practices.

In contrast to digital culture's translocalism, chapter 3 turns to a highly localized geopolitical aesthetic I call the Hong Kong Cantophone. As mentioned earlier, pandemic crisis epistemologies are often premised on a linear and presentist temporality that constructs each disease crisis as unprecedented and necessitating exceptional measures to avert planetary annihilation. The trope of human extinction is hence inveterate to many horror-driven outbreak narratives, its aura of urgency serving to camouflage ongoing historical structures of oppression. From the perspective of 2003 Hong Kong, however—the hardest hit global epicenter of SARS—what we find instead is a host of epidemic de-extinction texts. This chapter focuses on three filmic projects produced and released locally in 2003: *Project 1:99* (*1:99 din jeng haang dung/1:99 dianying xingdong*), a compilation of eleven shorts sponsored by the Hong Kong government and directed by fifteen top local directors; *City of SARS* (*Fei din yan sang/Feidian rensheng*), a low-budget movie with three interlinked story lines featuring an ensemble cast of local stars; and *Golden Chicken 2* (*Gam gai 2/Jin ji 2*), sequel to the award-winning comedy hit *Golden Chicken* from the year before, about a female sex worker with a zest for life who allegorizes the Hong Kong spirit of survival and resilience. Here, too, humor abounds, but the types of humor evoked are thickly tied to local history, local popular culture, and Cantonese inside references, with an enclave quality that solicits strong Hong Kong identification. In these multimedial texts, the pandemic is staged, not as a potentially terminal disaster that can end global and local life for good but as just one challenging event within Hong Kong's cyclical experience with disappearance and return, death and resurrection, extinction and deextinction. This unique aesthetic captures the local entertainment industry's sense of being a hitherto cultural subempire without sovereignty, one whose golden age of regional dominance has witnessed a slow collapse but that nonetheless perseveres in autoregeneration through Cantophone mnemonic stories and techniques. Alongside apocalyptic motifs of infection, illness, suicide, amnesia, bankruptcy, and so on are a host of companion deextinction tropes—the underdog comeback, the reversal of fortune, the eleventh-hour rescue, the overdue miracle. Hong Kong SARS films thus offer a key provincializing of pandemic crisis discourse by subordinating globally hegemonic agendas to the local concerns of small ex-colonial lives.

Finally, chapter 4 turns to nonfiction by delving into the anglophone archive on SARS index cases. I focus on three figures: Pang Zuoyao, the index patient of the Foshan outbreak and the world's first known case of SARS; Liu Jianlun, the index patient of the Hong Kong Metropole Hotel outbreak that internationalized the virus; and Esther Mok, the index patient of Singapore who was herself infected at the Metropole Hotel. As I will detail, the anglophone discourse around each patient, from mainstream news media to popular science journalism and even academic writing, repeatedly propagated inaccuracies and distortions that fed bio-orientalist and sinophobic perceptions of China and Chinese bodies. Even into the time of COVID, Pang has been mythicized as a village farmer with possible links to China's wildlife trade and "wet markets" who died of SARS after igniting a global pandemic— when in fact he was a local official with a desk job who transmitted the virus to only four family members, in a contained outbreak cluster with no fatalities and with himself surviving to tell his story ten years later. Similarly, Liu is often cast in a sinister light as the "patient zero" and "superspreader" who globalized SARS by carelessly or maliciously carrying the virus across the China–Hong Kong border and then killing everyone proximate to him— when in actuality he was a physician who unknowingly caught the virus while treating patients and was himself surrounded by family members throughout his illness until his death, with even his equally elderly wife surviving her infection by him. And Mok, salaciously vilified as a "modern-day Typhoid Mary" by the global press and publicly dubbed the "superinfector" who "infected the whole lot of us" by Singapore's health minister, lived through the tragic toll of SARS on her family to become an active church youth worker and spiritual role model. In all three instances, humanistic storytelling fell back on crisis-driven narrative conventions about disease and contagion that ultimately exacerbated georacial prejudices. By contrast, scientific literature, such as epidemiological studies on early outbreak clusters and medical documents on index cases, provides a trove of empirical tidbits from which to reconstruct each patient's disease experience and social world, allowing us to reclaim the ordinariness and goodness of their lives from a dehumanizing archive. Finally, this chapter's coda turns to the Singapore ghostwriter Russell Lee's *True Singapore Ghost Stories* series for a more heterodox account of the epidemic experience, via the crowdsourced ghost tale, as an alternative mode of indigenous folkloric transmission of interpandemic wisdom.

Despite these troubled years of COVID and the now almost certain prospect of future pandemics, I believe we can, per Leung Ping-kwan's plea in the epigraph to this introduction, grow to treat each other with greater humaneness—if we begin to tell better stories with better affects.

1

Pandemic Ordinariness

Epidemic Romances and Female Sentiments

Ugly Feelings in the Fallen City:
Eileen Chang's Affect Ordinariness

In her 1944 memoir essay "From the Ashes," Eileen Chang retrospects on her two-and-a-half-year stay in Hong Kong under Japanese rule, recalling in particular her stint as a part-time nurse in a makeshift hospital there. In this multiply biopoliticized space of wartime occupation and wounded colonial life, one would expect high drama. Yet, in Chang's rendering, "moments of drama were rare." Her patients were petty figures rather than revolutionary heroes or freedom fighters, "coolies hit by stray bullets and looters who had been injured as they were being arrested," and even they, in those slow humdrum days after the ceasefire, "began to grow fond of their own wounds" for amusement and distraction.[1] Meaningful drama, Chang implies, may be self-invented and interior, especially for small people caught up in big events. Chang's attention to these acts of self-regarding and self-valuing interiority can be read as a recovery of microagency amid macro chaos. This microagency may appear atomistic, even narcissistic. But, for Chang, it mediates individuals' enactment of survival as they sustain sentimental attachments to their own living bodies. Even an accidental flesh wound can become the source of tiny pleasure, of continued devotion to and desire for enduring, from hour to hour and day to day. For these patients, literal navel-gazing afforded greater comfort and interest in their still-breathing bodies and embodied world than any grand rhetoric of the nation.

We can turn to Chang today as one progenitor of the aesthetic of Lauren Berlant's crisis ordinariness. Famously, in this essay and elsewhere, Chang declares she had little desire "to write history," wishing instead that historians would concentrate more on "irrelevant things"—those "random and accidentally discovered moments of harmony" that yield a "sad and luminous clarity" within reality's "incomprehensible cacophony" and layers of "darkness."[2] Against what we would now term dominant or hegemonic narratives and what she describes as "monumental" writing, Chang unabashedly advocates an aesthetic of "trivial things," one that would illuminate the heterogeneities of "everyday modes of life."[3] As numerous critics have taken pains to show since Chang's death in 1995, the disdainful dismissal of her by mainland critics during her lifetime, as a frivolous Shanghai writer concerned only with the trifling affairs of women's hearts, unfairly overstates her dissociation from sociopolitical history and ignores her complex juxtaposing of gender politics with larger shifts in modernity and national politics. Leo Ou-fan Lee, for one, extols Chang for her "subversion of the grand narrative of modern Chinese history," and Nicole Huang adds that Chang offers "an alternative narrative of war, one that contradicted the grand narratives of national salvation and revolution that dominated the wartime literary scene."[4] Indeed, these tributes are part of a by now familiar critical rehabilitation of Chang in the canon of modern Chinese literature.

I will enlist this micropolitical understanding of Chang's aesthetic of the everyday for my reading of SARS romances and their affect-reshaping work vis-à-vis pandemic bio-orientalist and crisis discourses.[5] The central themes and plots of these texts—love, sexuality, domesticity, friendship—are often relegated to the realm of the sentimental or trivial and, during pandemic times, are all the more prone to be overlooked or derided, especially by global readers steeped in Western colonialist attitudes toward Chinese emotions. As Haiyan Lee notes, Western anthropology has historically constructed Chinese feelings as mere reflexes that operate on the level of the "twitch" rather than the "wink," as so many "involuntary muscle spasm[s]" rather than a purposeful force in social relations.[6] This quasi-animalizing framework, which voids Chinese subjects of agency over their emotions, assumes there is little to scrutinize in, and little to gain from scrutinizing, stories of Chinese sentiments. More pressingly, in the time of COVID-19, when Western feelings have coagulated around disgust and contempt toward Chinese bodies—as so many "illegitimate lives" unworthy of, to paraphrase Sara Ahmed, global love and grief even in sickness and pain—Chinese feelings can serve as a crucial site for affirming and deexceptionalizing Chinese humanity.[7] This chapter thus seeks to decolonize and deorientalize global affective forms toward pandemic China by showcasing Chinese lives in practices of love, as beings who love and are loved.

Additionally, the SARS romances selected here and the interpretive method I adopt aim to denaturalize pandemic crisis epistemologies by modeling an alternative paradigm of pandemic ordinariness. These narratives do not so much deny or trivialize epidemic disease as refuse to grant its destructiveness primacy of place in the narration of ordinary people's emotional lives. What Chang's writings validate is the significance of affect ordinariness at the epicenters of national and global crises, especially for female subjects. Her specific feminism works to open up the boundaries of sanctioned feelings for Chinese women, who often subsist under the crushing weight of historically congealed patriarchal and patriotic emotive norms and who are often derogated precisely on the basis of their improper feelings. Chang's oeuvre enables a reading of minor and ugly female affects without the imperative of moral recuperation, without the need to turn women into likable and sympathetic characters in order to have human worth. In effect, she propagates an ethos that vests Chinese women not just with affective agency but with affective sovereignty, even in the face of widescale devastation and injunctions of caregiving.

In narrating the Hong Kong hospital episode, for instance, instead of horror or trauma, tragic sorrow or profound pity, Chang plays up her own feelings of repulsion toward her patients. "There was one man whose tailbone was rotting with gangrene, exuding an evil stench," she recollects. "I was an irresponsible, heartless nurse. I hated him, because he was suffering terrible things. . . . The day the man died we were all happy enough to dance. . . . Selfish people such as ourselves went nonchalantly on with living." This scene of self-described selfishness, however, can be recoded along the lines of Berlant's lateral agency within crisis ordinariness. Tellingly, the nurses' celebration over the gangrene patient's death involved mundane activities such as cooking and eating, not a lavish feast but simply "some bread that tasted a bit like Chinese fermented rice cakes." In other small moments, they would find temporary relief and escape by sitting "behind a screen reading" or having "late-night snacks of specially delivered milk and bread."[8] Just as the patients found ways toward "self-continuity" and "life maintenance," so the nurses improvised means to go "on with living," for their own "reproduction of ordinary life" in a milieu of mass violence, disease, and death.[9]

Throughout this memoir essay, Chang deliberately accentuates what Sianne Ngai calls ugly feelings—boredom, irritation, disgust—"minor and generally unprestigious feelings" that do not culminate in radical political action or cathartic release and that are often attributed to women and minorities.[10] As Ngai points out, "'women's feelings' [are] often imagined as always easily prone to turning ugly," even as women are stereotypically expected to perform "compulsory sympathy."[11] Moreover, as Berlant emphasizes, the workplace is a deeply affect-normative gendered space, at once vertically "demanding deference" and horizontally "demanding collaboration" from women, who are routinely "forced, simply by convention and not by extraordinary monsters, to lubricate every situation of difference by magnifying the power source back to himself as twice his size." This, Berlant notes, is "femininity as a training in flattery and the going-underground of critique."[12] In the hospital scene, Chang highlights this patriarchal economy of emotional labor and expected deference at the very triage site of war and empire. On one side were the nurses, young women all, themselves displaced students trapped in the occupied war zone with neither power nor resources, and on the other were the male patients, who, their lower-class status notwithstanding, all pleaded for feminine care and sympathy with exhortations of "Miss! Oh, Miss!"[13] With her signature understated irony, Chang declines to perform. Rather than lubricating the narrative machinery by delivering to her patients and her readers an experience of female grace and healing touch, she compels a reckoning of affective gender norms, insisting on the right of her nurses to own and express their ugly minor feelings, even in the face of an open colonial wound.

36 CHAPTER 1

Sexual Agency in Shanghai:
Joan Chen's *Shanghai Strangers*

Among SARS romance fictions, Joan Chen's short film *Shanghai Strangers* (*Feidian qingren*), also entitled *Love in Shanghai* (*Ai zai feidian de rizi*) (2012), offers the clearest example of affect ordinariness in the tradition of Chang. A Shanghai native herself, Chen both wrote the script for and directed the film, describing it as her "love haiku" to her birth city.[14] The story interlaces the Shanghai of three epochs: the early 2010s of China's economic growth, the 2003 of SARS, and the 1940s of wartime.

The film opens in the present timeframe, in an upscale restaurant on Christmas Eve, with a boy's birthday party winding down. In the ensuing blackout, as everyone else leaves, the boy's mother, a sophisticated looking woman named Xiu Xiu, stays behind to wait for her receipt.[15] A lone Englishman is the only other remaining customer, and, in the dark, the two strike up a conversation, one they continue over coffee in a nearby café afterward. Because of the foreigner's "kind eyes," Xiu Xiu confides in him that her husband is not her son's biological father, and she proceeds to divulge a love story she has kept secret all these years. The film then flashes back to 2003, with a newly married Xiu Xiu riding her bicycle through a Shanghai *longtang*, looking much younger with a pageboy haircut and a pink face mask sporting a winking bunny. She narrates in voiceover that this was during the height of SARS in China, and, in her memory, hazmat-suited figures riddled the streets. The only person she remembers not wearing a mask at the time was a young man, a colleague's client and the potential buyer of a long vacant 1930s-era apartment building she had been tasked to show. Inside, the two discovered a trove of old photographs of the wartime Jewish ghetto, a postcard in German dated 1941, and a news clipping about the sinking of the ship *Goethe* in the Indian Ocean. In the days after, they separately pieced together that the apartment had belonged to a Viennese Jewish photographer named Viktor, who had waited three years for the arrival of his wife and son in Shanghai, the world's only open port city and a haven for Jewish refugees at the time. Yet he waited in vain, for his wife and son had both drowned in the shipwreck. This tragic love story touched Xiu Xiu and the young man deeply, and they agreed to meet one more time in the apartment, making love in Viktor's darkroom. From this sexual encounter she conceived her son, giving birth to him that Christmas Eve. She then resumed her conjugal life with a much-reformed husband turned doting father thereafter. She never saw the stranger again, but, in her growing son's face, she glimpses his. The movie ends not with some melodramatic revelation about the deadly cost of epidemic disobedience or illicit intimacy but with Xiu Xiu finishing her coffee and parting from the Englishman to return home, alone.

Shanghai Strangers exemplifies a narrative of pandemic ordinariness. Rather than frontloading SARS as the central plot element, the film embeds the outbreak within a longer timeline bookended by world war and global capital. Even within the SARS timeframe, the epidemic recedes into the background. The scenes of Xiu Xiu's recollections of public health workers spraying the streets with chemicals are tinged with a blurry unreality. Instead, what takes center stage and accrues interpretive weight are the micro sentiments and attachments that get lost in monumental history, requiring oblique postmemorial retrievals. The missed rendezvous at the wartime Jewish ghetto gets belated recompense in the chance encounter of two Chinese youths, whose brief passionate romance amid a global pandemic becomes the memory that lingers. Rather than scarred or debilitated bodies, the physical remnant and reminder of the SARS year for Xiu Xiu is the palimpsest of her lover's face in her son's aging one. What persists beneath historical ruptures of geopolitics and global disease is a substratum of female memory and illicit but unforgotten affect. Neither a bang nor whimper, SARS becomes a waning memory associated with the faded image of a former lover's silhouette.

Chen's film is highly redolent of Chang's aesthetics. The accidental rendezvous of strangers during a moment of suspended time, the opening up of romantic possibility for an unhappy young woman, muted female desire half played out yet lingering against the shadowy background of war and national collapse, the just as quick closing down of life possibilities through a moment's decision or withholding, and, of course, all these events unfurling against the atmospheric evocation of 1940s Shanghai—these elements are all trademarks of Chang's stories, signaling Chen's homage to the earlier writer. They share a trajectory, too, from Shanghai to the anglophone diaspora, encoded in Chen's film through its bilingual script. If Chang's feminism functions to legitimize a fuller range of female feelings, Chen's film opens up the allowable boundaries of female sexual agency and insists on female sexual sovereignty. Whether in the context of a global viral outbreak or transnational capitalism, the sexual intimacies of Chinese women are often scrutinized and policed or else fetishized in the light of day, and it is only in the metaphoric darkrooms and blackouts of public history that they, like Xiu Xiu, can exercise with social impunity their agency to act or not to act on sexual attraction. If Chen has Xiu Xiu ultimately decline the Englishman's tacit proposal for an affair, it is not to ratify her abstention as the proper response to racial and co-lonial gender politics but to stage the decision as her sexual choice, whether with or without sentiments attached.

The two novels analyzed below—Wuhan writer Hu Fayun's *Such Is This World@sars.come* (*Ruyan@sars.come*) (2004) and New York–based writer Chen Baozhen's *SARS Bride* (*SARS xinniang*) (2003)—likewise spotlight ordinary female affects and affections within macro crises. Like *Shanghai Strangers*, both novels attempt to restore female intimacy and attachment as guiding tropes for narrating life at epidemic epicenters. Against crisis epistemologies that construct pandemic milieus as terrifyingly poised on the cusp of disease emergency and species annihilation, these SARS texts reframe our imagination of pandemics by intertwining the exceptional with the nonexceptional, refusing to privilege disease disaster as the inevitable condition of globalization or dismiss the epidemic everyday as existentially inconsequential. From their configurations of pandemic ordinariness, we can distill a broader reading practice—one that attends to textual scenes of the ordinary alongside those of crisis rather than treating the two in isolation, that holds as equally important seemingly minor textual elements alongside episodes of high gravity. Moments of quiet mundane life, plotlines driven by small or personal dramas rather than national or global affairs, and details that may be deeply meaningful to individual characters but whose meaning is not reducible to a critique of macro power structures—these take on en-hanced significance. Alongside everyday affects, these novels also offer tem-plates for communal politics and ethics vis-à-vis pandemic living. In contrast to Chang's aesthetic of desolation that Chen partly inherits, both novels are surprisingly optimistic, anticipating not the falling away of civilization but the comfort of a homecoming or the spark of a new phase of vocational life, extending the hope of postcrisis optimism without cruelty.

Romance beyond Terror in Wuhan:
Hu Fayun's *Such Is This World*

To date, Hu Fayun's *Such Is This World* remains the most well-known Chi-nese fictional work on SARS, considered by some critics to be the "most important work of contemporary Chinese fiction to address the many social ramifications of the 2003 SARS outbreak."[16] First released online in 2004, the novel disappeared from public view when its hosting website was shut down a few months later, only to reappear in multiple versions over the next few years: as a popular internet novel on Sina, an abridged work in a regional journal, a bowdlerized edition by a Beijing publisher, an uncensored edition by a Hong Kong publisher, and an English translation based on the author's original manuscript. As A. E. Clark, Hu's English translator, points out, technically the novel was never banned since state officials insisted that any rumor about the book being on a list of eight censured works was a "misunderstanding," yet "this ban which was not a ban" achieved similar results, as it led mainland booksellers to discontinue advertising of the novel and Hu's prospective American translator to terminate the project.[17] In fact, the book's tortuous publication history is so well publicized that Jonathan Mirsky deems it a consummate example of the "anaconda in the chandelier," Perry Link's metaphor for the calculated vagueness of China's censorship regime that leaves everyone in its shadow adjusting through subtle self-censorship.[18] "Hu Fayun," Mirsky remarks, "must hear the anaconda shift its weight every day."[19] Elsewhere, I have compared the expurgated Beijing edition of the novel with the unabridged English translation to track the uneven and sometimes unpredictable practices of official censorship on a micro level.[20] Here, I focus on the ways Hu combines an explicit censure of the communist party-state's political repression with an equal emphasis on the continuities of daily life amid a global disease outbreak, braiding pandemic ordinariness into the very fabric of totalitarian history.

Set in an unnamed provincial capital and unfolding over the course of one year, *Such Is This World* intertwines two main story lines.[21] In the first, the eponymous protagonist, Ru Yan, a fortyish widow and single mother whose only son has gone abroad for graduate studies in France, adjusts to life alone in her city. The narrative opens with a backstory of the two things her son left behind: a puppy and a computer. The dog, named after her son, serves as a symbolic filial surrogate. The computer connects Ru Yan to an online community, particularly a forum called the Empty Nest where parents with children studying abroad gather. Here, she rediscovers her love of words and appreciation for good writing as well as her own stylistic talents. Before long, her online essays attract a following of admiring readers, including Liang Jinsheng, the local deputy mayor. Himself recently widowed and an Empty Nester, Liang is drawn to Ru Yan's old-fashioned sensibilities and poetic elegance and begins to court her. This female-centered domestic

40   CHAPTER 1

plotline—of a woman aging alone, caring for a pet, learning new technology, and rediscovering romance in middle age—functions as the text's opening and closing frame. But more than a framing device, it constitutes half the narrative focus of the novel, intersecting with yet also anchoring the other much more politically charged plotline in the small dramas of nonexceptional life.

For Hu, this spotlight on Ru Yan is far from incidental. As he writes in the Beijing edition's afterword, Ru Yan is modeled after his late first wife, Li Hong, who was battling stomach cancer during the book's composition and who died less than a year after its completion. Li was, as always, his manuscript's first reader and editor, and, upon the book's publication, he dedicated it to her memory.[22] This semibiographical dimension to Ru Yan's character might partly account for why, in the novel, Hu fixes his attention so sharply on her domestic life, almost to the exclusion of her professional one, which he addresses mostly in terms of office politics and romantic intrigue, despite her being a botanist at a state research institute. By all appearances, Ru Yan is competent enough to have contributed substantive scientific reflections on the virus, but, throughout the novel, she writes and thinks about SARS primarily as a mother and public citizen, from the standpoint of moral sentiment rather than specialized knowledge. The novel's construction of pandemic ordinariness is thus deeply mediated by a gender conservativism and male-oriented code of femininity. I will pick up on this gender politics at greater length later in this chapter.

The novel's other story line begins nearly midway through and revolves around SARS. In late 2002, Ru Yan calls her family in southern China and hears about the outbreak of a strange disease there. As Ru Yan's mother exclaims, "You get it, you die," yet authorities are restricting all epidemic information so that news circulates only unofficially via private cell phones (*STW* 178; *RY* 106). Before long, Ru Yan learns that her brother-in-law has been infected. Still finding no official news online, she composes an essay about his mysterious illness to warn her fellow Empty Nesters. Thus begins Ru Yan's political awakening as her post goes viral. As SARS spreads across the country and globe, including into her province, she is increasingly dismayed and then outraged by the government's response—first censoring information about the virus and covering up the epidemic, then implementing harsh public health measures that spawn brutality and abuse among local law enforcement. In the ensuing months, Ru Yan is spurred to write ever more damningly of these events, and she soon becomes the target of cyberbullying and internet censorship as well as, unbeknownst to her, government

PANDEMIC ORDINARINESS   **41**

surveillance. Meanwhile, she cultivates a small circle of dissident friends who foster her internet activism and deepen her political consciousness. Among them are Damo, the novel's other protagonist and a well-known activist blogger, and Teacher Wei, a respected elderly scholar who has emerged through decades of persecution with uncompromising moral integrity, courage, and wisdom. Precisely because of his influential role as the mentor to a group of independent youths, Wei falls prey to secret party machinations and dies a horrific death, falsely hospitalized as a SARS patient and then left to waste away alone in an isolation ward. Through the voices and fates of these two male characters, Hu conveys the novel's most direct indictment of the communist regime as a panoptic state seeking total control over biopolitical information, a self-preserving political structure that exercises absolute biopower over its citizens' lives and deaths.

To grasp the dual strands of *Such Is This World* and to contextualize the significance of Hu's treatment of pandemic ordinariness, we must first explore the novel's more overtly political and crisis-driven plotline. For Hu, it is impossible to understand contemporary China's epidemic governance without recognizing the persistence of its totalitarian legacy. Any consideration of the ordinary and the present would be inadequate, even foolish, he suggests, without a critical look at the long reach of communist history. Indeed, the novel strikes many observers in retrospect as a prophetic rough draft for COVID-19, insofar as Ru Yan's unnamed city is clearly Hu's native Wuhan, the original epicenter of the current pandemic. As Haiyan Lee puts it, revisiting *Such Is This World* in 2020 can give one a sense of "déjà vu," and even Ru Yan's character and online activism bear an eerily proleptic resemblance to the real-life Fang Fang and her digital *Wuhan Diary* during the city's lockdown, as I will discuss in the coda below.[23] By chance, Hu himself was not in China at the start of COVID. His current wife is Austrian Chinese, so he now spends a third of each year in Vienna, where her son's family resides. He was originally due to fly back to Wuhan in late January 2020, but, after hearing about the coronavirus outbreak from friends and family in-country, he decided to stay in Europe. For the first time in his life, he spent Chinese New Year outside his hometown.[24] Watching from abroad the epidemic unfold in China during those early months, Hu comments: "Many of the events today, compared to SARS years ago, are like an epic movie being remade and repeated, with many of the details, scenarios, and props being the same." He points to China's political system as a key factor for this repetition: "We can say that all natural disasters are fundamentally human disasters. If we don't learn our lesson, these disasters will keep happening, over and over again.... There's an old saying that even a stupid donkey won't fall down in the same place twice. But we are still looking on helplessly as [the Chinese government] tumbles into the same hole for the second time, and what's more, this time around the fall's even uglier." In fact, he notes, many readers feel that, compared to the SARS events recorded in his novel, the current situation is like an "upgraded edition." If Chinese writers themselves fail to document the continued instances of power corruption and abuse but instead "turn their backs and shut their eyes, pretending these problems don't exist, then Chinese literature will forever remain pseudo literature, accomplice literature."[25] For Hu, the costs of unchecked state power are borne above all by the people, with epidemic casualties and injuries representing one salient dimension. Far from being impervious to the suspension of rights under authoritarian disease governance—as some Western commentators implied about Chinese and Asian populaces vis-à-vis SARS, as I noted in the introduction—the characters in Hu's novel will bear gruesome witness to the multifaceted harm of exceptional disease biopolitics.

Crisis: Totalitarian Terror and Missing Bodies

In recent decades, political scientists have tried to dispel essentialist conceptions of Chinese authoritarianism as necessarily monolithic and top-down. Kenneth Lieberthal and Michel Oksenberg argue, for instance, that policymaking in post-Mao China is characterized by a structure of "fragmented authoritarianism," with extensive bargaining among bureaucracies at various levels. Rather than an absolute concentration of power at the top, with a coterie of autocrats relentlessly issuing coercive directives down the capillaries of the party system, authority is actually "fragmented, segmented, and stratified," with policy decisions occurring predominantly through negotiations and consensus building.[26] This paradigm shifts attention from raw power to institutional norms and practices, and from the cabal of top leaders to the country's vast bureaucracy and its multitudes of officials. As Lieberthal later qualifies, though, this model applies only to the political system "below the very peak" and does not illuminate the black box of leadership power since any such discussion is "bedeviled ... by the difficulty of gaining access to information."[27]

For Hu Fayun, however, party-state bureaucracy is merely a symptom whose root condition lies much deeper. In the political cartography of *Such*

Is This World, the source of power remains fixed at the country's political center, with raw power radiating outward as a lived effect for all Chinese subjects. Given the danger of censorship, Hu, like many antiestablishment writers, does not tackle this problem directly, but neither does he collapse sovereign power into institutional authority or cast totalitarianism and bureaucracy as opposing formations. On the contrary, these categories are utterly compatible for him, with one folded into the other in the cloth of everyday life. The state's sovereign capacity lurks just beneath the surface of bureaucratic normalcy, waiting to be sprung when a crisis erupts. No linear model of a political "post" can capture this sense of a persistent hidden matrix of totalitarian potentiality.

In his novel's political plotline then, Hu insistently characterizes contemporary China through the lens, if not language, of totalitarianism. The word *totalitarian* appears just once in the book, in a passage in which Wei laments the absence of an "untainted cultural vehicle" with which his generation can record their lives (*STW* 129; *RY* 75–76). In the Beijing edition, Wei's reference to "totalitarian countries like the former Soviet Union" is excised, so the word is altogether absent there. But beyond the literal level, and like many mainland writers critical of the communist state, Hu evokes totalitarianism in oblique ways. One common literary strategy is to establish a continuity between the Mao epoch and the post-Mao capitalist one so as to expose the falsity of contemporary state-driven propaganda about national prosperity and progress. Along this vein, Hu's novel proposes that, in the supposedly posttotalitarian present, individuals are motivated to embrace material comfort and social advancement as the ideal goals of an ordinary life, as China ostensibly moves farther and farther away from its tumultuous past toward a more liberal pluralist society. Yet beneath the veneer of national stability and wealth lies a general sense of terror, one that arises from historical memory and a recognition of collective bodily vulnerability. The novel thereby sketches out a biopolitical model of totalitarianism—one that shifts from complete ideological indoctrination to a biomedical state of exception where humans and animals alike can be reduced to, in Giorgio Agamben's term, supremely killable bare life, life that can be killed with impunity by all.[28] In Hu's portrayal, the 2003 epidemic serves merely as the party-state's pretext to declare a state of emergency and exert sovereign control over subjects' bodies. Against the crisis epistemology that naturalizes fear as the supremely proper response to pandemic threat, Hu reconstructs fear as the calculated product of a politicization of infectious disease. In doing so, the novel extends an alternative mode of ordinariness, one that compromises neither on personal ethics nor on communal politics.

To connect the biopolitics of communist history with that of SARS governance, and to resituate pandemic fear within the lineage of totalitarian terror, Hu makes use of a recurrent motif: the missing body. This motif first occurs in Damo's story line. In the year of SARS, Damo suffers the loss of a decades-long friendship, and, crucially, the cause is not disease but politics. Maozi, Damo's closest friend, was once a self-styled "dissident" philosopher who dreamed of recovering "the missing persons in the history of thought." Over time, however, he succumbed to both the pressures and enticements of the state, trading his ideals for career advancement and economic well-being. Now a respected senior professor at a top provincial university, Maozi writes best-selling academic books that bolster the legitimacy of party officials. This, Damo observes, is a "living specimen of the contemporary intellectual." He inwardly mourns the disappearance of the old Maozi, who has also "gone missing": "Lost without hope. They won't even find your body" (STW 216; RY 129). For Hu, Chinese intellectuals' complicity with the party-state lies at the heart of its continual rule by terror. Such a critique is not unique to him, but what is distinctive is his metaphor of the vanished body. Embedded within a larger story about SARS, this metaphor accrues biomedical resonance, as the terror over the missing body originates with not SARS but its political prehistory. Indeed, for a novel revolving around a pandemic, images of diseased bodies are surprisingly few. Instead, the motif of Maozi's missing body can be traced to another national emergency, one that lays bare the continual relevance of China's totalitarian inheritance: the Tiananmen massacre.

In the spring of 1989, Maozi had been an activist, signing petitions and joining marches, traveling to Beijing and enjoying the limelight there, and far more optimistic about the democracy movement than Damo. The massacre that ensued, however, drove him into despair, then temporary insanity, and, finally, resignation and compliance. In the wake of June Fourth, in words that echo numerous other Tiananmen narratives both historical and fictional, Maozi muttered to Damo: "It's too frightening, it's just too fucking frightening. China is finished, finished. . . . It's all over" (STW 202; RY 120). The novel's recollection of Tiananmen implicitly links Maozi's later figurative disappearance with those missing bodies of the massacre, the unknown number of bodies that were cremated in haste and in secret and that never made their way to any official casualty count. Hu insinuates that Maozi, too, may be deemed among those "missing persons in . . . history." After June Fourth,

Maozi "seemed to have forgotten a great deal" (*STW* 204; *RY* 121). It is in this passage linking political fear to historical amnesia that Hu embeds the implied titular proverb of the novel: at the moment Maozi begins to forget, Damo has the feeling the past is fading away like smoke (*wang shi ru yan*). By alluding to this proverb of a vanished past in the name of his eponymous heroine, Hu cues us into that past's enduring effects in the new millennium, with the long arm of the massacre casting its shadow onto characters' lives a dozen years later.

In those dozen years, Maozi joined the party and strategically built his career as a pro-establishment academic, writing books that dress up party officials' "scattered impromptu remarks" as systematic Marxist thought, in the process getting rapidly promoted through academe's ranks. When confronted by Damo about this political dishonesty and self-betrayal, Maozi resorts to the logic of survival in capitalist terms: "It's what they wanted. Gotta do what you gotta do.... It's how I chose to make a living. The assignment came down, you know? Plus there was a grant attached to it" (*STW* 197; *RY* 118). Later, with greater candor, he elaborates on his own Faustian bargain: "We're only human, all of us; we want normal lives, we want to provide for the wife and child. We'd all like to be better off; we deploy our little bit of time and energy in any grubby business that will improve our standard of living, even if it lacks a higher meaning, just as the construction workers and rural vegetable-peddlers do. You have no right to demand that everyone suffer for the sake of your ideals" (*STW* 211; *RY* 126). Significantly, this passage remains uncensored in the Beijing edition. Left in place, it conveys a portrait of Maozi as a pragmatist, someone who sees himself as having matured beyond the idealism and narcissism of the 1980s to become a responsible family man and well-to-do professional in the postsocialist era. By his own reckoning, he has not so much traded conscience for material comfort as outgrown youthful zeal and narrow pride in favor of paternal duty and familial security. In this self-portrait, the intellectual's professionalization is a positive historical development and political good, exemplifying the choice to abandon violent revolution of whatever cause, democracy included, for the gentler ordeals and more modest rewards of a steady career. No longer a separate class of the nation's self-proclaimed moral elite but normalized like everyone else, the intelligentsia can finally and simply "make a living." Maozi's example supposedly demonstrates the transformation of the intellectual into a jobholder and bureaucrat. He has the capacity not only to survive history and bloodshed but to thrive in their aftermath, so that even if "China is finished" and "it's all over" by 1989, posthistory under authoritarian rule turns out to be entirely livable, even cozy.

Beneath the surface of social acquiescence and cheerfulness, however, lies ongoing terror and trauma born from witnessing firsthand state-executed carnage. It is in this context that Damo characterizes Maozi as having "gone missing." Before SARS takes center stage, the metaphor of the lost body is raised via Tiananmen. In a moment of didactic exegesis, Damo diagnoses Maozi as an exemplar of a terror regime's effects: "Damo knew that Maozi's case was all about fear. . . . It inspired another of Damo's essays: *The Power of Fear*. To terrify people, he wrote, is more effective than to kill them. Killing disposes of the dissident's body. Terror can transform his soul, turning the most troublesome rebel into a docile slave who will serve as an example to others" (*STW* 203–4; *RY* 121). Maozi ultimately remains rooted in this fear, unable and unwilling to give up the safety of his current life to join forces with Damo. As the latter observes toward novel's end: "These days there were an awful lot of people like Maozi. . . . [He] was not a wicked man. He wasn't even a mean-spirited man. But over the course of an era he had been molded, slowly, into who he was," for "terror still haunted his mind" (*STW* 414–15; *RY* 250). Hu would agree with Hannah Arendt that terror is a key instrument of totalitarian rule, and, in his novel, it snakes through the whole of communist history.[29] In the Beijing edition, the word *terror* or *fear* (*kongju*) appears for the first time in the above passage. But in the author's manuscript, the word is used much earlier, in a chapter that harkens back to the Maoist period. Tellingly, just as Maozi embodies the impact of political fear on the post-Tiananmen intellectual, so prior historical manifestations of it are attributed to his predecessor and mentor, Teacher Wei.

In their youth in the early 1970s, Damo and Maozi belonged to a group of freethinking iconoclasts called Qing Ma or the Young Marxists. Wei was their intellectual and spiritual leader, a teacher who had been denounced in the 1950s and then again at the beginning of the Cultural Revolution but who has since been rehabilitated with a relatively prestigious academic position. In 2002, former members of the Qing Ma group gather to celebrate Wei's eightieth birthday. It is at this gathering that the word *terror* first appears in the original manuscript, as Wei recollects the Maoist years and laments the absence of a totalitarian artistic tradition in modern China. According to Wei, unlike other countries, even other totalitarian ones, China has no literary or artistic tradition to draw on for genuine expressions of suffering under tyranny. Whereas "terror didn't stop [the Russians] from creating great art to enshrine their memories," the Chinese of his generation produced only hymns to the party and to Mao. As a result, "even private emotional memories have been alloyed with a quicksilver ideological culture that pervades everything," and what remains is "something paltry and preposterous," the bankrupt artifacts of power (*STW* 129–30; *RY* 75–76). In a few key lines of devastating criticism that are deleted from the censored edition, Wei bewails: "But look at us: a whole army routed, a mass surrender, and with one command, all individual voices vanish. We live like pigs and dogs, without sorrow, only terror. Without courage, only frenzy. Without dignity, only arrogance. Without reverence for life, only obsequiousness to power" (*STW* 116).[30] Wei's disquisition reverberates with Damo's later assessment of Maozi, allowing Hu to connect the persecuted Mao-era intellectual with his latter-day prosperous heir as both victims of totalitarian terror.

Thus contextualized within Maoist history and the Tiananmen massacre, the missing body motif then returns with stark literalness in the SARS plotline. Where political persecution fails to terrorize and subjugate Wei, SARS steps in to finish the job. Soon after his birthday party, Wei contracts pneumonia and is hospitalized. The timing of his illness proves fatal. With the Chinese government coming under intense international scrutiny by the spring of 2003, each province's handling of the outbreak turned into a political crucible. Hu is keenly aware of this global backdrop to SARS's local impact: at one point, in several lines deleted from the censored text, Ru Yan's son emails her from France that the "Chinese government has come in for heavy criticism" over its handling of the domestic outbreak and that "it's been humiliating" for overseas Chinese students (*STW* 309). Wei is at first given an optimistic prognosis by his doctors and slated to be released after a few days of antibiotic treatment, but, amid the panic aroused by SARS, he is transferred to an isolation ward that houses several other suspected SARS cases. From this point on, his body disappears from the text. Within a few days, his friends learn he has again been transferred, this time to a university hospital, where he gets classified as a suspected SARS patient. After weeks of isolation, he is declared dead. His body is promptly cremated, his personal effects disinfected and bagged, all accomplished narratively off-scene, "behind closed doors," by functionaries of the state. Upon receiving his ashes, his widow pronounces his "the loneliest of deaths . . . the most miserable way a man can leave this world" (*STW* 377; *RY* 227). Ru Yan, too, ponders "the extreme brutality of letting a man die this way . . . on the white sheets of a hospital bed . . . no better than dying in an unlit dungeon" (*STW* 373; *RY* 225).

Hu further shifts our attention from the biopolitics of life to the state's necropolitics, to death as a means of perpetuating power. Officially, Wei's family and friends are told he was never given a "definitive diagnosis" since his condition "had many complications." "It's actually better for the family members this way," they are told, because of the stigma around SARS. Out of supposed consideration, Wei's death is ruled a case of not viral contagion but pneumonia-induced heart failure. Conveniently, this medical decision allows authorities to subtract Wei from the national SARS fatality count, even as they press upon his widow the importance of not probing too deeply into the cause of death: "We hope that, together with members of his family, at a time when the whole country is united with one heart and one mind in the struggle against SARS, we can contribute to the stability and the larger interests of the nation" (*STW* 379; *RY* 229). To die for SARS, if not of it, can be branded a patriotic act, and to accept the official medical verdict without question can be a demonstration of political loyalty and good citizenship. The "larger interests of the nation"—that is, China's global credibility—is built on this internal compliance by the surviving and a gray zone of indeterminate cause for the deceased. Wei may or may not have died from SARS, but what matters is that he was sacrificed for the nation's health security and international reputation. The logic of public health dictates that victims suspend personal judgment, that the public forego its desire for transparency and accountability. Hu's implication is clear: at the pandemic epicenter, maintaining global health security entails this fate for totalitarian subjects. Biopolitically, the isolation ward converges with the prison cell as the millennial state's new space of death, now sanitized as the ostensible place of sustenance and care, a specially demarcated space that presumably strives to save infected lives but where in fact ailing unruly bodies go to die unseen. In Wei, the metaphor of the missing body becomes literalized, lost in the state's labyrinth of isolation and quarantine zones.

The novel also cues us to the problem of a specifically *Chinese* missing body in the context of a global pandemic, a problem at the intersecting operations of totalitarian state power, the biopolitics of disease containment, and the geopolitics of global health governance. In these overlapping circumstances, Wei's missing body takes on global, not just domestic, significance. For China itself, Hu highlights SARS as a biopolitical event in which a totalitarian history of sovereign biopower gets reactivated. At a transnational level, he registers the global forces bearing down on the Chinese government at the height of SARS. As Wei himself observes at one point, "Actually, there are all kinds of pestilence in Nature; it's a perfectly normal phenomenon at every period of history and in every country. In the history of Europe, there were terrible plagues that wiped out half the population, but they're OK now. I don't know why these things become a political matter when they happen in our country" (*STW* 253; *RY* 152). Echoing Kyle Whyte's critique of the language of unprecedentedness in crisis epistemologies, Hu has Wei posit here the unexceptionalism of human pandemic experience. What is truly exceptional is the communist state's mode of epidemic governance. Despite Wei's singling out of China, we can extract a larger critique of global disease epistemologies that likewise exceptionalize pandemic events for political ends, and Wei's fate exemplifies what happens when totalitarian biopower is validated in the name of maintaining and saving global lives. And when local bodies are made to disappear, they cease to speak. When Wei first submits to his hospitalization, he is an optimistic and willing patient, ignorant of the death that awaits him. Only posthumously do his last words make their way back to the outside world, in a final notebook, akin to prison jottings. On its last page is an "almost indecipherable" riddle, as though written in "a child's scribble": "When it is not, they say it is; / When it is, they will say it is not" (*STW* 381–82; *RY* 230–31). Despite his lifelong yearning for an authentic totalitarian literature, Wei fails to leave behind a record of his own suffering; at most, his veiled aphorism alludes to the official falsehoods around SARS. Up to the novel's last page, no document of life or death in the isolation ward manages to reach us.

Worse yet, what Wei's family and friends never discover, but what the novel goes on to reveal, is that his death was politically plotted. As a "sensitive figure" (*STW* 313; *RY* 189), Wei had been closely watched by the provincial party cadres for years. One of his political enemies happens to be the father of Jiang Xiaoli. Jiang, a coworker and romantic rival of Ru Yan's, shrewdly took advantage of the epidemic to pull strings behind the scenes and arrange Wei's transfer to the university hospital where he would eventually die. So, while Wei's friends were desperately appealing to the authorities to release him during his initial isolation, Jiang had ensured he would be lodged ever more deeply in the network of quarantine facilities, in effect guaranteeing his chances of catching SARS. She is as close to a villain as the novel gives us, and her single-minded machinations are certainly chilling. Yet her motives are neither extravagantly malevolent nor base. If anything, she seems driven by traditional values—by a sense of filial piety to prevent political storms from "shatter[ing] the peace of her father's declining years," by genuine love for a man whose career she hopes to protect and advance, and at her most venal, by a distaste for dissident upstarts who threaten to dismantle the political status quo and humiliate "children of people like her father" (*STW* 395; *RY* 238). Jiang is a portrait of the ruling elite's next generation or *guanerdai*, but Hu highlights not so much the depravity and greed of this new elite as its tenacious belief in its prerogative to rule. Jiang readily acknowledges the rampant corruption and incompetence within the party, yet she sees these as problems to be solved by cadres and their children, not "outsiders": it is not a matter of "right and wrong" but one of "winning and losing" (*STW* 422; *RY* 255). The elimination of political opponents is simply a prerequisite for securing the interests of those in power, and an infectious disease outbreak conveniently legitimizes exceptional means to this end. More than just an emergency public health measure, the isolation ward can serve these political calculations, emplacing an invisible execution ground where political death sentences can be carried out untraceably, where germs do the work and no human hand or surgical scalpel, much less a gun, need ever be lifted. The novel is meticulous in relocating the primary site of terror from disease to power, from SARS to its secret governors and the political environment in which they operate. Much more than the virus itself, this insidious power structure constitutes the true horror of the contemporary epoch for Hu.

Ordinariness: Romance and Domesticity

While many elements in the novel's personal plotline are entangled with the political one, the former is not reducible to the latter. That is to say, ordinariness is not crafted by Hu trivially, as life allowed to live through a temporary suspension of sovereign power or a mere reprieve from an underlying permanent state of exception. Such are indeed the escalated terms of Wei's, and sometimes Damo's, diagnosis of modern China, but, significantly, these grand pronouncements play off of the less dramatic details of Ru Yan's domestic life, the novel's other core narrative.

Scholars have singled out the themes of the animal and the internet as exemplary of the novel's representation of crisis politics, but we can equally recast these within a matrix of crisis ordinariness. Chapter 55, for example—arguably the book's most graphically violent and terror-saturated chapter—opens with haunting scenes of animal carnage. When SARS spreads into Ru Yan's city, her housing development comes under quarantine and residents are forbidden to keep their pets, which are deemed potential viral carriers that must be surrendered to the authorities. Ru Yan manages to hide her dog at home by cowing it into silence, but she often hears the howls of animals being beaten to death in the streets. On one occasion, she witnesses a group of security guards gleefully tearing a small dog to pieces with hooked poles. She photographs the episode with her camera and posts the pictures online, denouncing this sanctioned torture and public execution of animals as "a city's disgrace" and comparing it to Auschwitz. "The days we are living through," she writes, "have laid bare things more dreadful than SARS" (*STW* 363–64; *RY* 219). Haiyan Lee aptly reads these scenes in biopolitical terms, as reflecting a state of exception in which human and animal life alike have been reduced to the "degradation of bare life."[31] As she notes, "Since animals often bear the brunt of the biopolitical regime, they become a powerful trope for disclosing the state of exception that undergirds modern sovereign power."[32] This resonance between human and animal precarity is further reinforced by the chapter's concluding announcement of Wei's death.

Yet, despite the prominence of these scenes of horrific animal violence, Ru Yan's own dog survives both SARS and the official pet ban. What's more, while the creature is somewhat traumatized by that period of house confinement and pet slaughter, it emerges from epidemic crisis with its intuitions and empathy intact. The novel's final reference to the dog shows it perched on the edge of Ru Yan's bed, anxiously waiting for her to wake up after her breakup with Liang Jinsheng—ultimately the more faithful and caring companion. Ru Yan is "deeply moved" by the dog's love and concern, and it is in this moment of human-animal mutual attention and affection, as "she reached out from under her blanket and caressed the dog's head," that she decides she is "okay" and ready for "a fresh start" (*STW* 442; *RY* 268). Animal life, then, does not materialize in the text as solely or even primarily a trope of crisis biopolitics or bare life. Instead, the lingering image of Ru Yan as much as her dog after the pandemic is that of two resilient beings, each keeping the other company with body and heart unbroken. Similarly, Ru Yan's brief career as a cyber personage ends on a note of understated resolution. On the one-year anniversary of her initiation into the internet, she revisits the Empty Nest forum after a long hiatus and lurks there, browsing messages and even coming across nostalgic posts about her "lovely prose." But instead of plunging into another cycle of online activism and spiteful backlash, she decides to remain a lurker, "to keep these friendly feelings" and "let the acrimony fade into the past" (*STW* 443; *RY* 268–69). Rather than bitterness and cynicism or even melancholy and regret, the affect that lasts for her is the residual memory of friendship.

Above all, Ru Yan weathers the abrupt dissolution of her relationship with Liang Jinsheng without any profound scarring of spirit or psyche. Nor is this relationship a minor component of her narrative, for nearly half the novel is dedicated to meticulously tracking its growth and the gradual reawakening of her sexual desire. A series of episodes centers on Liang's attentively orchestrated dates with Ru Yan. In one, he drives her to an artificial beach in a new quarter of the city so they can better moon-gaze on the Mid-Autumn Festival. In another, after being incommunicado for almost a month while he attends the Party Congress in Beijing and is then sent to the United States, he returns with a gift-wrapped box of hot dogs, "fresh out of the oven" from America, per Ru Yan's jesting request (*STW* 140; *RY* 82). Even after SARS hits the city and Liang, as the deputy mayor responsible for public health, is put in charge of epidemic management, he remembers Valentine's Day and treats Ru Yan to a banquet of rare delicacies at a private restaurant owned by a descendant of imperial chefs. In the culminating scene of their romance, he leaves the quarantine center to visit her unannounced one night, intending to simply look up at her window from his car so as not to expose her, but she rushes down and drags him upstairs into her apartment. They have sex for the first (and only) time, passionately and with abandon, until they are spent "like two wild animals that have been shot" (*STW* 345; *RY* 207). Afterward, with fastidious attention to the intricacies of Ru Yan's inner life, the narrative follows her reveries as she contemplates her uncharacteristic indifference to the disorderliness in the room and her unselfconsciousness about their nudity. Then, in a seemingly gratuitous passage, Liang wakes up in the middle of the night and says, to Ru Yan's delight, that he needs to "pee-pee"—not "To use the bathroom" or "I have to relieve myself," she muses lovingly, almost maternally, but "to pee-pee," "like a drowsy child talking to his mother." She stands and watches over him as he urinates, and the text does not neglect to mention that she flushes the toilet for him (*STW* 346–47; *RY* 208). Veering far from the disaster-filled political plotline, this scene zooms in on details of bodily life that are not so easily subsumable under the rubric of totalitarian biopower but are instead saturated with sentiment. If Roland Barthes names by "reality effect" those "superfluous" or "futile" textual details that have no significance except to induce a sense of reality, we can call this passage part of the novel's ordinariness effect.[33]

To be sure, each of these romantic episodes can readily be read as encapsulating some direct or implied sociopolitical commentary—on the scarcity of unpolluted lakes in China; the culture of secrecy around party proceedings; the continued privilege of officials to dine, literally like royalty, amid an epidemic outbreak and its animal bans; and the unrestricted mobility of VIPs like Liang versus the conspired imprisonment of undesirable elements like Wei. Nonetheless, we are led to view Liang's courtship of Ru Yan not as the superficial or deceitful performance of a political villain, much less the prelude to a relationship fatefully doomed by totalitarian power or epidemic death, but as the mature affection of an older widower who has learned to value love and companionship after repeated loss. His devotion to Ru Yan is depicted as sincere, if ultimately not deeper than his political ambitions. Tellingly, their breakup occurs as the result of a reluctant but voluntary decision on Liang's part, not as the inevitable tragic fallout of a totalizing external force. Toward the novel's end, Liang has successfully checked SARS in his city and is poised to be promoted through the party ranks. In order to preserve and advance his career, he chooses to sever ties with Ru Yan, who has become suspect for her internet activism and friendship with Wei. His is a bureaucrat's decision, made out of pragmatic self-interest and moral weakness. Just as June Fourth broke the spirit of the dissident youth in Maozi and remade him into an obedient civil servant, so SARS dashes the hopes of the chivalric adventurer in Liang and remakes him into the party's rising star. Through Liang's character, Hu allows us to imagine real-life officials who are likewise promoted up the ladder of governmental or institutional power through small personal acts of surrender. His betrayal of Ru Yan rises to the level of villainy only insofar as he fits Arendt's notion of the banality of evil: he is merely a cog in the political machine, his greatest failure being an incapacity to think—and feel—more deeply. Even so, Liang is no Eichmann. He does not fail to consult his own conscience before consenting to carry out the commands of his superiors, and he sacrifices his relationship with Ru Yan with full self-awareness, even regret and self-disappointment.

Liang's decision transpires, however, without Ru Yan's knowledge, and the narrative diligently traces her private torment as she waits, week after week, for him to get back in touch. So politically innocent is she that she never realizes it is her own heartfelt writing that "might have harmed the standing of a man in the world of officialdom" (*STW* 428; *RY* 259). She deals with her heartache not through any grand gestures but by having a conversation with another woman, Wei's widow, in one of the novel's rare scenes of genuine female bonding. It is the latter who identifies the root problem of the relationship: Ru Yan "seeks the overarching values in life, its ultimate meaning," while Liang is "unable to detach . . . from worldly fame and power" (*STW* 435; *RY* 264). By the novel's end, Ru Yan, too, makes a decision, albeit a relatively undramatic one: "to begin life anew and live one's days well" (*RY* 268).[34] For her, this means a return to routines, the first of which is walking the dog.

Were Hu more invested in rendering a wholesale totalitarian dystopia, he could easily have maximized the disastrous ramifications of SARS and its governance effects, perhaps with the death of Ru Yan's dog, the arrest of Damo's group, or the breaking of Ru Yan's spirit. Instead, the novel ends modestly, uneventfully. Rather than heroic acts of resistance or bold declarations of a transformed future, the story's quiet conclusion recasts the terms of ongoing life in contemporary China from an exceptional politics of sovereign biopower and bare life, state repression and grassroots protest, toward an ethos of everyday endurance. Taking a walk, closing a web page, even deciding not to respond to an online post become the daily acts that constitute survival, whether from postepidemic traumatic stress, cyberbullying, romantic disappointment, or political betrayal. These acts have no large-scale or long-term sociopolitical impact, but neither do they represent forms of quietism or futility. They instantiate a kind of experiential self-acknowledgment and life maintenance: to recognize recent events of calamity without alarm, to regulate personal memory without denial, and to sustain livable life beyond the emergency, without escalation and with conscious intent. They epitomize Berlant's notion of lateral politics: "valuing political action as the action of not being worn out by politics," valuing commonplace agency beyond "melodramatic" spectacles of resistance, and "reinvent[ing], from the scene of survival, new idioms of the political."[35] Insofar as Hu depicts contemporary Chinese life as also steeped in neoliberal malaise, most clearly manifested in the trope of Maozi's missing body, we can read this concluding note of lateral agency as the enduring substratum of postsocialist life when revolution and protest die.

Like Berlant, Hu seems engaged in a kindred project of theorizing crisis ordinariness, but with more straightforward optimism. Even in the wake of a global pandemic and in the shadow of panoptic state power, Ru Yan is anything but a victim of debilitating desires or slow death. She remains wholly herself at the novel's close, ever the loving mother and compassionate moral citizen, ever full of dignity, self-respect, and cautious hope for the future. The last scene sees her throwing out the wrinkled suit worn by Liang after their night of passion and the new slippers meant for him, not into the trash bin but out her window, for the scrap collector passing by below. This minor deed converts into nothing spectacular on the macro stage of history, but, for Ru Yan, it is at once a step forward from her failed relationship, a small civic gesture toward the poor, and an ecological act of recycling—no more, no less. It expresses an instance of everyday ethics, not as antihegemonic opposition or radical rupture but as action carried out in the spaces of prosaic home life.[36] Rather than a nonbiopolitical act, we can read it as nonexceptionalist biopolitics. Through Ru Yan, Hu retrieves from the catastrophic scene of terror and disease an alternative affective realm for more mundane and nonelitist forms of sentimental attachment. Enacted as self-care, human-animal companionship, and sexual desire, these attachments do not ineluctably feed back into the theater of national and global politics. The novel leaves Ru Yan and the reader with a feeling of returning to a familiar domesticity after living through an extraordinary time, where the postcrisis world does not have to be postapocalyptic but can offer a modest homecoming.

Gendered Receptions and Grassroots Shifts

Interestingly, while Western reviewers tend to emphasize Wei's and Damo's sections of the novel, often by quoting their more grandiose critiques of China's history and politics, enthusiastic responses on the Chinese internet initially concentrated on Ru Yan's character. According to Perry Link, Chinese readers "adored Ru Yan for being 'what China needs' and 'the way a person should be,'" with her "simple virtues" of "modesty, integrity, and common decency."[37] As one reader writes in an online post, "While I'm skeptical whether there really is a Ru Yan in China, I'm hopeful. Perhaps many ordinary people in China are Ru Yans."[38] Though Chinese readers comment abundantly, too, on the macropolitical aspects of Hu's book, its outstanding feature for them is not the wise victimized patriarch or the uncompromising dissident intellectual but its spotlight on the sheer ordinary goodness of the female protagonist. As noted earlier, Hu's emphasis on Ru Yan's moral sensibility to the near exclusion of her intellectual or professional competence may appear somewhat misogynistic. Indeed, most of the novel's explicitly politics-oriented dialogues occur among male interlocutors, with Ru Yan only an occasional and peripheral presence in those exchanges, and only too obviously positioned as an acolyte being tutored by older male figures. As Hui Faye Xiao observes about *The Fourth-Generation Women*, an earlier piece of reportage literature by Hu on marital conflicts in contemporary China, his commentary there subscribes to a "fantasized timeless image of a feminine homemaker situated in a binary structure of family versus market," where women are praised for their "'natural' attachment to family life" and the feminized domestic space is tasked with "guard[ing] modern men's emotional well-being by acting as an antidote to the alienating forces of market capitalism." In effect, "women are abstracted as the embodiment of the pure feminine interior uncontaminated by the 'dirty' politics and money of the masculine outside." For Xiao, this trend toward redomesticating the woman reflects a specifically Chinese response to socialist history, as postsocialist writers struggle to "resist the hegemony of a male-centered master narrative of socialist revolution" but ironically "give birth to a new master narrative that renders women as prediscursive and apolitical creatures situated at the heart of the domestic interior."[39] So, even if Ru Yan's domesticated virtues are not yoked to a telos of male happiness, Xiao's insight raises the question of whose gaze her character satisfies, and what gendered desires the novel buttresses vis-à-vis neoliberal anxieties. If Western responses to Hu's novel fixated on the male critiques of communist power, the Chinese internet's enthusiastic embrace of Ru Yan may be symptomatic of a postsocialist desire for female redomestication.

Yet the novel is not entirely blind to its own skewed gender representations, and we may view its heavy-handed paternalism as Hu's marking the limits of a masculinist intellectual tradition. While he may take up this discourse as a vehicle for delivering his own political exegeses, he also shows an awareness of the changing landscape of the public sphere, where, after the failure of the Tiananmen protests, liberatory narratives of democracy and national salvation seem increasingly dubious and vain. Hence, old-school intellectuals such as Wei will continue to speak in the terms of earlier grand narratives and regard themselves in the new millennium as moral advisers and guardians of the nation—an elitist posture that Hu flags as such, even if he does not wholly reject it. But these male figures are also dramatized, literally in the case of Wei, as past their prime, lacking social efficacy during recent crises such as SARS and entirely naive and defenseless against the maneuverings of state power, even by a younger cadre like Jiang Xiaoli. Through Wei, Hu submits a sincere and trenchant critique of totalitarian resilience, but he also hints that this is the lexicon used among men, a style of thought and speech arising predominantly between self-perceived elites. Sebastian Veg would call Wei a paragon of the "universal intellectual," the high-minded man of justice who traffics in universal ideals and ends.[40] That his character occupies the limelight in Western reviews of Hu's novel but receives shorter shrift in Chinese internet discussions likely reflects Chinese readers' skeptical attitude toward this outdated mold of the male intellectual.

Damo, by contrast, personifies a new class of what Veg calls the "grass-roots (or *minjian*) intellectual," who breaks from that older tradition by focusing less on saving China and more on solving concrete problems, especially in relation to marginal social groups.[41] Hu's portrait of Damo reveals not only his cognizance of the rise of the blogger in the early 2000s as an influential social actor and grassroots intellectual but also his esteem for the type of anonymous nonelite blogger who is "of the folk" in his livelihood, as opposed to celebrity bloggers such as Han Han who claim anti-elite status but exhibit "residual elitism" toward the masses.[42] Unlike Maozi and Wei, Damo is not affiliated with any academic institution and hence preserves a degree of intellectual autonomy. A handyman by day and a blogger by night, he does not depend on the state for an income or the market for his writing. As Hu explains, people like Damo "haven't sought out great success inside the system, or profit by being in the mainstream. They want free knowledge and a proper reflection and expression of themselves as their highest goal. This group is the greatest force in the past decade toward liberating thinking and criticizing society. It's precisely because these people have independent professions that they aren't afraid of the government smashing their rice bowl. Many have very simple lives, even to the point of poverty, but can make a living and take care of themselves and their family."[43] When Ru Yan meets Damo in person for the first time, he is introduced as someone "sprung from the common people of this city," as part of its "genuine home-grown people." For Ru Yan, he embodies authentic indigeneity—evocative of Hu himself, who has spent his entire life in Wuhan except for two sent-down years during the Cultural Revolution.[44] Hu brings out the class disparity between them by having her muse with inward embarrassment that "large swaths of this city, and most of the people who lived in it, were not much more familiar to her than a country in Africa" (*STW* 175; *RY* 104). As Damo jocularly admits, he does not have a diploma but is an autodidact, in his trade as an electrician as much as his sideline as a blogger. While Ru Yan admires his essays for taking up "big questions," he insists they are "little questions, extremely practical and specific," aimed at making interventions into concrete daily issues that confront "us ordinary people," such as "workers who've been laid off, medical care, housing, temporary residence permits." On SARS, his assessment is couched in equally matter-of-fact terms, focused on tangible outcomes rather than abstract principles: "They say a virus is no respecter of persons . . . and both rich and poor will get sick: but when it comes to treatment, it's going to make a big difference whether you're rich or poor. . . . The poor are more likely to get sick when an epidemic breaks out" (*STW* 186–87; *RY* 110–11).

Suggestively then, while the hospital represents a nightmarish biopolitical space of contagious death for Wei, it retains the quality of a nonexceptional place, even a place of new life and familial joy, in Damo's domestic story line. In a scene of consummate pandemic ordinariness, Ru Yan calls Damo on New Year's Day and learns that his daughter had given birth to a baby girl the night before. "Eight pounds, six ounces," he gleefully tells Ru Yan over the phone. "Natural birth; mother and child resting comfortably." Fearing the spread of SARS into the city, Ru Yan cautions Damo to be "careful at the hospital" (*STW* 241; *RY* 144). This remark, rather than serving as narrative foreshadowing, transpires as a passing note of concern between friends, and SARS never erupts into Damo's home life, most of which takes place off-page. For Hu, ordinariness may be a largely feminine configuration, but it is not exclusively so.

Female Fellowship in Guangzhou: Chen Baozhen's *SARS Bride*

If *Such Is This World* is well-known among Chinese readers but relatively little-known in canons of world literature, *SARS Bride* is a truly obscure text, in both sinophone and anglophone realms. Written at the height of SARS by the New York–based Chinese American writer Chen Baozhen, the novella was published by Cosy House Publisher in New York in 2003. The story of the press itself is relevant here. Established in 2000 by the longtime immigrant couple Chen Wenqiao and Zeng Bihua, Cosy House was a small noncommercial press dedicated to publishing overseas Chinese-language writing by nonprofessional writers. Its motto was "to publish books on behalf of ordinary people and to record the achievements of common folks."[45] Booklovers both, Chen and Zeng recognized the need for such a press, since Chinese-language writing by immigrants, especially nontechnical writing, frequently falls between the cracks of both mainland Chinese and American publishing. In China, aside from the many stages of official and unofficial vetting, authors face high printing costs, whereas, in the United States, commercial sales drive the publishing industry, a factor that hugely disadvantages non-English writers. Cosy House set out to help those unknown Chinese aspiring to publish the odd book, writers who are not big names but who desire to leave behind some record of their voices, often for very humble and personal or familial reasons. By customizing each book based on authorial need and readerly interest, the press produced small initial runs and kept costs low for authors.[46] In their way, Chen and Zeng may also be considered grassroots intellectuals, laboring with an ethics of ordinariness on behalf of Chinese diasporic communities. Unfortunately, after Chen passed away from cancer in 2005, Cosy House ceased to operate. Meanwhile, the Chinese internet has taken off, opening up more sinophone platforms than ever before for overseas Chinese to connect with each other and with mainland readers by publishing works online—the nascent stages of which Hu traces in his novel when he describes Ru Yan discovering, with shock and delight, the "great many [internet] works that had never made it into print" (*STW* 134; *RY* 78). But *SARS Bride*, as one of Cosy House's sixty-six titles, remains a book with only a handful of printed copies in circulation, with no translated editions and almost no online presence. It embodies a mode of diasporic creativity that ekes out an existence in the untimely gaps of ascendant technologies and majoritarian cultures.

Still, while Chen Baozhen may not be a widely known writer in either China or America, neither is she an amateur one. Over the past two decades, aside from *SARS Bride*, she has published three novels, a playscript, a poetry collection, an essay collection, and a literary biography, all in Chinese, some by Cosy House and others by mainland presses, in addition to numerous poems and articles online.[47] Born in Guangzhou in 1936, Chen immigrated to the United States in 1982. She started writing creatively in high school but did not become a full-time writer until 1999, after suffering a hand injury at the clothing factory where she worked and after supporting her husband and three children through graduate school.[48] She thus writes out of her experiences as a working woman as much as a wife and mother, and *SARS Bride*, much more so than *Such Is This World*, exudes a strong feminist ethos by centering not just the professional lives of but also the intimate fellowships among women.

Epidemic Care Work and Frontline Feelings

Despite its name, *SARS Bride* centers not on male-female romance but female-female camaraderie, paying especial homage to the courage, resourcefulness, and professionalism of female medical workers during SARS. It is a women-centered bildungsroman and medical drama, tracking the growth of the spirited heroine, Wu Li, from an inexperienced rural migrant to a seasoned frontline nurse at the epicenter of a global pandemic. When the story opens, Wu Li is around seventeen years old, newly arrived from Yunnan at an unnamed seaside city in southern China. As with Hu's novel and Wuhan, the anonymous setting here clearly suggests Chen's native Guangzhou, the capital of the province where the SARS virus first appeared in late 2002. Wu Li is accompanied by Yue E, her friend from the village, and the two girls quickly get recruited for domestic work at separate households. Wu Li is engaged to be married the following spring, and her original plan is to earn some money for the wedding while her fiancé, Song Wei, does the same as a factory floor supervisor in another city. Over time, her employer, a retired Chinese opera diva named Hong Xing, or Aunty Hong, grows fond of Wu Li and comes to regard her as a goddaughter, encouraging her to become a nurse and even funding her training. A middle school graduate, Wu Li had always wanted to further her education but lacked the means to do so, so she jumps at Hong's offer. Her ambition at this point of the story remains modest, her desire shaped around the prospect of becoming a more suitable wife to Song Wei, a vocational school graduate, so that he would not be looked down on by their fellow villagers. With Song Wei's support, she postpones their wedding and begins working as a nurse at a city hospital, where she becomes the protégé of the head nurse, Su Weiling, in the lead-up to SARS. From there, Wu Li's devotion to and friendship with Su takes center stage, transforming her sense of self from a rural migrant bride-to-be to an independent professional at the vanguard of the nation's epidemic control efforts.

From this perspective, SARS Bride may be read as epidemic sentimental fiction that reorganizes female affect away from patriarchal kinship structures toward a new space of professional female sociality, one prompted by the crisis of SARS but that endures beyond it. As the novella progresses, Chen shows Wu Li increasingly shifting her allegiance from her marriage engagement to her medical work, and more specifically, to the "sisterhood" of nurses by her side. On the eve of moving into her hospital's dormitory, which has been designated a quarantine zone, Wu Li firmly tells the worried Hong and Yue E that she must go and continue her work, since "the country's in trouble!" (17).[49] But privately, beneath this patriotic bluster, she has a moment of indecision, as she muses: "She thought of how she had originally set out to become a nurse so as to learn a skill and gain a livelihood. Come next spring, after getting married, for better or worse she'd still be a nurse, and Ah Wei would be able to stand a little taller in front of other people. Who would've thought that being a nurse these days means risking your life. It's not too late to turn back now and leave this hospital, but then I can forget about being a nurse ever again" (18). Ultimately, it is the thought of disappointing Hong and Su, of dashing these female mentors' faith in her, rather than some abstract self-judgment about letting down the nation, that seals Wu Li's resolve to join the frontline medical staff.

Two months later, the epidemic rages on. One day, Wu Li stumbles onto a secret scene of tearful reunion between Su and her family, who are allowed to converse briefly through a glass partition. Unbeknownst to Wu Li and the rest of the nurses under her charge, not only has Su volunteered herself for frontline duty despite having an eight-year-old son at home, but even her husband, a medical school professor, has volunteered to be assigned to another quarantine hospital in the city, leaving their son in the care of a teacher. Wu Li has hitherto regarded Su as the archetypal socialist strong woman, a successful and inspiring boss who is warmhearted and approachable but discloses no weaknesses or dependencies. But in this moment, she realizes with surprise that Su "can cry too! . . . She's human too, and a woman besides! And with a family like this to fret over." Then, speaking to herself in a silent monologue: "Ah Wei, you know why I keep deferring our wedding date? I don't want to abandon Boss and my group of sisters here. The life here is hard and also dangerous, but we can't leave each other. There's a force of genuine feeling that binds us together. . . . How then can I sneak off alone for personal happiness when all my sisters are still in the midst of peril?" (38). Through Wu Li, Chen dramatizes a woman's transfer of primary emotional attachment away from her future husband to a female community of colleagues. Her sense of professional and sororal solidarity overrides her sense of conjugal obligation, and the novella may be read as validating this shift in female sentiment especially for a generation of migrant women who may believe that their most secure prospect is marriage. It also seems that Song Wei's character is present not to raise the issue of female sexual agency as a vehicle of modern urban womanhood along the lines of Joan Chen's film but to make chaste the medical sisterhood and mark it as nonqueer and socially proper. The novella's portrait of female community hence affirms women's decision to defer marriage even as it regulates their sexuality along heteronormative lines.

In contrast to Hu's domestication of Ru Yan, Chen uses the SARS narrative to propel her female characters into the limelight of the emergency state's public sphere. Whereas Ru Yan has no close female friends and only male mentors, embodying a kind of sui generis ideal woman in Hu's novel, Wu Li is surrounded by female companions, whether friends or coworkers, mentors or supervisors, guardians or parental proxies. A number of these characters are also rendered with affective complexity, each with her own moments of focalizing interiority, from the tough-minded and valiant Su Weiling to the timid but loyal Yue E to the shrewd and generous Aunty Hong. Collectively, they populate Chen's epidemic text with a heterogeneous spectrum of female perspectives across age, class, and background. The novella thus offers not a singular narrative unified around the central heroine but a polyphonic panorama of female social life. Significantly, in contrast to the biopoliticized and mostly off-scene space of the hospital in *Such Is This World*, the hospital is the pivotal place for Wu Li's development as a gendered subject. It functions as a space of alternative domesticity for women, literalized by the trope of the quarantine dormitories, and also a domain of female professional guidance, growth, and mutual nurture, where women look after not just their patients or the nation's health but each other.

The novella brings this theme home in the scenes of its first and last SARS casualties: both victims are female, emphasizing the special bodily vulnerability of women due to their reproductive and caretaker roles. On Wu Li's first day in the SARS critical care unit, her first patient is a seven-months-pregnant young woman. After a successful caesarean delivery, her condition worsens. Wu Li feels helpless in the face of the young mother's pitiful yearning to see her newborn, but Su has the presence of mind to have the staff take a photograph of the child. In the final moments before the woman's death, Su orders a nurse to bring the infant over in a biohazard suit so the mother can see her child through the glass partition. This is the first time Wu Li has seen a patient die in front of her eyes, and beholding "the newly birthed alongside the newly dead makes her realize how fragile life is, and how fearful SARS is" (22).

A few months later, Wu Li herself contracts the virus. In her semiconscious state, she recognizes Su attending to her after working hours, gently cleaning her body and patiently spoon-feeding her when she gets irritable. Under Su's assiduous care, Wu Li recovers and is released from the hospital. By this point in the novella, Aunty Hong has all but adopted Wu Li and gladly takes her home to convalesce, with Yue E's help. But Wu Li soon learns that Su has caught SARS, most likely from Wu Li herself. Deeply anxious and mortified, she gives up the chance to follow through on her wedding plans and returns to work. Over the next few weeks, she dedicates herself to Su's care between shifts, washing the older woman's fevered body and changing her diapers, reciprocating the loving attention she herself had received. After Su's emergency surgery, she stays by Su's bedside all night, turning off her cell phone so that Song Wei's calls would not disturb Su's sleep (137). As one character later comments, theirs is an "emotional bond of life and death" (*sheng si qing*) (151)—one that supersedes feelings of romantic love, even as it stands guard over and blesses that love. Tellingly, Chen does not reinscribe this female sentimental bond within the terms of the *oikos* by allegorizing Su and Wu Li's relationship as a mother-daughter one. Instead, Su remains to the end Wu Li's most cherished and venerated "Boss" (*tou'er*), at once teacher and adviser, friend and guardian spirit. After Su dies from her illness, she is awarded the Florence Nightingale Medal and bestowed the posthumous titles of "martyr" and "model party member," with a bust in her likeness erected in front of the hospital (143). It is before this statue that Wu Li and Song Wei finally get married toward the novella's end, to honor Su's wish in life to officiate at their wedding.

Aside from these grand ceremonious gestures, however, quieter tributes are paid to Su by her fellow nurses. In the breakroom, they leave anonymous tokens of remembrance, such as roses and azaleas and pine leaves picked from the hospital garden, "all of which happened without coordination, in silence." When this makeshift memorial is relocated to the new head nurse's office, Su's former mentees "would come and silently salute her, with a 'I'm here, Boss' and a 'I'm leaving now, Boss.' These habits, formed during Su's lifetime, carry on, unchanged" (140). Akin to Ru Yan's return to prosaic routines at the end of *Such Is This World*, the nurses carry on their customary greetings to Su after her death, small acts that sustain a communal rapport and ritual and that include her in spirit and memory. The accent, as in Hu's novel, is on quiet endurance and resilience amid and despite SARS, not its destructiveness. Yet the ending here is markedly less solitary. In the novella's final scene, with the outbreak relatively contained in southern China, we see Wu Li, now newly married, preparing to travel north to Beijing with a contingent of volunteer medical workers. Far from being debilitated by loss and sickness, Chen's heroine appears as heartily galvanized as ever to continue her work alongside fellow "white-robed warriors" (154).

As this ending scene intimates, revolutionary rhetoric surfaces periodically throughout Chen's novella and indexes another key difference between her and Hu. In sharp contrast to the latter's novel, SARS *Bride* offers no political critiques of the party-state. Su, for example, is depicted as a loyal party member in life and a willing national martyr in death. While there is no overt ideological glorification of socialism, every state-affiliated character is portrayed as upstanding, responsible, and hypercompetent, from the local party secretary to the anticorruption police investigator to the provincial public health official. Moreover, Chen is not averse to appropriating the narrative codes of Maoist revolutionary drama for her SARS tale, and for the most part, she presents a black-and-white moral universe with clear heroes and villains. Per its title, the novella repeatedly suggests that Wu Li is bride not to Song Wei but to the national fight against SARS, thus retrieving her from what Xiao calls "bourgeois conjugality" only to return her to socialist nationhood.[50] More than once, the text raises the comparison of Wu Li to a revolutionary bride and of Su's team of nurses to the "red detachment of women" (47). In one especially conspicuous passage, in a conversation with the hospital's party secretary, Su analogizes the frontline nurses to soldiers on a battlefield, surrounded on all sides by unseen enemies, at which point the party secretary, nostalgically recalling his own wartime experiences, heartily agrees (46). As Hong Zhang notes, the deployment of communist war rhetoric was an official strategy of the Chinese state during SARS, when "the government repackaged Mao-era rhetoric to rally the nation for a patriotic 'people's war'" against the virus. State media frequently used "words such as 'warriors' (*zhanshi*), 'brave person' (*yongshi*), and 'martyr' (*lieshi*) to extol people fighting on the front line against SARS," and "medical workers who died or fell sick when treating SARS patients were eulogized as heroes who were sacrificing their lives for a heroic cause."[51] It might be tempting, then, to read Chen's novella as a pro-establishment work, either deliberately or naively parroting state propaganda. Especially alongside Hu's novel, *SARS Bride* gives us an exact reversal of the liberal humanist expectation that every Chinese writer is only too eager to leverage her political freedom of expression in the West to deliver an anticommunist dissident treatise.

Yet we must be careful not to overly polarize Chen and Hu, lest we feed the orientalist reductionism of Xiaobing Tang's dissidence hypothesis, whereby any noncondemnatory invocation of Maoist language signals a straightforward subscription to state ideology. In fact, *SARS Bride* is a much more heteroglossic text than meets the eye. It is important to notice that revolutionary rhetoric constitutes just one discursive strand within the novella's larger linguistic fabric, not the central ideological language that subsumes all others. Even in the scene mentioned above, Su's analogy of SARS to the Sino-Japanese War and the party secretary's nostalgic remembrance occur not as the rousing thesis that explicates the whole book but as a chance metaphor, in a casual and destressing conversation between friendly colleagues in the midst of disease management, and as one historical comparison that provides meaning to an older generation's epidemic experience. Clearly, this citational practice is not the same as political indoctrination. We can interpret Chen as attempting to capture the diversity of social idioms around SARS—which entails refusing to banish all traces of socialist speech from the postsocialist present. In a later scene, the revolutionary past resurfaces again in a debate between Wu Li and Song Wei, but, this time, it serves not as a historical parallel to the present but as the present's ambiguous precursor. With Su still hospitalized, Wu Li has again delayed her wedding, telling Song Wei that she intends to wait until "there is no more SARS," even if it means waiting another ten years. Frustrated, Song Wei snaps, "During the Long March, didn't some old revolutionaries get married anyway?" To which she replies, "That's not the same. That was wartime." He then rebuts, "Didn't you yourself say this is also war?" (132). The conversation ends with a sheepish Wu Li neither agreeing nor disagreeing with Song Wei's proposal that they get married on her next leave. For this younger generation coming of age in the early 2000s, the revolutionary past may be summoned as an expedient figure of speech and a pragmatic courtship tactic, not spoken out of nostalgic idolatry or smug disparagement but leveraged to score argumentative points when couples bicker. For and among them, there is little need to take on the posture of blanket rejection or denunciation as a banner of enlightened modernity. One might feel embarrassed at being called out on inconsistency as Wu Li does, but there is no illusion that recycled old rhetoric determines one's present choices.

In this respect, Chen is much less invested than Hu in probing the haunting legacies of China's past and, by extension, incriminating all party members as cogs in the totalitarian machine. Instead, she opts to focus on professionals like Su for whom party membership is subsidiary to their daily work and affective bonds. The novella's positive portrayals of authority figures seem aimed to promote not political trust in the party-state system but public confidence in the possibility that some individuals, including those in power, will put citizens' welfare above political and material gain. Thus, in one of the novella's few explicitly political passages, the provincial official who heads infectious disease control adamantly calls for transparency of information and public education about SARS. He does so against multiple objections raised by voices that go unnamed in the text—that "escalating the situation will affect the city's economy," that "it's a political question," and that "the upcoming March meeting in Beijing is a critical time of leadership changeover, so we cannot stir up chaos for the country" (16). Obliquely alluding to the fractures in governmental attitudes toward SARS management at the time, including those that leaned toward political self-interest and economic stability, the novella retains optimistic faith in the presence of public-minded officials inside the party-state system.

Chen's subtle deviation from the party line can be discerned more clearly if we probe further into the uneven official discourse on SARS at the time. In her preface to the novella, written in late June 2003 near the end of the global outbreak, Chen recalls watching televised coverage of the epidemic within China from New York, "being intensely worried about the country and the people," and finally breaking down in tears when she saw interviews with Chinese medical workers. Tellingly, she saw all this not on American news channels but on China Central Television, the premier state-controlled station.[52] By her own account then, *SARS Bride* has its genesis in her diasporically mediated encounter with SARS through China's state media and its transnational outlets. Indeed, medical narratives celebrating the heroism and altruism of doctors and nurses circulated profusely on both official and unofficial Chinese media during the pandemic. These stories built social morale and deterred mass panic by focusing on medical workers' bravery and self-sacrificing public service, precisely the themes highlighted in the novella. Yet Chen's handling of this source material is a considered one. As I will elaborate in the next chapter, in the early months of SARS, as part of the government's effort to suppress negative news about the domestic outbreak, Chinese mainstream media co-opted the voices of medical professionals so as to create a narrative of successful viral containment. Not only did these expert reports attempt to reassure the public by selectively spotlighting recovery stories, particularly those of frontline medical workers, but some went as far as to downplay disease risk and inflate treatment results, projecting that an otherwise healthy person would recover from an infection in just two weeks' time, or declaring that "doctors were capable of killing any type of virus" and did not even need to wear face masks outside the emergency room.[53] In contrast to these overly buoyant and downright inaccurate accounts broadcasted by state media outlets, Chen's novella provides a modest corrective: doctors and nurses may be heroic, but they are not invincible, and they do die from SARS. The ones who most boldly and selflessly throw themselves into the line of contagion may also be the ones whose immunity stands to become most compromised through repeated exposure, overwork, and exhaustion, and they are the ones least likely to recover. Su's death is not just a conventional plot element in a medical drama or a purely sentimental device aimed at producing tragic pathos; it can also be read as a counterpoint to the sanitizing imperative of official discourse, political by virtue of what it does not reiterate.

For comparison, we can look to the volume *The Storm That Tests the Grass* (*Ji feng jing cao*), released by Guangdong People's Publishing House in June 2003, in a parallel publishing timeline to *SARS Bride*. This book compiles dozens of vignettes by medical staffs at Guangdong hospitals recounting their personal experiences with SARS in intensive care units. There is even an essay by a real-life "SARS bride" with the surname Wu, a nurse at the Guangdong Traditional Chinese Medical Hospital who remembers being called back to work the morning after her wedding day and spending her honeymoon in the quarantine wards.[54] The collection as a whole concentrates on the positive aspects and outcomes of the epidemic, and the essays in homage to or by infected medical workers, including a chief nurse very much resembling Su Weiling, all end with the patients' recovery as well as their ardent return to work. The editorial apparatus even emphasizes how SARS has served to buttress the ranks of the party, how a number of medical "comrades have gloriously joined the Chinese Communist Party while in the line of fire even as others now await approval on their applications." The reasons behind this application trend are not explored, leaving readers with the impression that party membership represents a lifelong dream and a kind of bucket list item for these "white-robed warriors."[55] *SARS Bride* may not strike a stridently discordant tone toward party membership from this volume, but it also pointedly does not trumpet the self-congratulatory rhetoric of party-state organs.

Endemic Violence and Subaltern Survival

In the novella's other major story line, Chen further insinuates her subtle departure from the state imperative toward economic development. Here, SARS is crucially tied to endemic social issues in reform-era China. The main villain is Li Kejun, an unscrupulous businessman who owns the clothing factory where Song Wei works. With SARS dealing a heavy blow to his business, Li decides to profit from the outbreak by switching to producing face masks, and when his supply line runs dry, he secretly authorizes the use of rat-bitten gauze at his factory, unbeknownst to his workers. Song

Wei inadvertently stumbles across this scheme, and under Wu Li's shrewd direction, he becomes a whistleblower and trial witness, successfully bringing Li to legal justice. With this thrilleresque plot, Chen situates SARS within ongoing social problems in the capitalist era, taking up in particular public concern over the safety of fake consumer goods. Her novella is prescient in anticipating the string of toxic food incidents that would erupt over the next few years and that would culminate in the notorious melamine-tainted milk scandal of 2008. Like Hu, Chen deflates and displaces pandemic terror, redirecting fear from the disease itself to everyday instances of entrepreneurial corruption with direct impact on people's health. Rather than political obedience and self-preservation, her novella emphasizes the importance of individual agency and communal ethics over socioeconomic benefit and political apprehension, instructing readers to take civic action against those who jeopardize public safety, even at the cost of one's job. It is a pedagogical text, but one that works to reconstruct and repair communal trust in ordinary people as much as authority figures. Indeed, Chen is not so unlike Damo in Hu's novel, a grassroots intellectual whose medium is feminist fiction rather than the internet essay.

Chen's novella further interlocks this corruption plotline with another on sex trafficking and the exploitation of female rural migrants, spotlighting again women's distinct exposure amid and beyond the disease outbreak. Where Wu Li is the fortunate heroine who meets with good-hearted helpers throughout her journey, Yue E is her shadow double, the female migrant beleaguered by predators from the start. Rather than a fairy godmother, her first employer in the city is none other than Li Kejun, who also happens to be a pedophile and serial rapist. Li is one of the many clients of Madame Zhou, a pimp and sex trafficker who lures rural migrant women into domestic servitude and sexual slavery for wealthy city men. Misled by Madame Zhou to believe that Li has a wife, Yue E soon discovers he is in fact a bachelor with a sexual appetite for young virgins. Herself only about fourteen at the time, a lone migrant without resources in the city, she helplessly submits to repeated rape but manages to run away during one of Li's business trips. She wants desperately to confide in Wu Li, but she is afraid that news would travel back to her parents in the village, so she lies about being fired. Taking in Yue E out of pity and compassion, Aunty Hong detects the girl's pregnancy and guesses the truth. At the urging of Hong and Wu Li and with help from Su, Yue E gets an abortion, though she remains too scared to bring criminal charges against Li, despite the other women's encouragement. With usual foresight,

Su obtains Yue E's permission for a DNA test for both her and the fetus, keeping a record of the test results that would later prove essential in the trial against Li. Through this plotline, Chen constellates the four main female characters in a collective effort, one that provides not just domestic support and emotional comfort but also professional expertise and even legal counsel for the rape survivor.

By a twist of fate, Li later contracts SARS and becomes Wu Li's patient. She is consumed with rage on Yue E's behalf and almost carries out a revenge killing, stopped only by Su's timely intervention and severe reprimand. It is this near act of medical murder on Wu Li's part, driven by fierce sisterly loyalty, that finally moves Yue E to public testimony. As Yue E reasons inwardly:

> Aunty Hong is right, my whole life has been ruined by [Li Kejun]. Would anyone still want me in the future? If my parents find out, I'd rather die. But if I die, who'll take care of them? If I wanted to die, I should be dead by now. What am I waiting for? Wu Li is so loyal [*gou yiqi*], she'd even take revenge for me. As for me, why am I so scared? I really don't have to be afraid of his retaliation anymore, so what am I still scared of? Who knows, maybe when that Madame Zhou was being interrogated, she already disclosed everything about me. And if I am to be outed anyway, why not come forward myself? I can even claim damages, and the money can be used to help make my parents' old age more comfortable. Isn't that better than ending up empty-handed after he's already destroyed me? (105–6)

We can read Yue E's interior monologue as an instance of lateral politics, of life that does not resign itself to victim status even if it does not blare out its protest. Her decision to testify against her rapist does not arise from abstract principles of feminist justice, not even from a general sense of solidarity with other women victims, but from concrete and practical reasons concerning those she loves and cares for: her best friend's steadfast friendship and the cost of elder care in the countryside. This passage illuminates the unique vulnerability of young female migrants in the early 2000s. Even amid a global pandemic and even at one of its original epicenters, the migrant woman's greatest calamity is not infectious disease but sexual violence enabled by wealth disparities, a much more endemic kind of health insecurity in the era of global capital. Furthermore, Yue E must combat social shame and anxiety as an unmarried woman who has lost her virginity and aborted a child, as well as the cultural stigma around rape, all while balancing filial duty to a poor family and her own assault trauma. Whereas Wu Li and Su represent socioeconomically secure subjects who feel empowered to assume a feminist stance outright, who moreover are in stable relationships with supportive partners, Yue E is the precarious migrant who possesses none of these advantages. The language of frontline heroism and bold sacrifice may blast through Wu Li's story line, but it is a restrained ethical calculation that characterizes all of Yue E's interior scenes.

Yue E's story line may be read as showcasing the rise in gender crimes in the postsocialist period as well as concomitant transformations in feminist activism. As Qi Wang details, China's economic reforms have led to a resurgence in "traditional gender ideology and male chauvinism," so that "gender discrimination had become widespread . . . women's conditions in general had deteriorated," and domestic violence and abuse are "pervasive." At the same time, these developments have prompted the flourishing of a younger generation of feminist activists who "have little tolerance for gender discrimination and social injustice," who "react spontaneously to gender discriminative actions and language," and who mostly work outside the state system through informal networks. Chen sketches one early moment of this new formation, where women of "diverse ages and backgrounds are drawn together" into a "political generation" of gender activism.[56] Yue E may not stand out as a poster child of this new feminism and Chen may not give pride of place to her in the author's preface, but her character's inclusion reminds us to heed the contributions of minor actors, in the quiet spaces even of preyed-on subaltern life. For Yue E, the sentiment that matters, that ultimately motivates personal action, is not romantic love or love of country, not self-righteous anger or vindictive hatred but female *yiqi*—the spirit of loyalty between friends, traditionally cast as a male affect securing social brotherhood but relocated here in the zone of female fellowship. While Wu Li feels the much more classically feminist emotion of anger at her friend's sexual assault, anger alone would not have brought Li Kejun to justice. The novella dramatizes how it takes a village of women to engineer the right outcome, along with a diverse range of female affects circulating among multiple subjects both high and low. Yue E's character highlights this central role of emotions in feminist politics: as Ahmed theorizes, feminism is constituted not so much by a purely rational commitment to a set of ideals and positions as by one's emotional attachments to them, whereby "one becomes attached to feminism," and whereby emotions form "one's response to the world" and precipitate "a reorientation of one's bodily relation to social norms."[57] Yue E's affect may not rise to the level of Ahmed's "feminist wonder" with its passionate "radicalization of our relation to the past," but her change of heart suggests a definite reorientation of her emotional relation to the social world and its history of unjust norms, as she rejects the acceptability of what has existentially congealed for her into an injury-induced shame ordinariness.[58]

Not every thread of Chen's novella is loaded with such social and moral weight, however. In fact, its overall tone tends toward the lighthearted, with moments of pandemic ordinariness buoyed by humor, even for Yue E. Early on in the outbreak, when people are still figuring out how to live with SARS, Yue E and Aunty Hong go shopping one day. First, they discover that their face masks are made with runny dye, streaking their faces like those of Chinese opera performers, giving Yue E a good laugh. The reference to "unethical merchants" in this scene does not escalate into anything more than a gruff complaint (30), and the pair proceeds with their shopping. Recalling that vinegar kills germs, they scour the city for it, but all the stores except for two have sold out. These two stores have in turn inflated the price from three yuan a bottle to five and ten yuan a catty. At the traditional herb store, many beauty and health products now have SARS-prevention labels, and people flock to buy these up. When one woman asks the shopkeeper about her phlegmless, dry cough, one of SARS's telltale symptoms, the whole store suddenly empties, with all the customers scattering in cartoonish panic "like marble balls in a child's game" (31). Even the owner disappears from the counter, and, as soon as Yue E and Hong step outside, the door bangs shut behind them. The next day, they return to the store, having seen on television a new kind of "anti-SARS" herbal medicine. Smelling something burning, they alert the shopkeeper, who is appalled to find his wife disinfecting hundred-yuan bills by toasting them in the backroom microwave. He briskly gathers up the money and heads for the bank, again leaving Yue E and Hong stranded. Tired out by all this ado, the two decide to eat out, choosing a higher-tier restaurant for food safety. To their annoyance and ire, the price for wonton noodles has also skyrocketed. When Hong confronts the owner, he pleads bad business and a disinfection fee. At this, Hong scoffs, "You mean you don't normally disinfect?" Once home, Hong is determined to try the herbal medicine. She dutifully follows the instructions and consumes it three days in a row; on the third day, she wakes in the middle of the night with chills, covered in sweat and fearing for her life. Only later does she realize she should have consulted a physician rather than pin her hopes on some magic panacea. "Sure, go ask a doctor," she mutters grouchily to herself, repeating the television mantra. "But who dares go these days?" (32). Through Yue E and Hong's peripatetic adventures, Chen catalogs some of the quotidian effects of SARS, from exploitative business practices to media equivocation and misinformation, from irrational mob panic to potentially dangerous attempts at self-medication. But all this is narrated comically and unhistrionically, with gentle rather than riotous laughter, and humane rather than contemptuous satire. At the end of the day, Yue E and Hong tease each other and chuckle at their own foibles while grumbling about their fellow citizens' petty lapses in the face of an epidemic. And then they move on with their lives. This pandemic small humor will be the focus of the next chapter.

Coda: Wuhan Lockdown and Fang Fang's COVID Diary

In the initial days of COVID-19, when the city of Wuhan went into massive lockdown on January 23, 2020, Hu Fayun, as noted above, was in Vienna and could only follow events in his hometown from abroad, much as Chen Baozhen did during SARS from New York. This time around, the author who emerged as the emblematic voice of China's early pandemic experience was an uncanny real-life counterpart to Ru Yan: the writer Fang Fang, who began to record daily life under lockdown just two days later in her online *Wuhan Diary*. Her posts, uploaded nightly onto various social media platforms and "offering real-time responses to and reflections on events and news reports that had transpired just hours earlier," soon gained a huge readership, with some posts getting up to ten million hits within a few days.[59] Fang Fang had lived in Wuhan for over sixty years, since age two, so this diary was, in the words of her English translator Michael Berry, "her love letter to Wuhan"— not so unlike Joan Chen's film of SARS Shanghai.[60] In keeping with this female lineage of SARS narratives, Fang Fang's COVID chronicle, too, captures the ordinary routines and affective flux of quarantine life, enfolding small gestures and small feelings into the milieu of macro crisis, yielding an epidemic form quite different from the international media's reportage of China's coronavirus situation at the time.

For one exemplary moment, we may recall the death of Li Wenliang on February 7, 2020. An ophthalmologist at Wuhan Central Hospital, Li had

PANDEMIC ORDINARINESS **73**

sent a warning message to a WeChat group of colleagues in late December 2019 about a possible SARS-like viral outbreak in the city, only to contract the virus himself from a patient several days later. Upon his demise, global news media lionized him as the "whistleblower doctor" who spoke truth to power and "warned the world" about COVID, even though Li initially told his colleagues "not to share the information outside the WeChat group."[61] In a further re-iteration of Xiaobing Tang's dissidence hypothesis, global coverage of Chinese reactions to Li's death fixated on the "fury on social media," especially the trending hashtags "I/we want freedom of speech" and their subsequent censorship.[62] This early discourse on pandemic China, before the corona-virus spread west, remained mired in the binary terms of oppression versus resistance, heroic martyrs and freedom-loving publics versus authoritarian state harassment and silencing. If one prominent Western view is that "you don't have any social media" in China because "social media are not free in [authoritarian] countries," as the French president Emmanuel Macron avowed that year, Chinese social media is nonetheless ostentatiously exhib-ited when saturated with antigovernment rage.[63]

In contrast, Fang Fang's diary reveals how people navigated the disease outbreak and the city's lockdown in the day-to-day, showcasing social media as a space for prosocial solidarity and comfort in the depths of crisis and mourning. Her post on February 7, for instance, opens with an homage to Li and a sharing of her personal grief: "Dr. Li Wenliang died overnight and I am broken. . . . Tonight the entire city of Wuhan is crying for Li Wenliang." In her recounting, there was certainly rage in the city that day, but this feeling was just one among many, as millions of residents endured day sixteen of quarantine with "depression, sadness, and anger in their hearts." "Perhaps this is why Li Wenliang's death broke the entire city's heart?" she ponders. "Perhaps all they needed was an opportunity to let it all go and just cry out? Perhaps it also has to do with the fact that Li Wenliang was just like the rest of us—he was one of us," rather than some exceptionalized hero or victim. As Fang Fang makes a note of recording, someone was heard yelling, "The people of Wuhan will take care of Li Wenliang's family!" that afternoon. In this moment, posthumous honoring and mutual caring did not necessitate grand actions, and small gestures when multiplied became the fabric of daily pandemic survival as well as the balm for social pandemic grief. "To com-memorate Dr. Li," she reports, "tonight everyone in Wuhan plans to turn off their lights, then at exactly the time he passed away overnight, we will shine flashlights or cellphone lights into the sky while whistling for him. During this dark, heavy night, Li Wenliang will be our light."[64] This quiet communal remembrance recalls the nurses' makeshift memorial for Su Weiling in *SARS Bride*. Here, the intended audience was not just Li and the heavens but also the residents of Wuhan themselves, as they communicated care and support for each other. And then, like Yue E and Aunty Hong, they moved on with their lives, just as Fang Fang does in this post: "Everyone has been locked up in their tiny, cramped apartments for too long," she muses, and "you can only surf the internet for so long before you get bored of that, too. Besides that, everyone is facing their own set of problems in life."[65] She then goes on to worry about her two diabetic brothers and their lack of exercise during quarantine and her own dilemma of whether to pick up medication from the hospital the next day. Rather than a constant state of heightened political anger, ugly feelings of boredom and micro decisions about endemic issues defined the smaller pockets of daily lockdown life.

Jana Fedtke, Mohammed Ibahrine, and Yuting Wang have analyzed Fang Fang's diary in terms of *sous*veillance: if "surveillance occurs when citizens are watched by the state apparatus . . . sousveillance occurs when individual citizens watch their environment . . . in an unofficial way from the bottom up."[66] *Wuhan Diary*, they suggest, can be read as a "performance of sousveillance" that seeks to "keep officials accountable," with its "micro stories" challenging "the pervasiveness of the COVID-19-related macro-stories by the Chinese government."[67] As they rightly underscore, however, Fang Fang is far from a dissident writer and repeatedly expresses support for government policies in her diary. At most, hers is a "humble act of sousveillance," one aimed not at revolution but at making space for experiential self-witnessing and an online community oriented toward "compassion and hope."[68] Fang Fang herself would agree with this assessment. Some ten days after Li's death, she meditates on one reader's question about why she records mostly "little details of everyday life and not important things like the People's Liberation Army entering the city." In language reminiscent of Eileen Chang's, she responds: "I . . . as an independent writer, only have my own perspective on things. The only things I can pay attention to and experience are those little details that are happening around me and those real people I encounter in my life. And so that's all I can write—I provide a record of those trivial things happening around me; I write about my feelings and reflections in real time as things happen in order to leave a record for myself of this life experience."[69]

The defense of "little details" and "trivial things," the appeal to "feelings and reflections in real time"—these themes of pandemic ordinariness and affective sovereignty run through this chapter. If Fang Fang has been criticized by some dissident writers as a voice of "inband sousveillance" who is "much too soft" on state power, perhaps what needs redress is not her politics but the tyranny of politics without sociality.[70]

2

Pandemic Humor

Digital Prosociality for the Epidemic Socius

Humor and the Mass Socius

"China's modern literary history," writes Christopher Rea in *The Age of Irreverence*, "is one of lost laughter." In his study on humor in early twentieth-century China, Rea notes that official communist historiography has largely erased the rich comic cultures of the pre-1949 decades, so that "the Old Society" gets narrated as purely "a time of tears and sorrow." Such monumental histories (as Eileen Chang would call them), reconstructing the past as a series of grand events identified in hindsight, "tend to focus on the traumatic and the dramatic, rather than on everyday moments of communal or private amusement." To tell the story of modern China from the perspective of laughter, Rea suggests, is to offer "a 'new' history."[1] Likewise with SARS: pandemic crisis epistemologies tend to project tales of high trauma and drama, tears and sorrow, onto epidemic epicenters. Yet if we attend to the microsociality of life amid SARS within sinophone realms, we, too, discover everyday moments of communal and private amusement—manifesting, in one prominent cultural form, in a surprisingly voluminous and heterogeneous body of digital SARS jokes.

Throughout the months of the 2003 outbreak, pandemic humor was pervasive across the then budding world of Chinese digital media, and, crucially, the magnitude of this humor culture was enabled by new communication technologies. By the end of that year, China had 87 million internet users and over 200 million mobile phone users.[2] During SARS, usage of these technologies skyrocketed. Over the Spring Festival period alone, when rumors of the virus began to spread from southern China across the country, a total of seven billion text messages were sent.[3] After the epidemic became officially acknowledged by the state media, internet use in Beijing and Guangdong allegedly doubled, with Sina's SARS news website receiving three million hits per day.[4] Huiling Ding calls these digital platforms "guerilla media," which played a pivotal role in disseminating informal disease information within China during the outbreak.[5] Shaohua Guo further sees these digital platforms as exemplifying people's everyday microagency, "forging politically minded citizens at a micro level" as "diverse agents . . . compete for discursive legitimacy."[6] In the preface to her study on the evolution of the Chinese internet, Guo traces her own emerging identity as a netizen as well as the rise of digital community within China to the time of SARS. She recollects: "For the first time, surfing the web became a 'full-time job' for students. Confined in my dorm, I worked remotely as a part-time translator for Sina, the then dominant news portal in China, while frequenting bulletin board systems to gather information about life in the US. . . . SARS cultivated a special emotional attachment to the Internet for a large number of Chinese. This is not only because online media challenged the state's initial cover-up of SARS but also because this moment of national crisis fostered a strong sense of community among early netizens. I was one of them."[7] SARS was thus a key event in the formation of a Chinese digital mass socius.

Hong Zhang, one of the earliest scholars to explore the relation between Chinese digital technology and the "virtual public sphere" it fostered, was also the first to recognize that among the "new forms of sociality" emerging from this dynamic was a subculture of joking about SARS online. In May and

78   CHAPTER 2

June 2003, she conducted a "virtual ethnography" of the Chinese internet and amassed 150 SARS jokes, many of which appeared on popular websites in major cities such as Beijing and Shanghai and were then cross-posted on other regional websites, testifying to their widespread appeal across the country and perhaps beyond.[8] A more permanent and eclectic record of this comic culture can be found in the anthology *Laughing at SARS* (*Xiao dui SARS*), published by the Petroleum Industry Press in Beijing in June 2003. Collating over a thousand jokes and humorous expressions, this volume contains some of the pieces analyzed by Zhang but captures in addition a diverse array of cultural tidbits, from holiday felicitations and daily greeting text messages to poems, songs, anecdotes, vignettes, and cartoons. In its heterogeneity, the book resembles what was fast becoming an established genre of popular entertainment on mainstream television by the early 2000s: the team-hosted variety show, featuring an ever-changing cast of guest stars and filled with small segments of performances, chats, skits, and games, all intended to produce lighthearted and heartwarming laughter for mass audiences. The weekly series *Happy Camp*, for instance, debuted in 1997 and is still on the air today as one of China's most widely watched shows. One hallmark of this mainstream media culture is its ability to expand the realm of the enjoyable within safe political limits, accommodating the rapidly diversifying modes of mass entertainment and their humor forms. *Laughing at SARS* can be situated squarely within this milieu. On the surface, many of the anthologized pieces do not appear funny at all, but, precisely so, their inclusion in SARS joke compilations attests to an expansive understanding of what counted as humor during the epidemic.

In light of this archive of pandemic humor texts, in this chapter I adopt a broad approach to the concept of humor. I bring into consideration here not just conventional modes of laughter-oriented joke-telling but a fuller spectrum of social expressions around SARS, with special emphasis on everyday messages that may seem too trivial or banal for serious analysis but that vitally mediated a sense of collective crisis ordinariness, of a society enduring and smiling its way through SARS together. Extrapolating from Lauren Berlant's theory of lateral politics, I treat these humor practices as enactments of pandemic microagency. They may have been carried out in the privacy and seclusion of one's home, on the little screen of one's personal computer or cell phone, but, insofar as their products—which I will call SARS jokes as a shorthand—came to circulate on sundry social media platforms, they brought into being an enactive mass public, materializing in action people's shared psychic worries and hopes about the epidemic. I first examine political and parapolitical SARS humor as well as the politics of SARS humor before turning to what I call nonpartisan SARS humor—humor that does not have politics as its central engagement. I focus on the communal aspects of this nonpartisan humor and the often overlooked but richly complex affective dimensions of humor culture. Building on the recent burgeoning of scholarship on Chinese humor, this chapter illuminates not only that contemporary China is funnier than it has been given credit for, as several scholars have argued of late, but also that postsocialist Chinese humor can be profoundly animated by a concern with the socius rather than just the polis. Beyond mockery and critique, the humor spotlighted here more often than not aimed to restore frayed social connections during SARS, exemplifying practices of pandemic prosociality by circulating positive small affects for a socius in crisis. Giving this humor due attention is yet another way to "reinvent, from the scene of survival, new idioms of the political, and of belonging itself."[9]

As a corpus, SARS jokes represent a distinct type of mass culture. Most are of ambiguous origins and lack authorial attribution, spreading anonymously via private and informal social and digital networks. Characterized by roving linkages and unlocalized multiplicities rather than a unified, fixed, or hierarchical reception structure, they belong to an unofficial mediascape reminiscent of Gilles Deleuze and Félix Guattari's rhizome: "always in the middle, between things," with "no beginning or end" and with "any point . . . connected to anything other."[10] In this regard, they differ significantly from the previous chapter's epidemic novels, the transmission of which remains largely tied to systems of professional authorship. Chen Baozhen's *SARS Bride* had a limited print run and distribution circuit and is long out of print, while Hu Fayun's *Such Is This World@sars.come*, for all its internet origins, has been repeatedly censored and curtailed. By contrast, by eschewing formal affiliations and authority structures, and by virtue of their brevity, digital SARS jokes were highly elusive and eminently replicable, managing to reach much bigger audiences within shorter spans of time. Anonymity meant no one gained authorial credit or shouldered authorial blame. Though reliant on consumer technology, these jokes emerged outside of the commercial production process and were closer to uncommoditized ephemera. Along Xudong Zhang's Jamesonian formulation of Chinese postsocialism of the long 1990s, they may symptomize the "contradictions and chaos" of a "Chinese everyday world and mass culture" with its "mixed economy and its overlapping political and cultural (dis)order."[11] But in Hong Zhang's Habermasian view, they reflect a more deliberate attempt by China's rising urban middle class to create new spaces for public citizenship.[12] And along Huiling Ding's even stronger de Certeauian definition of guerilla media, they can serve as "weapons of the weak" that tactically intervene on the Chinese government's totalizing strategies of power.[13]

Still, laughter may seem a counterintuitive mass response to large-scale pestilence and death, and less innocent than the sentimental novel's appeal to romance, domesticity, and friendship. As a then unknown and lethal virus that struck down thousands, SARS was hardly suitable material for comedy, especially among those living within its global epicenter. When the ethnic burden of disease morbidity and mortality was so disproportionately Chinese, one might expect humor to arise only remotely, from non–Chinese majority sites. That is to say, one might be predisposed to treat pandemic laughter as indicative of georacial distance and privilege, mediating schadenfreude, defensive relief, or displaced fear about the sick and contaminating other—Freudian explanatory models for many theorists of disaster humor.[14] With SARS, though, disease humor was most abundant and visible precisely in the sinophone digital sphere, flourishing by repetition as much as invention. This comic sociality, I argue, was at heart more prosocial than antisocial or critical, insofar as it built a care-based cultural ecosystem and affective economy. My reading thus departs from prevailing paradigms in humor studies that privilege satirical, oppositional, or insubordinate modes of humor. Instead, I advance a model of pandemic humor beyond crisis epistemologies, one I will theorize as small humor—humor that deliberately revels in bathos rather than pathos, that channels a gentle and generous laughing alongside rather than a spiteful or angry laughing at, that ultimately works to cohere people into a feeling of shared everyday living within recurrent but survivable strife. As with the sentimental narratives and love practices highlighted in chapter 1, showcasing China's SARS humor culture may help reshape COVID-era Western bio-orientalist feelings toward Chinese subjects as somehow not fully human, partitioned off from what Sara Ahmed calls a "sociality of pain" but on a global scale, as so many unlovable and ungrievable "illegitimate lives." Against the backdrop of our current pandemic, resurfacing these small humor practices during SARS can illumine epidemic Chinese lives as those deserving of not just life and care but companionship, as people one might want to share a laugh, a joke, a tender moment with, in healing communion.

PANDEMIC HUMOR   81

Political SARS Humor and the Politics of SARS Humor

In her taxonomy of SARS jokes, Hong Zhang identifies five major themes: those that offered "comfort and advice in dealing with the crisis"; those that "ridiculed overreaction" and "mocked the overvigilant and scrupulous"; those that "focused on romance and sex, reflecting the current openness on matters of intimacy"; those that revealed "the excesses of the new commercial economy" and its "dark side"; and, finally, those that were explicitly political and satirized official party ideology.[15] As she explicates, "Since the post-Mao thaw in the late 1970s, political humor has resurfaced with a vengeance.... In the SARS crisis, the government's initial secrecy and subsequent recourse to Maoist-style mass mobilization sparked another round of political jokes using SARS as the topic."[16] The most daringly explicit of political SARS jokes used the outbreak as an occasion not just to poke fun at top leaders but to enumerate the many hypocrisies and failures of the party throughout communist history. One example is "What the Party Has Failed to Do, SARS Has Succeeded":

> The Party failed to control dining extravagantly, SARS succeeded.
> The Party failed to control touring on public funds, SARS succeeded.
> The Party failed to control having a set of meetings, SARS succeeded.
> The Party failed to control deceiving one's superiors and deluding one's subordinates, SARS succeeded.
> The Party failed to control prostitution and whoring, SARS succeeded.[17]

Jokes such as this one "may not rally political action, but they circulate political critique that would otherwise be suppressed or silenced." For Zhang, politics suffuses the bulk of SARS humor. Even jokes that lampoon seemingly apolitical social foibles such as sexual vanity and material greed are construed parapolitically as indirect critiques of the state, signaling the myriad ways people venture into new virtual spaces to explore the reform era's loosened boundaries around previously tabooed topics. While she acknowledges the stylistic differences among SARS jokes, their fundamental spirit for her is defiance, their bottom line a political reckoning. Yet she, too, reads SARS humor as ultimately "connecting everyday life with political agency" and "activating a sense of ordinary and efficacious citizenship" for "ordinary people."[18]

Zhang is not an outlier in prioritizing the political. The field of cultural studies is centrally preoccupied with the subversive potential of humor, and many studies treat laughter as a means to upend, disrupt, or contest authority structures. Humor is typically theorized as oppositional and iconoclastic, as the perfect tool for undermining hegemons, with emphasis on the target being pulled down through laughter rather than the multitudes united through it. This template especially dominates studies of Chinese humor. Perry Link and Kate Zhou, for instance, zero in on the class of "rhythmical satirical sayings known as *shunkouliu* (slippery jingles) or *minyao* (folk rhymes)" that have roots in early twentieth-century folk ditties and that proliferated in the 1980s and 1990s, with an "overwhelming majority" of them expressing political or social criticism, whether about official corruption, the market economy, or the party-state.[19] As a "countermedium to the official media," Link and Zhou endow *shunkouliu* with a "corrosive effect on the legitimacy of the Communist Party and Chinese state institutions" in the long run.[20] Similarly, Tao Dongfeng draws on Mikhail Bakhtin's theory of the carnivalesque to explicate the late 1990s trend of "canon-mocking literature" (*dahua wenxue*), which he sees as channeling the "jubilant, chaotic, subversive energy of parody" to "temporarily resist and subvert the ideological constraints of the dominant culture" in a posttotalitarian society.[21] For Tao, this literature's humor constitutes an indirect "weapon of resistance," displacing people's oppositional energy from open attacks on the regime to the ridiculing of relatively safe literary targets.[22] This argument is echoed by Liu Xiaobo in his analysis of 2000s internet *egao* (wicked-making) culture. Likewise citing Bakhtin, Liu traces *egao* to "grassroots wit" and invests it with radical insurgent potential: "In a post-totalitarian dictatorship, the grins of the people are the nightmares of the dictators."[23]

Other scholars analyzing postsocialist Chinese humor largely follow this framework of political critique, subversion, and resistance. In the most utopian formulations, Chinese laughter is said to tap into a reservoir of revolutionary energy. The flip side of this comic utopianism, however, is the constant dismissal of laughter that falls short politically, a looking askance at any humor that might be "merely" destructive, nihilistic, or complicitous with state power. This binarist impasse, whereby the assessment of a Chinese cultural form's legitimacy is caught between the rigid poles of rebellion and subservience, recalls once again Xiaobing Tang's dissidence hypothesis. We may also recall Stuart Hall's caution against romanticizing the popular via a "dialectic [of] containment/resistance," especially in colonial and decolonial settings.[24] In studies of postsocialist China, a similar problem confronts analyses of *egao* practitioners. As Rea points out, these cultural producers remain "poorly understood... because commentators have tended to strike a moralizing tone—either celebrating their perceived political subversiveness or wringing their hands about how they represent a symptom of grave decline in public decency"; as a result, *egao* culture is often portrayed as the realm of "either heroic dissidents or cyber-schoolyard bullies."[25] In effect, the political albatross hanging around the neck of Chinese humor entraps it within a reductive moral universe.

In this context, the anthology *Maoist Laughter* provides an important corrective by sketching out the socialist prehistory to postsocialist humor. In her introduction to the volume, Ping Zhu overturns the widespread perception of the Mao era as solely one of violence and tragedy, "a gloomy period incompatible with laughter as a genuine expression of happiness and freedom." Too often, she notes, humor becomes reified as "a weapon of defiance" that "should be pitted against the Mao era." This myopic view, she argues, not only fails to recognize the diversity of humor's forms and functions but overlooks how humor was historically institutionalized by the Maoist state itself, as "a crucial social practice for the reproduction of socialist ideology, state-building, and subject-making."[26] Rather than puritanically opposed to humor on principle, the party was in fact guided by Marx's suggestion that "the final phase of world-historical form is its comedy." For Mao, socialist laughter was also a potent weapon that could serve, in his words, to "unite and educate people, attack and annihilate enemies."[27] Superior to bourgeois laughter, which was deemed capable of only hypocrisy and deceit, socialist laughter was posited as "cheerful, hearty, genuine, and healthy," reflecting the "euphoric, rhapsodic, and optimistic" nature of the socialist spirit. Hence, laughter was neither a "universal human vocalization" nor an element "external to Maoist discourse" but "an integral part" of it. Subversive and satirical laughter was disavowed by socialist humor, projected onto the United States as a cultural form unique to capitalist and imperialist societies with unequal class and race relations.[28] In this light, the dominance of subversive critique paradigms in contemporary humor studies may actually symptomize the intellectual hegemony of neoliberal imperialism.

Given this lineage, it becomes entirely logical that the Chinese state would attempt to co-opt popular jokes into a framework of socialist humor during SARS. Far from censoring the profusion of SARS jokes, the government, cannily recognizing the political sensitivity of a domestic infectious disease outbreak and also the malleability of its meanings, took steps to publicize and promote these jokes in the state media.[29] By May 2003, the website of the party's flagship newspaper *People's Daily* was reporting with approval a host of irreverent practices around SARS, posting reader op-eds with headlines such as "'Atypical' Humor for 'Atypical Pneumonia' Times."[30] The website also published a short compilation of trendy SARS jokes, divided into rubrics such as "tender and warmhearted," "bizarre and weird," "funny and zany," and so forth.[31] Chinese Central Television also ran a contest asking the public to vote on their favorite SARS-related text messages, and, when the winning entries were published on the CCTV website, seven of the top ten pieces contained some comic component.[32] While explicit political satires were predictably excluded, several jokes interpreted by Hong Zhang as illustrative of parapolitical censure were included in both forums. Both, for instance, published a version of the popular "ways of dying from SARS" joke:

> Several ways of dying from SARS: suffocated by a face mask; poisoned by Chinese medicine; scared to death by a coworker's infection; tired to death from avoiding public transportation and walking to and from work every day; depressed to death by friends' and family's neglect after returning from a trip to an infected zone; cured to death by a mistaken diagnosis; cursed to death for spreading rumors; beaten to death for sneezing in public.[33]

The interpretive battle over SARS humor becomes especially evident here. Zhang reads the many variations on this death-by-SARS joke as making fun of disease phobia, which she sees as fanned by the government's draconian quarantine measures.[34] But if authorities felt at all uneasy about this joke's implied political discontent, their response was to control its meaning through promotion and pedagogy rather than suppression and erasure. The CCTV website included pedagogical devices after each winning entry, such as the reason for its recommendation and a brief exegesis, in order to shape each piece's reception. While the above death joke might seem too sarcastic or disparaging of the government's containment efforts to be safely listed, the official exegesis here was that the joke used comic exaggeration and "benevolent ridicule" to call out human selfishness and timidity but fundamentally allowed for healthy laughter so people could "release repressed gloominess and resume a positive attitude."[35] In this way, even borderline risqué gallows humor was recuperated and assimilated into the rhetoric of socialist humor—as morally beneficial, spiritually uplifting, and socially wholesome humor that serves the people. More subtly, the government might have been signaling its growing tolerance of certain cultural forms of irony, even those with a slight cynical edge toward the sociopolitical present, thereby insinuating its intolerance of what crossed that line. This effort to appropriate and resignify SARS humor, as Zhang observes, showcases the state's ability to adapt to new communications technology and respond to the emerging virtual public.[36] We can also read this cultural responsiveness as indexing the government's authoritarian resilience in the postsocialist era. At the end of the day, political SARS humor and the politics of SARS humor yield neither a radical break from nor a noteworthy culmination of modern China's humor history.

Nonpartisan SARS Humor and Epidemic Chatter

The vast majority of SARS jokes, though, are nonpolitical in content. They can certainly be deciphered along political lines as parapolitical humor, so rather than calling them nonpolitical and installing a false binary, I will designate them nonpartisan, insofar as they do not have the spoofing of the party-state as their principal concern. This nonpartisan or extrapolitical character becomes especially salient when we define jokes in the most capacious sense to encompass indigenous varieties such as folk rhymes and clever wordplays as well as anything considered funny, amusing, or inane. As scholars of Chinese humor often point out, the generic Chinese term for humor, *youmo*, is a modern import, a loan word transliterated from English in the 1920s. Before that, no one Chinese term offered a unified idea of humor or treated it as a universal humanist rubric. Instead, classical texts had a rich lexicon that captured the many shades of the comical or laughable, and many of these terms have no exact English equivalents: *xue* and *paidiao* both connote joking, *ji* and *chao* are both forms of ridicule and derision, and *xie* and *guji* or *huaji* all evoke glibness.[37] The contemporary word *xiao*, also of ancient roots, contains a host of meanings and can be used "as a verb (to laugh, to smile, to mock), as a descriptor (laughable, ridiculous, derisive), and as a noun (laughter, smile, joke, jest)," further highlighting the nonequivalence between Chinese and English vocabularies of humor and the need, in comparative cultural studies, to heed context.[38]

Additionally, as Jocelyn Chey points out, the Chinese language is a "particularly apt vehicle to convey humour, being rich in homophones that have great potential for punning," "linguistic plays on words and *double entendres*."[39]

During SARS, this Chinese-specific linguistic humor abounded. One subgenre of SARS jokes comprises a host of droll anecdotes that turn on the phrase *wo feidian* and pun specifically on *feidian* (atypical pneumonia), the name SARS was most commonly known by in Mandarin on the mainland. In the many permutations of this joke, someone who naively uses the phrase would be mistaken for a SARS-infected person and briskly carted away by health authorities. One example:

> I took my client to dinner. That damned guy insisted on ordering a crab dish [an expensive meal]. I advised him not to do so as it was not the season. He would not listen to me. Picking his teeth while flipping through the menu, he shouted at me: "I have never eaten that dish before. You are not going to stop me. *Wo feidian! Wo feidian!* [I must order that]." All of a sudden, three face-masked men sprang out from the soup bowl and took him away.[40]

The *wo feidian* jokes exemplify a class of SARS humor that encapsulates at once political criticism, parapolitical parody, and nonpartisan linguistic play. The scenario of unsuspected arrest due to an unintended linguistic slip carries haunting echoes within communist history, recalling the intense ideological policing of everyday language during the Cultural Revolution. The tacit connection between the Maoist past and the postsocialist present, and the very repetition of the joke scenario across different mundane situations in contemporary life, further raise the specter of a totalizing surveillance state, with government monitors lurking around every corner, ever ready to pounce on the poor soul who happens to misspeak. Zhang ascribes the popularity of this joke during SARS to a general public disgruntlement toward the state's massive quarantine measures that were perceived as "excessive and arbitrary."[41] At the same time, the exorbitant outcome to the client's profligate banqueting ties the comedy here to a kind of revenge fantasy directed against the wealthy elite's material excesses during the capitalist era. Finally, these anecdotes require a certain amount of linguistic as well as storytelling skill and can serve to showcase a teller's wit, cleverness, and social savvy. As Zhang points out, "Being able to tell jokes has become associated with being cool, smart, rebellious, and independent," and during SARS, joke-telling was for some "an opportunity to demonstrate their intellectual prowess, independence, and rebelliousness," especially among the rising urban middle class.[42] Linguistic humor, then, can go hand in hand with political satire and social parody.

Yet a great deal of SARS humor does not aim for that level of cerebral prowess or flashy wit, and it is precisely the more mundane and modest comical expressions that the anthology *Laughing at SARS* becomes an archive for. Many linguistic jokes recorded in the volume are much shorter, and they make their puns in much more prosaic and predictable ways. One example of an amateurish *feidian* joke:

> Many people are afraid of *feidian*, but actually there's no need to be afraid! Isn't it just a matter of wearing a face mask that's a bit thicker [*hou dian*], sleeping a bit longer [*duo dian*], going out a bit less [*shao dian*], and shaking hands with a pretty girl a bit more carefully [*zhuyi dian*]? (Jiang et al., 23)[43]

Unlike the more self-consciously elaborate *wo feidian* stories that turn on surprising and sharp-witted double entendres, this joke makes its pun on *feidian* with a noticeable laziness, by repeating just one rhyme word for *dian*—and the most obvious word at that—as if to play up its teller's lack of creativity and effort. Beyond wordplay, many of the linguistic jokes toy with tone and diction, and, again, many play up their own prosaicness and flat-footedness. The following text message, for instance, may not seem funny at all at first glance, but, on closer scrutiny, we can see it donning the guise of a philosophical musing only to gently mock its own lack of crescendo:

> Who can say how many random flukes make up human life? All the joys and sorrows brought to you by each coincidence are also your greatest riches. Maybe people are the same, and maybe "SARS," too, is a kind of fluke. (297)

Instead of culminating in some shrewd nugget of wisdom or clinching with some slick turn of phrase, this text message seems to wallow in its dulled affect by drifting off into a half-baked thought, in mild self-mockery and chagrin. That it, too, was taken up as an instance of SARS humor underscores the capaciousness and flexibility with which humor was interpreted during the outbreak. Superficially, much of this everyday SARS humor seems trivial or hackneyed, sometimes not even that droll or jocular, just part of the evanescent flotsam of mass culture and daily life. But this nonpartisan humor needs to be understood as performing community building, on the one hand, as I will elaborate below, and mediating epidemic chatter, on the other.

To understand the epidemic chatter function of these joke pieces, finer-grained attention to the timeline of SARS information is key. Contrary to broad-strokes accounts about SARS-era China, the central government did not shift overnight from blanket censorship to comprehensive control of SARS news. Instead, throughout the epidemic period, both state and public knowledge about the disease varied greatly across levels and regions, as Yanzhong Huang and Huiling Ding have separately chronicled.[44] The first known case of SARS appeared in mid-November 2002 in the city of Foshan in Guangdong, and, by mid-January 2003, the virus had spread to three other cities in the province. On January 27, an investigative team of health experts from both the provincial and national government completed a top-secret report on the outbreak and sent it to the Guangdong Health Administration and likely the Ministry of Health in Beijing. This document, though, remained unopened for three days due to the absence of personnel with adequate security clearance. When it was finally read, a notice was issued to hospital heads across the province, but, by that point, most of them had gone on vacation for the Spring Festival break. Thus, it was not until over two weeks later, on February 11, that Guangdong health officials held "the first and only press conference to release official statistics about the SARS situation in the province."[45] One problem thereafter was that the disparate organs of the country's public health sector tended to operate independently, with municipal governments and various health ministries not sharing disease information with one another. As a result, the general public's as much as state authorities' knowledge about SARS was highly uneven across the country. Huang thus attributes the overall delay in the central government's acknowledgment of SARS not to any nefarious scheming on the part of top party leaders but to the "fragmented authoritarianism" of China's political system, with its "fragmented and disjointed" bureaucracy leading to multilevel "coordination problems" in policymaking.[46]

Another major impediment to the timely and accurate disclosure of SARS data was the climate of political fear and self-interest. The virus's sudden appearance coincided with a particularly tension-filled period for officials all over the country, as this was the lead-up to the March meeting of the National People's Congress in Beijing, the quinquennial forum for the changeover in national leadership and a decisive time for the career fates of many cadres down the chain of command. Hence, at the February 11 press conference, Guangdong officials were keenly aware of the urgency of placating public fears and preserving social stability when they announced that "all patients [had] been effectively treated and the outbreak [had] been brought under control."[47] In order not to disrupt local economies or fan social panic, various local authorities preemptively implemented a news blackout on SARS, one that lasted from late February to early April. State secret laws further discouraged transparency on the part of lower-level cadres since all public health information on infectious diseases was classified as state secrets at the time and any unauthorized reporting was punishable as treason.[48] Huang thus speculates that top party leaders themselves were kept in the dark about SARS's true scale because lower-level officials actively "intercepted and distorted the upward information flow" to downplay the outbreak until after the People's Congress meeting had concluded.[49] Even then, during an April 3 national press conference, the first held by the central government and televised live, the health minister reassured Premier Wen Jiabao and the national public that SARS had "already been brought under effective control" and that China was "safe to visit" for foreigners.[50] Ironically, on that same day across the international date line, the WHO issued its first ever travel advisory against Guangdong and Hong Kong.

The temporary lack of top-down directives and institutional coordination, however, did not prevent local governments from establishing a common rhetorical front to the public. As Ding details, news censorship meant not a total silencing of SARS-related topics but a strict policing and crafting of disease information by official media outlets. As word of the virus spread through private unofficial channels, and as international news started to aggressively report on the rapidly globalizing pandemic, panic buying broke out across several provinces, threatening social and economic stability precisely during the sensitive time of the People's Congress meeting. When local authorities could no longer rest on silence or denial, they fashioned a politically safe "containment narrative" to reassure the public that SARS was "under control," that governmental efforts at fighting the disease were successful, and that people should continue to "live normal lives." As noted in chapter 1, in lieu of hard data, state media concentrated on the heroic self-sacrifice of medical professionals, feel-good recovery stories of infected patients, generic prevention tips and healthy living advice, and the "social side effects" of the epidemic such as panic buying and price inflation.[51] In this period, the public was not so much kept in total darkness as flooded with human interest stories about SARS. It was not until April 20—after the whistleblower Jiang Yanyong, the chief physician at the People's Liberation Army General Hospital, exposed the cover-up of a major Beijing outbreak in a letter leaked to the international press—that the central government at last revealed that the domestic SARS count was ten times higher than previously claimed and that the country needed to mobilize an all-out "people's war" against SARS.[52] Thereafter, the central government began to adopt "a more transparent approach to the release of information" by providing daily updates and granting media outlets "greater autonomy" in their epidemic reporting.[53]

It is against this fluctuating backdrop of official silence, containment discourse, warlike propaganda, selective coverage, and the ever-present threat of an eventual relapse into information crackdown that we can grasp the chatter function of nonpartisan SARS humor. While the internet jokes examined by Zhang cropped up, by her estimation, between late April and early May 2003, many of the pieces compiled in *Laughing at SARS* date to as early as the first days of February, perhaps earlier, given the section on text greetings for the Chinese New Year, which fell on February 1 that year.[54] Indeed, some of these messages do not explicitly mention SARS but only allude to it via an emphasis on health or sickness, and we can infer that they were composed before *feidian* or "atypical pneumonia" became the official name used by authorities in the first days of February (and certainly before the name "SARS" was coined by the WHO in mid-March).[55] These SARS-inflected greetings thus surfaced over a week before the Guangdong press conference, several weeks before the proliferation of containment narratives in mainstream media, and over two months before the central government's official policy response. During those weeks of a void in reliable information about the domestic outbreak, or what Ding calls a "risk communication vacuum," unofficial media exploded with warning messages.[56] As she details, guerilla media—technology-assisted communication channels outside of state outlets such as personal phone calls, mobile phone text messages, internet discussion boards and chat rooms, and personal blogs—allowed people to "circumvent state surveillance" and "distribute and receive unauthorized risk messages" about SARS.[57] The first messages were likely sent by medical workers at affected hospitals to their immediate social circles; these then dispersed outward, multiplying and transforming along the way, sometimes into rumor and gossip. Indeed, a putative 80 percent of Guangzhou residents had already heard about the virus through unofficial channels by the time of the February 11 Guangdong press conference.[58] If the jokes discussed by Zhang struck her as predominantly satirical or critical in orientation, it may be that, by late April and May, popular humor had taken a sharper turn, as people became increasingly frustrated and embittered by the reversals in official media coverage and, perhaps, also emboldened by the surfeit of authorized SARS stories.

The appearance and proliferation of nonpartisan jokes, meanwhile, testify to a type of epidemic talk that falls not only between official and anti-official discourse, between passive reiteration and outright dissent, but also between truth and lies. While these jokes did not come into being outside of politics, their humor introduced new epidemic styles—new ways of chatting about SARS and feeling about epidemic life. Rather than the restrictive dyads of data/rumor and knowledge/cover-up, these jokes filled the chasm of the articulable with a broader array of everyday speech and affects, inventing as it were new subgenres such as the SARS greeting, SARS sweet-talk, SARS folk recipes, SARS mimic poems, and SARS fanfiction.

Before I analyze these SARS styles and forms more closely, it is worth noting the disjunction between the myriad pieces gathered up in *Laughing at SARS* and the volume itself as a textual product of state discourse. Even as the former circulated innumerable private and unofficial ways of talking about SARS during the outbreak, the latter aimed to consolidate and control their meanings within a state-compliant framework after the outbreak's end. Most saliently, none of the anthologized pieces are overtly political or censorious of the party-state, and we can well imagine the book's team of nearly three dozen editors working diligently to weed out negative, disruptive, or inappropriate material. The book's many layers of paratextual apparatuses also attest to how the editors went to great lengths to bring pandemic joke-telling within the bounds of socialist humor. The annotated table of contents didactically glosses each section with a message on healthy and cheerful laughter, at times repeating almost verbatim the state media's exegeses of SARS jokes. In his afterword, the editor-in-chief Jiang Zuohao further stresses that the volume is intended to promote and restore public health, especially mental health, on the heels of SARS, and his language echoes the Maoist construction of comedy, per Zhu's formulation, as a "crucial social practice for the reproduction of socialist ideology, state-building, and subject-making": "To adopt humor toward 'SARS' is to demonstrate an optimistic and positive attitude," Jiang writes, "one that expresses our faith and courage in defeating 'SARS' while also displaying our indomitable ethnonational spirit [*minzu jingsheng*] in the face of a catastrophe."[59] The editors also emphatically marshal the authority of science, with the book cover and dustjacket prominently featuring Hong Zhaoguan, flagged as a cardiovascular specialist and the medical director of Beijing Anzhen Hospital at Capital Medical University, as the project's principal health consultant. In his foreword, Hong expounds on the adverse physiological effects of fear and advises readers to maintain a calm and happy state of mind, for which "humor is key."[60] The book co-opts this biomedical discourse as if to suggest that Western science has at last caught up with what socialist doctrine has always known about human laughter. By situating SARS jokes within this updated socialist humor framework, *Laughing at SARS* not only ensures that the jokes stay safely within official bounds, as expressions unequivocally reflective of the Chinese people's ethnonational vigor and moral courage in the face of epidemic disease, but also tries to preempt alternative reactions to the jokes themselves.

Yet no archive, however micromanaged, can entirely foreclose the horizon of interpretation and meaning. It is in the spirit of prosocial community-building amid COVID-19 that I now turn to this small humor archive, not just to academically excavate it but also to affectively share with my readers its range of prosocial microaffirmations and ordinary fun. Above all, I want to highlight that, in the milieu of SARS China, even between the crisis poles of politics and pandemic, people concocted countless microagentive acts to mediate and sustain human warmth—which may yet touch us across the decades and continents if we open our hearts to it.

Small Humor and New Epidemic Subgenres

SARS Greetings

> Making friends requires 30% chivalry, and good conduct requires integrity. In our time together, let's act with sincerity and heart. When *feidian* is attacking us, all the more should we face it hand in hand, heart to heart. My friend, please hold these things dear. (239)

On the face of it, this text message, included under the section on greetings and felicitations in *Laughing at SARS*, does not seem funny at all. If anything, it seems to merely recycle corny clichés. Yet it typifies the tone and spirit of a host of text messages that circulated during SARS, little electronic notes that relay affection, support, or cheer between friends and strangers, during the holiday season and beyond. Those that do not explicitly mention *feidian* allude to it but put the emphasis on self-care, with reminders about the importance of good health and well-being. Many open with the formulaic address "My friend" and go on to offer simple life advice, such as "work is never done, your health is your own, comradeship is priceless, and power is fleeting. However busy you are, remember to prioritize your health" (238–39)

PANDEMIC HUMOR 93

or "come out from that fog of worry! Life is calling you, knowledge is calling you, urgent and meaningful work is calling you" (241). We imagine the speaker as a gently nagging but caring friend, sending out a microaffirmation in an odd moment to convey they are thinking of you. Today, we would equate these messages with emojis, virtual smiles of encouragement or remote squeezes on the arm. At a time when people were acutely conscious of the need to maintain social distance and avoid unnecessary gatherings, these small and gratuitous communications, imparting neither important disease information nor salacious epidemic gossip, stitched together a social zeitgeist of supererogatory mutual care.

These texts distill what I call small humor. In contrast to sardonic, scornful, judgmental, or cruel humor, small humor channels the laughter of smiles and grins, chuckles and giggles, groans and eye rolls. It may be the appreciation of wit and clever trickery, but it may also be the half-grudging acknowledgment of deliberately bad jokes, forced puns, nonsensical buffooneries, or mock displays of emotion. It can be impish and playful, but it is mischief without injury or offense, rather than the uproarious mirth of the carnivalesque or the wounding derision of satire. In colloquial terms, rather than a laughing *at*, it is a laughing *with*. Small humor is sympathetic and generous; it is, in a word, good-humored. Its laughter propels participants toward cohesion, however momentary, shoring up a quick sense of a shared world. It is less about tearing down or lashing out at despised targets than holding on to something or someone precious to care for. And it is less about conjuring up a community ex nihilo than sustaining a socius that is imagined as already there. It assumes people to share a joke with, to laugh alongside, without having to provide explanations or justifications. Put another way, it assumes personhood on the receiving end, without the other party needing to prove their humanity, intelligence, or worth. Small humor does not necessitate laughter as an outcome but often routes through smaller feelings and gestures, such as a brief flash of cheer or quick warming of the heart. It does not even have to be funny but can simply aim toward boosting mood and morale. What matters is that, in its telling, it makes more affectively real one's connection to an imagined affable community.

From a bioevolutionary standpoint, small humor may actually be closer to our species' need for positive companionship than louder forms of humor. According to the neuroscientist Robert Provine, people laugh about thirty times more when in the company of others than when alone, and laughter all but vanishes when individuals are solitary and, crucially, without media stimulation. In fact, "most human laughter takes place during ordinary conversations, rather than in response to structured attempts at humor, such as jokes or stories," so it is ultimately "more about relationships than humor."[61]

During SARS, this prosocial dimension of digital humor is not to be underestimated, given the many exaggerated disease-risk messages that circulated over unofficial media. As Ding points out, although guerilla media was instrumental in raising people's viral awareness, it also facilitated the spread of panic-inducing rumors. In the early months of the outbreak, a legion of anonymous text messages fueled mass paranoia about the virus's deadliness. One message claimed that "any face-to-face meeting or even taking the same bus with a patient may result in getting the same disease"; another related how medical workers who contracted the virus in the morning died by the evening; yet another reported a 100 percent viral death rate, with the whole of Guangzhou having been turned into "a dead city." Other messages misidentified SARS as avian flu, the bubonic plague, or the mutation of a pollen strain, and some even attributed the epidemic to a bioterrorist attack by the United States or Taiwan. Many recycled inaccurate and potentially dangerous information about folk remedies, herbal cures, and disinfecting products, all of which were exploited by opportunistic merchants who sold rice, salt, vinegar, and other household goods at inflated prices.[62]

In this chaotic informational and affective environment, the smaller the humor, the more effectively it down-regulated high-pitched emotions and diffused social mistrust. Rather than portraying neighbors and fellow citizens as potential sources of contagion or rivals in the scarcity economy of pandemic survival, these seemingly trite SARS texts emphasized the sharing of a common lot, the value of camaraderie, and the persistence of goodness beneath crisis. They fostered the reproduction of prosocial feelings, and they did so without top-down pronouncements or stern warnings, modeling instead humble and lighthearted lateral affirmation. They restored heteroglossia back into SARS discourse, validating everyday idioms and minor voices excessive of governmental and biomedical jargon, allowing people to sustain a fuller spectrum of affective relations toward epidemic life and each other. The reliance on clichés, stale proverbs, and bad genre conventions is not insignificant, for these literary devices can quickly provoke not just a sense of the familiar but also a shared comfort in nonaggressive and nonideological laughter. It may be that, in the face of an enigmatic disease threat and a supposedly zero-sum survival game, what reassured more than the fire of confrontation was the endurance of the pedestrian, the silly, the schmaltzy—and the knowledge that there remained people who would continue to indulge in the nonhurtful fun of little snickers, giggles, and snorts, and who would be generous enough to share these with strangers online.

We can find a plethora of small humor in *Laughing at SARS*. The insider quality of these pieces runs the gamut, from the personal and intimate to the broadly cultural. Yet they mostly take for granted an audience that already exists in overlapping linguistic and cultural worlds, that would immediately recognize the references and get the joke, or else groan at the gag or pun.[63] They invite collective empathy precisely through this heightening of insider idioms and allusions. At heart, their humor is about keeping familiar company, making absent but already existing ties viscerally and gut-warmingly real. In content, they do not so much ignore larger power structures as temporarily suspend the thinking of and deep engagement with those structures, holding them at playful bay. During SARS, these humorous tidbits made manifold and porous the gateways through which individuals could enter into a cultural commons and exercise microagency over shared cultural goods, even if only by digital replication and recirculation. Put another way, small humor lowered the bar for what counted as cultural agency within the epidemic crisis milieu. It opened up a realm of small acts—composing a short nonsense rhyme, sending someone a brief mushy message, sharing a bad joke or *not* sharing a bad joke—that could carry meaning for both oneself and others, concretizing intentions of self-care and social solidarity. In staying ephemeral and anonymous, spontaneous and unorganized, these pieces ebbed and flowed in a zone of the unco-opted, as ends in themselves rather than means to grander ends. As such, they could not be easily weaponized, by either the state or its critics, as instruments of either socialist propaganda or intellectual dissidence.

Small humor can be related to the concept of *huaji* in Chinese humor history. In contrast to the early twentieth-century neologism *youmo*, coined by Lin Yutang and theorized by him as a civilizing comic sensibility and moral ideal, the ancient term *huaji* refers to the "quick wit" of jesters and clowns, the "funny stuff of dirty jokes, slapstick and nonsense."[64] As Jocelyn Chey notes, "We tend to over-estimate the importance of types [of humor] favoured by the literati and the elites," when surely, she speculates, "voiceless and unrecorded ordinary people throughout history" also had their cultures of "subaltern humor."[65] While *huaji*, too, had its roots in imperial court politics and originally connoted the "sharpness of intellect" of state advisers and operated to "consolidate in-circle relations between scholar/

officials educated in the Confucian classics," over the centuries it came to be appropriated by popular print culture and helped blur the line between high and low comedy.[66] By the time *youmo* became the standard modern term for humor, *huaji* had narrowed in meaning, with some defining it as wordless or lowly humor such as "clowning, joking, funny actions/behavior and ridiculous speech," as opposed to *youmo*'s more intellectual and language-oriented laughter.[67] "Nowadays," Rea comments, "*huaji* is more often used to denote the silly, ridiculous, or farcical," part of the legacy of 1920s Shanghai farce culture.[68] "Funny Shanghai," as Rea dubs this milieu, popularized the upbeat and mischievous comic modes of pranksters and tricksters. By "invest[ing] mundane experiences with comic potential," *huaji* "affirmed the common person's ability to survive, and even have fun in an adverse environment."[69]

Farther afield, small humor can be compared to what Wendy Gan calls "amiable humor." Digging into the Anglo-American cultural archive, she uncovers a body of little-known comic texts from the late nineteenth century onward that depict China not in the yellow peril terms of racist humor but as a site for forging cross-culturally inclusive communities of laughter. These works offer readers a "more innocent and benevolent source of amusement, based on incongruity instead of ridicule as the trigger for laughter," marked not by feelings of superiority over the exotic and primitive other but by "a consistent attempt to create comic parity between self and other, foreigner and Chinese, transforming Occidental and Oriental into friends, neighbors, equals, and allies." This amiable humor, Gan argues, played a key role in affectively structuring Western modernity's encounter with China, a buried archive in the history of empire and its orientalisms that can usefully be reclaimed today for building playful yet respectful relationships across racial, national, and imperial divides.[70] In COVID times, discerning this affinity between Western amiable and Chinese small humor may be more important than ever for a global dismantling of dehumanizing othering mentalities.

SARS Sweet-Talk

Baby, my tooth has started aching recently. It must be because I think of you at night all the time. This feeling is so sweet it gives me a cavity. (280)

Another subgenre of text message jokes consists of what we might call SARS sweet-talk—sappy love notes that express yearning for an absent partner or romantic crush. Here, too, SARS is often not mentioned directly, but the thematic refrain of separation and distance hints at epidemic conditions of quarantine, isolation, and restricted travel. Some have the quality of conjugal banter, some play on the conventions of the love confession, and some adopt a more flirtatious carpe diem tone. Some feign the self-pitying plea of the forlorn spouse, some the rhapsodic rapture of the lovesick suitor, and some the wretched moaning of the sexual supplicant. Whatever roles and situations are invoked, these sweet-talk messages all articulate their attachments in deliberately and identifiably nonserious ways, whether by adopting maudlin clichés or histrionic hyperboles, forced rhymes or painfully bad puns. As the example above self-reflexively plays up, the language used to convey its sentiment, like the feeling itself, "is so sweet it gives [one] a cavity." Other examples:

> I am a helpless little bird with one wing missing. Will you be my pillar? (325)
>
> You are a serene harbor, and the vessel of my longing willingly moors itself wherever you are. (245)
>
> You once said that, no matter if we are separated to the ends of the earth, there will be no distance between us, as our longing is the prime mover pulling our hearts toward each other. However enormous the sky and earth, there is only you. (244)
>
> Come back soon [*lai*], because I can't cook alone [*lai*]. Come back soon [*lai*], because the dinner table lights up for you alone [*jingcai*]. Don't let my stomach be empty as the sea [*hai*]. (314)

The humor here arises not just from the messages' playful tenor or wordplay but also from their unabashed corniness. They seem to self-consciously acknowledge that, in ordinary times, one would not resort to such cloying declarations, but, because of SARS, one would let go of false airs and false pride—because the recipient is worthy of schmaltz. There is a hint, too, that times are not so extraordinary as to merit going overboard with truly profound end-of-life statements. The affective structures of this particular scene of crisis ordinariness are the cheesy, the mushy, the sappy. As private jests and private jokes, these love messages likely injected small doses of humor back into the fabric of lived domesticity and intimacy. We can imagine the senders half sheepishly and half impishly sending these messages off and the faraway recipients recognizing the underlying affection with a chuckle or smile, a groan or eye roll, a blush or flutter of the heart.

SARS Folk Recipes

> Don't be afraid, don't be panicked [*huang*],
> *feidian* pneumonia can be prevented [*yufang*].
> Clean and sweep, get hygienic, dry your clothes and bedcovers in
>   the sun,
> ventilate indoors and open your windows [*kai chuang*].
> Dress up or down with the changing weather,
> exercise outdoors is important too [*zhongyao*].
> After coughing or blowing your nose,
> don't forget to wash your hands right away [*liao*]. (213)[71]

If SARS sweet-talk messages intimate personal ties, the subgenre of SARS jokes patterned after folk prescriptions or medical formulas suggests a broader sociality. *Laughing at SARS* contains a section of about thirty pieces in this category, many of which circulated digitally at the time; some were even staged as public group performances as a service for seniors, such as the "SARS Prevention Song" above, composed by Shanghai Zhongshan Hospital's Professor Qin Yingyun.[72] Ostensibly, these pieces outline recipes for good health and long life by promoting wholesome lifestyles, diets, habits, relationships, mindsets, and so forth, and they seem aimed particularly at children and the elderly, populations that might have needed the extra mnemonics to remember all the SARS-related public health guidelines. Copying the stanza structures of Confucian primers such as *Three Character Classic* and *Thousand Character Classic*, these folk recipe songs made epidemic hygiene rules easier to recall and more game-like to practice. However, their yoking of classical form to distinctly modern, sometimes hackneyed, and often eclectic and arbitrary content about health and hygiene can create a kind of humorous clash. In Qin's "SARS Prevention Song," for instance, interspersed with straightforward SARS conduct rules—such as avoiding crowded spaces, seeking prompt medical attention for symptoms, and wearing face masks—is an assortment of basic hygiene facts and fitness tips, such as dressing according to changing temperatures, exercising outdoors, and washing one's hands after blowing one's nose. This last piece of advice in particular seems to play on a trope of children's disgust, in the spirit of playground humor, injecting an element of bathos into the everyday scenes of epidemic protocols.

This humorous template was then taken up by digital users for more overtly parodic pseudomedical ditties, including ones that impersonate

PANDEMIC HUMOR   **99**

the idiom of traditional Chinese medicine. One "Congee Cure Song," for example, contains eight rhyming couplets of five-character lines, with an opening couplet that rhymes insomnia (*shimian*) with white lotus (*bailian*): "If you don't want to have insomnia, when cooking congee add white lotus." The jingle then goes on to list random congee ingredients for various ailments, such as longan for low self-confidence, chrysanthemum for headaches, chestnuts for backaches, lotus root for constipation, mung beans for heat stroke, and, most preposterously, brown rice for athlete's foot—in that order (219–20).

Read against the backdrop of official SARS discourse, these pieces of folk medicine mimicry may have served to reaffirm the everyday agency of a lay *socius*. In the early months of SARS, as Ding notes, the reassurances of biomedical experts in mainstream news outlets could not be trusted since many physicians "chose either to passively obey administrative orders of censorship or to actively comply with the official ideology of stability by reinforcing the official 'no risk' narrative."[73] Traditional Chinese medicine and its practitioners, too, came to be co-opted by the state campaign against SARS, leading to rampant misinformation about and panic buying of herbs such as *banlangan*, as Chen Baozhen portrays in *SARS Bride*.[74] In this context, the corpus of pseudomedical ditties might have circulated as tacit mockery of state-engineered medical discourses. Yet we detect little malice or anger in them. Instead, they deliver their own symbolic reassurances, as if proposing a set of nonspecialized homeopathic alternatives. The advice they put forward seems banal and obvious, but the banality and obviousness of folk wisdom may be precisely what was being conjured for the sake of dispelling social paranoia and resuscitating social self-reliance, individual self-confidence, and mutual trust. For all their levity and occasional absurdity, these folk recipes broadcast the prosocial message that the intelligent layperson can fall back on what they already know in the face of a pandemic: eat well, exercise, get enough sleep; take care of oneself, take care of others, be considerate; wear a mask, wash one's hands, make congee. These are ordinary know-hows that the average person can pursue without the questionable expertise of doctors, whether traditional or modern, these jokes imply: don't rely on miracle herbal cures, don't let predatory merchants exploit your desperation, and remember the small routines of daily self-care that will carry you through even an epidemic.

SARS Mimic Poems

> Not seeing you for one day, I lower my head [*di xia tou*].
> Not seeing you for two days, my sorrow deepens [*chou gen chou*].
> Not seeing you for three days, I'm ready to jump off a building [*yao tiaolou*]. (252)

To any reader of classical Chinese poetry, the above SARS joke will immediately summon up Li Bo. The first two lines conjure two well-known conceits and much-memorialized phrases from the famous Tang poet: lowering one's head with homesickness, from the last line of "Quiet Night Thoughts," and deepening sorrow despite wallowing in wine, from the penultimate couplet of "A Farewell to Secretary Shuyun at Xuanzhou's Xietiao Villa." This SARS mimic poem borrows the elevated and dignified aura of classical poetry as well as its verbal condensation to rapidly sketch a contemporary scene of someone worrying about and missing a loved one during the epidemic. The last line, however, abruptly turns this high poetic lexicon of lament into coarse modern slang, crescendoing not with philosophical insight but a vulgar punchline. Echoing the first couplet's trisyllabic finish, the final trisyllabic rhyme is at once deflating in diction and exorbitant in sentiment, even as it flaunts its own tongue-in-cheek melodrama. Still, the specter of suicide, while a disproportionate reaction here, was likely not unthinkable in the midst of SARS (as I will discuss in the next chapter). In just three short lines, this poem conveys care and attachment, loneliness and dejection, even as it impishly apes and meshes the stock tropes of classical verse and chuckles at its own verbal trickery. Notably, it does all this by assuming an audience that can instantly pick up on the puns and echoes, someone who would get the joke without exegesis.

Classical poetry provides a useful template for digital humor, not only because its brevity and simplicity lends a ready-made linguistic structure for short compositions on new media platforms but also because its association with high literati culture lends itself to mimicry and play. In the early months of SARS, when people did not know much about the virus or the extent of the outbreak, they also could not have known the proper attitude essential for survival and health. It may be tempting and even necessary eventually to scale up one's emotional response to disease threat, but, equally, it may be foolish and foolhardy to do so. Should one then imitate the persona crafted by ancient poets, that of the refined gentleman scholar who faces the trials and tribulations of life with deep feeling and existential acceptance? Or should one laugh at the romantic and vain desire for this transcendent deportment, flipping it inside out and reveling at least in one's own minor acts of word-play and roleplay? In that equivocal atmosphere, classical poetry offered a fitting vehicle for compacted linguistic humor, complete with a culturally shared reservoir of exalted language and lofty sentiments crying out for bathetic treatment.

Laughing at SARS collects numerous joke pieces in this vein, comic verses that mime famous canonical poems and retrofit them with SARS-related situations and affects. Most are relatively short, no more than a few lines. In one longer and especially ingenious example, Su Shi's "Prelude to Water Melody," a famous Song lyric from the eleventh century, is reworked from a wistful meditation about brotherly nostalgia and human vicissitudes into a whimsical lamentation on SARS:

> When will there be no more SARS? [*feidian jishi wu*]
> I lift my medicine and ask the blue sky. [*ba yao wen qingtian*]
> I don't know when this situation [*bu zhi ci fan guangjing*]
> will persist until. [*chixu dao he nian*]
> I wish I could leave quietly, [*wo yu qiaoran liqu*]
> but I'm afraid that in every part of China [*you kong shenzhou gedi*]
> there's nowhere without transmission. [*wuchu bu liuchuan*]
> Rather than being alarmed and anxious, [*huanghuang wu ning ri*]
> I might as well just calm down! [*buru ba xin an*]
> Don't skimp on handwashing, [*qin xishou*]
> exercise more, [*duo duanlian*]
> don't lose sleep. [*mo wu mian*]
> I should have no regrets, [*bu ying you hen*]
> since all things will be shouldered by the people! [*wanshi dou you
>   renmin dan*]
> Heaven has unpredictable weather, [*tian you buce de fengyun*]
> humans have ups and downs, good and bad fortune, [*ren you danxi
>   huofu*]
> and nothing's perfect since the beginning of time. [*ci shi gu nan quan*]
> Let's just hope we all live a long life, [*dan yuan ren changjiu*]
> let's join hands to get through this crisis together! [*xieshou du nan-
>   guan*] (29–30)

By Su Shi's own account, he composed his verse on the Mid-Autumn Festival in 1076, after a night of drinking, to commemorate his younger brother, whom he had not seen in years, as they held official posts far from each other. The SARS mimic poem, anonymous and untitled, makes no direct reference to Su Shi, yet a reader familiar with classical poetry would readily recognize the echoes. The exact stanzaic structure of the original is preserved, and key words are retained in the same positions. The opening couplet, for instance, repeats the five-character lines of the original, swiftly cuing the reader into the syntactic form of the question "when will there be x?" (. . . *jishi* . . .) followed by the iconic gesture of "lifting y to the sky" (*ba . . . wen qingtian*). The humor arises from the intertextual punning and the unexpected substitutions. Instead of the moon, a well-worn literary symbol of the paradoxical vagaries and constancy of human bonds, the poem inserts *feidian*. It then changes the last word of the line from "having" (*you*) to its inverse of "not having" (*wu*), deflating the high sentiment of melancholic dispossession into an irritable complaint, a frustrated grumble. The tone then quickly shifts from what the classical structure initially sets up, in a poetic sleight of hand, and the posture of the lyric poet as a philosophical and brooding man of feeling is dislodged by the voice of a cranky but slightly self-mocking and embarrassed patient, someone who holds not his delicate wine cup up to the moon but maybe a paper cup or plastic tumbler up to his window.

Genre mashing is often a technique in fanfiction, and this SARS poem deftly mimes and mashes a number of incongruous genre codes, from classical poetry to socialist rhetoric. Given its reference to the magnitude of the outbreak, we can guess that it was composed after the central government's April 20 announcement. Its worry that "there's nowhere without transmission," however, is not couched in the panicked language of epidemic rumors. Instead, the poet eschews alarm and anxiety, bringing the reader back to daily routines with bits of down-home hygienic wisdom like those in the folk recipes above: washing one's hands, exercising regularly, getting enough sleep. Rather than the authoritative or sanctimonious voice of the health expert, the poet affects the pose of the little guy—someone, almost always coded male by default, who frets about contracting the disease, whose concern for others stems from his personal sense of grievance, and who shuns the lofty oratory of self-proclaimed selfless public servants. To underscore this point, in the poem's one moment of political mockery, the poet parodies official rhetoric about "the people" and their burden of responsibility. But his sarcasm is fleeting, and the poem concludes by returning to the mildly self-taunting voice of the resigned little guy. He knows enough Su Shi to recite a famous poem, he has enough literary cleverness to rescript it vis-à-vis

SARS, but he does not feel inspired, privileged, or bestirred enough to create beautiful proverbs for posterity amid the crisis. So, Su Shi's most celebrated lines—"We have sad and happy partings and reunions / The moon has bright and dark fullness and waning"—are anticlimactically replaced by the hackneyed "heaven has unpredictable weather / humans have ups and downs, bad and good fortune." The axiom that "nothing's perfect," while not rejected outright, takes on the quality not of an elegant and timeless truth but of a pragmatic outlook of last resort. In the final rousing couplet, the poet rallies enough to exhort everyone to take heart and find small comfort in epidemic solidarity. The poem gives an overall impression of an extended pep talk to oneself, though the poetic persona does not seem to mind if others eavesdrop with sympathy too.

Significantly, the closing revision of Su Shi here is neither an angry attack on the Song poet's canonical authority nor a merciless lampoon of the moral universe he occupied and propagated. Indeed, the ending chord of hopeful well-wishing and social camaraderie, even if edged with irony against officialese, harmonizes with the original poem's ending. As with the Li Bo mimic poem, this piece projects someone impersonating Su Shi within an environment of ambiguous affect—where it might or might not be expedient ultimately to assume the composure of ancient poets. Those poets, after all, though belonging to the ranks of intellectual elites, had to survive the caprices of imperial courts and monarchs, including suffering repeated exile to far-flung outposts as well as protracted separation from friends and family, a condition imagined here as not so dissimilar to epidemic isolation and social distancing. One might not be Su Shi, but, in some respects, one might not *not* be Su Shi either. It is in this aspect, too, that the poem's canon-mimicking humor most departs from the carnivalesque. Its parroting is aimed more at self-soothing than other-antagonizing. The rebellious trickster might scoff at any serious and abiding identification with the big man, but the little guy would not refrain from wallowing in that fantasy. Where the trickster guffaws, the little guy smiles rueful, hangdog smiles. Where the trickster invites rollicking and riotous laughter, the little guy shakes his head and sighs exaggerated sighs. Where the trickster thumbs his nose at the higher-ups, the little guy pokes gentle fun at himself for even this ephemeral act of mimicry.

We can call these SARS jokes that variously imitate or recycle traditional forms canon-mimicking humor, as distinct from Tao Dongfeng's category of canon-mocking literature. While canon-mimicking humor also makes use of collage and pastiche to repurpose canonical texts for amusement, it is not fixated on a disobedient assault, whether overt or covert, on power structures. It is less intent on destabilizing moral and social codes than on reconstituting and reaffirming, if only transiently, moral and social connections, and it is fundamentally oriented toward the socius rather than the polis. These little-guy jokesters do not even rise to the level of the classic trickster, who is often regarded as a conduit to "the social consciousness of all the people."[75] By contrast, small-humor jokesters make no pretense to representing "the people." They offer neither a cultural form embodying the ideal of social responsibility nor a scathing rebuke of this ideal's tired rhetoric. What they hold on to is the trickster's belovedness and, through that belovedness, the imagining of a community temporarily united in fondness and fun. They are not bothered by their suspended macroagency, taking for granted their own microagency, aspiring to nothing more large-scale or long-lived than the spark of merriment in the moment.

Returning to the Su Shi mimic poem, let us note that the cultural commons it imagines is much broader than a literary elite and includes the listening publics of contemporary Chinese popular music across sinophone locales. Su Shi's "Prelude" has been multiply adapted into song, first made famous in the 1980s by the Taiwanese singer Teresa Teng, then repopularized, upon her death in the 1990s and in homage to her, by the Hong Kong pop queen Faye Wong. By the time of SARS, even if readers failed to trace the mimic poem to Su Shi, they would likely recognize the lyrics of the pop ballad, aided by the fact that the one and only line repeated verbatim from the original poem—the penultimate "wishing we all live a long life"—is also the title of both renditions. The commercial music industry thus plays a key role in recycling classical poetry for contemporary mass consumers, so that a canon-revising text rarely refers to its premodern precursor in a strict one-to-one correspondence; more often than not, the echo chamber is already richly pluralized. The SARS poem may be mimicking Teresa Teng and Faye Wong as much as Su Shi, and this intertextual web makes its joke comprehensible to those in sinophone regions beyond mainland China. In this sense, the poem can be considered a transnationally convivial text, one that unites through shared cultural humor rather than dividing through dialect, politics, or location, constructing communities of epidemic laughter across geopolitical and ideological differences not so unlike Gan's amiable humor archive.

SARS Fanfiction

> To find an effective cure to SARS, West Lake Hospital expressly hired two specialists in traditional Chinese medicine from Mount Emei Hospital— Bai Suzhen and Xiaoqing. Bai Suzhen worked night and day, putting in many hours of overtime, and finally developed a TCM prescription formula that helped the people of the West Lake region regain their peaceful and happy lives. . . . (4)

Another subgenre of SARS canon-mimicking jokes achieves a similar effect: those comical vignettes that renarrate classical legends and historical tales within the terms of SARS—in effect, SARS fanfiction. Like Su Shi's poem, the original source materials are widely recognizable, not only because they belong to a classical canon passed down through the centuries both orally and textually but also because they have been repeatedly adapted into film, television drama, and other popular cultural forms across mainland China, Taiwan, Hong Kong, Singapore, and the wider sinophone diaspora. These well-known legends and tales saturate contemporary popular media and readily lend themselves to online fanfiction. In addition to Su Shi, who makes an explicit appearance in one vignette, historical figures such as Cao Cao, Liu Bei, and Zhang Fei—all staple characters in historical dramas on television and in film—are revived in the milieu of SARS, in a high-spirited hodgepodge that pays no heed to historical or biographical accuracy. In one piece, Zhang Yimou's 2002 movie *Hero*, based on the much-adapted historical account of Jing Ke's assassination attempt on Qin Shi Huang in 227 BC and featuring an ensemble cast of megastars, is exuberantly rescripted. The assassin No-Name is renamed No-Sickness, the secret weapon deployed becomes a flying droplet of coronavirus-infected saliva that cuts through US military-grade surgical masks, and the Qin emperor's infamous burning of the books is explained as an act of frustration at the ancient texts for failing to deliver a remedy to his SARS-crippled health (11). Modern classics are also reworked. In one cartoon, the hero in *wuxia* novelist Jin Yong's *Legend of the Condor Heroes*, Guo Jing, is portrayed in iconic profile with bow and arrow drawn, but, instead of giant birds, he takes aim at two condor-size germ particles hovering in the sky, with one shaking in fright and the other wearing a mean scowl, both labeled "SARS" in English (10). By virtue of their textual brevity and visual iconicity, these comic SARS fanfictions could be drafted and consumed quickly, allowing netizens to perform and share little bursts of creativity and glee amid the epidemic. Their creators seem invested in fanfiction not so much as a mode of "interpretation of the source text" or "sociopolitical argument," not even for "individual engagement and identificatory practice" or "audience response," but primarily as "a communal gesture"—to make oneself and others feel a sense of convivial joy and fun about beloved cultural stories, during and despite SARS.[76] As Karen Hellekson and Kristina Busse point out, fans are not just "enthusiasts" but "affective agents," and fan affects can be powerful forces for imagining and affirming community.[77]

Among the vignettes compiled in *Laughing at SARS* is an inventive sequence on "Four Major Classic Love Stories: The SARS Edition." One story retells the tragedy of Liang Shanbo and Zhu Yingtai, the so-called Butterfly Lovers: here, Liang dies from SARS and a grief-stricken Zhu dies from heartbreak, both bequeathing their bodies to medical research (4–5). Another story rewrites the tragic final scene of the opera *Farewell My Concubine* by placing Xiang Yu the Western Chu warlord and Consort Yu in a train station in an epidemic zone. She has a fever that hovers just below thirty-eight degrees Celsius, a clinical sign of SARS infection, while he worries about being quarantined as her close contact and delayed in returning to his company headquarters. But, instead of a double suicide, just as Consort Yu is about to slit her wrist with a paring knife, Xiang Yu stops her, and the two spend the night locked in each other's arms (6). The most upbeat story in the series is a revamping of *Romance of the West Chamber*, in which the scholar Zhang Sheng happily elopes with his lover Cui Yingying after they both recover from SARS, and after her disapproving father dies from the virus and her infected mother fails to intervene. The story ends with the newlyweds appearing as guest stars on an episode of a television show called *SARS Couples*, where they revel in retelling their love marriage's many travails to a fan audience (7).

The first story, the SARS edition of *Legend of the White Snake*, opens as excerpted above, with the green and white snake spirits, Bai Suzhen and Xiaoqing, as modern-day TCM specialists tasked with finding a SARS cure. The vignette then continues:

> During this time, Bai Suzhen also fell in love at first sight with the reporter Xu Xian, and they promptly got married. The CEO of Jinshan Temple Pharmaceutical Co., Fahai, wanted to buy Bai Suzhen's formula so he could monopolize the supply lines of SARS drugs in the West Lake region. Bai Suzhen forcefully resisted, and the two became mortal enemies. Using Dr. Bai's recurrent exposure to SARS patients as an excuse, Fahai had her isolated in Leifeng Pagoda. The docile Xu Xian, afraid of

PANDEMIC HUMOR 107

being infected, was too much of a coward to stand up to popular opinion and rescue Bai Suzhen. In the end, it was Xiaoqing who smashed the iron door to the isolation ward to save her. Bai Suzhen, much saddened, divorced Xu Xian and resumed her honorable work as a white-robed angel, helping the dying and healing the sick. (4)

As with other SARS canon-mimicking jokes, the humor here derives partly from the mashup of classical material with contemporary contexts and lingo. The two mythic heroines, instead of snake spirits, are medical scientists; the fainthearted scholar Xu Xian is updated to a meek and craven reporter; and the pious Buddhist monk Fahai is remade into a villainous boss of corporate greed and abusive power. Dynastic landmarks are modernized as bureaucratic institutions, fantasy and magic are converted into the banality of slander and brute strength, and the elevated lyricism of classical prose gets eclectically mixed with proverbs on overtime work, inflated rhetoric from revenge melodramas, and propagandist clichés about the glories of medicine. Despite its clear critiques of the capitalist era, this spoof does not end with moral punishment or vengeance, nor does it culminate in a heteronormative romantic ending, as in some popular versions of the legend. The concluding tone here, and the community being imagined, are akin to the Su Shi mimic poem's—lighthearted resignation by the little guys, who sympathize with the injustices and treacheries endured by heroic women but who have insufficient means to intervene on their behalf, even fan-fictionally. There is a similar posture of acceptance that nothing is perfect, that the allotment of power and suffering has remained relatively constant from antiquity to the present. Still, there lurks a hint of a feminist queer subtext, and fan readers so inclined may fantasize that Bai Suzhen, beyond her angelic white robes, now returns home each day to her devoted Xiaoqing, in a fulfillment of the lesbian happy ending that is nowhere visible in sanctioned media but that has fortuitously been enabled by SARS. And this domesticity they keep private, between the lines, away from erotic spectacles.

In this fanfiction vignette, SARS is a mere backdrop, one passing circumstance against which a timeless theater of good and evil, love and betrayal, loyalty and cowardice plays out. In the other fanfiction legends, too, SARS constitutes a subordinate or substitute plot element, not the crisis that steers the course of age-old scripts toward unprecedented catastrophe. Despite their genre differences, all four stories resituate the outbreak within long-standing narratives and reassuringly archetypal conflicts. They intimate that there will always be Bai Suzhens and Xiaoqings, Fahais and Xu Xians, Liang Shanbos and Zhu Yingtais, Xiang Yus and Consort Yus, Zhang Shengs and Cui Yingyings. And they propose that SARS, however mysterious and supposedly novel, presents nothing that Chinese cultural myths cannot narrate and make sense of, whether in high tragic or low comic terms or both. The familiar cast of characters, and the revivability and repeatability of their lives and dramas, provide a sense of continuity and endurance—as if SARS, too, will soon pass into the stuff of legends, in a cycle of the spiraling eternal, with its own eminently imitable and mashable canon.

Coda: COVID Digital Prosociality and Quarantine Humor

If the Chinese internet was still in its fledgling phase in 2003, by 2008 China had the world's biggest internet user base, and by 2012 this base more than doubled America's.[78] Between the SARS and COVID outbreaks, China's internet population increased more than tenfold, from 87 million at the end of 2003 to 989 million by the end of 2020.[79] The rise of new social media platforms such as Weibo, WeChat, and Douyin means that, this time around, unofficial media are much more integrated into people's lives. As Shiqi Lin observes, COVID has fostered a pervasive "documentary impulse" among professional chroniclers and amateur social media users alike as they archive daily pandemic experiences.[80] These mundane digital activities "operat[e] on quotidian levels of micro-fixing," as people's "small gestures of care" and "modest forms of companionship to help each other pull through moments of disorientation and breakdown." As she further points out, "During the peak weeks of the coronavirus outbreak in China, precisely at the high point of the spread of misinformation, xenophobia, and infrastructure breakdown there was a simultaneous boom of mutual support on social media," where the very act of reassembling "disarticulated pieces of online postings [worked] to construct an alternative space-time for communication and cohabitation."[81] The digital mass socius that emerged with SARS can thus be said to have gone supernova with COVID, along with microagentive acts of online prosociality.

Guobin Yang highlights one form of this pandemic digital prosociality vis-à-vis netizens' countercensorship practices during the early phase of COVID. About a month after the death of "whistleblower" Li Wenliang, an online interview surfaced about "whistle-giver" Ai Fen, a Wuhan Central Hospital physician who had likewise been censured for alerting her colleagues to a SARS-like virus in the city. This story was quickly censored, but netizens kept it alive through an "online relay" as they "posted and reposted remixed versions of the original censored story on social media," impishly rearranging words into foreign languages and local dialects, oracle-bone scripts and Morse code, Braille and emojis, all in an effort to circumvent computer censorship programs.[82] "Such a 'game,'" Yang writes, "invited massive participation ... expos[ing] censorship to more people than ever before." Fang Fang, too, he notes, discussed Ai Fen's story in her *Wuhan Diary* and thereby "gave the relay a major boost," allowing readers to comment on and share their "anger, helplessness, and sympathy." By expressing these "negative emotions [that are] out of tune with the mainstream ideology of positive energy," people enacted "a refutation of the mainstream discourse."[83]

In the same pandemic period but in less politically dramatic fashion, small humor also exploded on the Chinese internet. As with SARS, COVID has spawned new genres of humor online. These digital humor practices expand the range of rhetorical styles and permissible affects around epidemic disease, often veering toward the silly and the ridiculous as they playfully capture people's microadjustments to pandemic life. During the Wuhan lockdown especially, memes of quarantine boredom and stir-craziness abounded. Netizens recorded themselves singing the lockdown blues by rescripting classic popular tunes, whimsically reanimating the canon-mimicking impulse via live home videos. They exhibited themselves fishing from home aquariums, playing mahjong with plastic bags over their heads, playing solo mahjong, playing mahjong with pets, staging mahjong games among pets, playing living-room badminton, and choreographing wacky dance moves, among countless other new home routines of comic survival and creative endurance. People also showcased their sartorial flare by venturing out to neighborhood convenience stores and parks in over-the-top inflatable costumes of T-Rex dinosaurs, green aliens, and Christmas trees, all filmed and shared for the amusement of their fellow netizens. When they ran out of face masks, some half-jokingly substituted with bras, sanitary pads, and fruit rinds, and these droll photographs went viral too.[84]

As Manya Koetse remarked in Beijing at the time, these social media trends allowed people to "mock neighbors, their friends or family, or even themselves in the extreme and sometimes silly measures they are taking to avoid the coronavirus."[85] But more than mockery, the rampant relays of these memes beg to be read as constructive and healing acts. In times of high stress and distress, social isolation and separation, to sustain these virtual communities is to deliver shared recognition, concern, and laughter. Oriented toward the socius rather than the polis, and promoting cheer rather than bile, these digital practices of small humor epitomize the care economy of lateral agency and pandemic prosociality. To understand them properly, we must grasp their affective intentions—and grasping these, we may be educated in a better mode of pandemic living. For even as Western social media users fanned global disgust and fear by fixating on sinophobic images of Wuhan "wet markets" and bio-orientalist accounts of Chinese consumption of bat soup and wild pangolins, as I will detail in chapter 4, Chinese netizens were already modeling a reparative way of being and feeling within crisis, treating each other, as Leung Ping-kwan had hoped in his SARS poem, with greater humaneness.

Pandemic Resilience

Deextinction and the Hong Kong Cantophone

Alternative Resilience

In March 2020, in the early days of COVID's entry into Europe and America, Benjamin Davis and Jonathan Catlin noted the prevalence of the word *resilience* in English's rapidly evolving pandemic vocabulary. Implicitly echoing Kyle Whyte's critique of crisis epistemology, they write in "Theses for Theory in a Time of Crisis": "Catastrophe is not 'to come,' but here and now. Before the current pandemic, our way of life was already killing life on earth," so we should "contest the rhetoric of a return to normal," which exceptionalizes the pandemic present by romanticizing a prepandemic status quo. Moreover, they argue, we should "avoid the rhetoric of resilience," harnessed as it is to notions of "latent normalcy" that "place the burden [of resilience] on those already burdened."[1] Yet, since then, the language of COVID resilience has only proliferated. In neoliberal co-optations of the word especially, public health success is often equated with national economic success, exemplified by Bloomberg's Covid Resilience Ranking that tracks "the best and worst places to be during the pandemic," as if offering mobile cosmopolitans a global relocation guide for escape hot spots.[2]

Rather than reject the concept altogether, I turn in this chapter to SARS-era Hong Kong to delineate an alternative model of pandemic resilience, one that the Western world seems to have forgotten or never noticed in the first place. Seventeen years before COVID raised the question of collective adaptation and recovery for Europeans and Americans, Hong Kongers weathered a novel coronavirus outbreak and found ways to live with and beyond it. This vitality was due in no small part to the ex-colony's long-standing experience with threats of political and cultural dissolution and, in turn, to local cultural agents' creative responses and survival practices. Long before 2003, local popular media had cultivated and entrenched an image of Hong Kong as a place of perpetual revivification capable of rebounding from any crisis—an ethos I will trace throughout this chapter under the rubric of deextinction. Rather than the top-down dream of neoliberal elites, this model of resilience is saturated with peopleness and locality, bubbling up from the creative life force of local culture, local vernaculars, and local sounds. In finding Hong Kong as its global epicenter, SARS fortuitously hit a city long practiced in self-deextinction.

I borrow the concept of deextinction from biology, where it refers to the process of bringing extinct species back to life through technologies of selective breeding and genome editing, often for purposes of restoring biodiversity and regenerating ecosystems.[3] Biologists have long known that concepts of species and extinction are "fluid," with "gradations" that account for evolution, hybridization, hierarchy, and locality.[4] But in the popular imagination, extinction is a terminus, with no return and no reversal, with all members of a species perishing permanently from the face of the earth. The idea of de-extinction is compelling for me precisely because it overturns this linearity principle. In cultural studies of Hong Kong, one prevailing trend has been to treat the decline of its media industry as a one-way street, a linear trek toward metaphorical extinction. This fixation on themes of death and disappearance misses the many ways local popular culture imagines its own extinction as always fused with deextinction, and the dynamic ways this culture creates tales of extinction as protein for self-perpetuation and auto-regeneration.

PANDEMIC RESILIENCE 113

Extinction and deextinction are thus, and have been for decades, two sides of the same coin.

In the context of 2003's successive tragedies, when apocalyptic feelings ran high and deep, it is not surprising that the extinction/deextinction dyad became the central narrative structure for Hong Kong's SARS texts. To understand these texts, we must first understand the central role played by the city's entertainment industry, and we can start by tuning in to one of its keystone events: the annual Hong Kong Film Awards ceremony.

Assembling at the Apocalypse

In 2003 this ceremony fell on April 6. Typically a grand star-studded affair, a visual feast for local television viewers as well as a moment of cultural pride for the city's globally renowned cinema, it was uncharacteristically somber in mood that year. Like the American Oscars a month prior, which had canceled its customary red carpet parade due to the Iraq War, the Hong Kong ceremony replaced its red carpet star walk with low-key tributes to local healthcare workers on the frontline of SARS. By that point, the city was in its third month of the outbreak and entering what would become its most severe phase, as the virus spread beyond hospitals into the community.[5] Just that past week had brought a series of grim developments. On Monday, March 31, over two hundred cases of infection erupted at the Amoy Gardens housing estate in Kowloon, the highest daily surge in infected cases in the world thus far, leading to the mass relocation of an entire block of residents to two "holiday camps" in the New Territories the very next day.[6] On that same day, April 1, an article using the *Ming Pao* newspaper logo and layout circulated on the local internet claiming that the government had declared Hong Kong an "infected port," that Chief Executive Tung Chee-hwa had resigned, and that the stock market had collapsed. The story turned out to be fake news, an April Fool's prank by a fourteen-year-old boy hacker who was later arrested on criminal charges.[7] But before officials could clarify the rumor, panic had broken out across the city, as thousands of residents mobbed banks and supermarkets and fought over food supplies.[8] Heightening public fear that day was the real news that the US State Department was evacuating all nonessential personnel from its Hong Kong consulate office.[9] A day later, on April 2, WHO followed with its first-ever travel advisory against Hong Kong and Guangdong Province.[10] A day later still, on April 3, the first Hong Kong

114 CHAPTER 3

medical worker, the pediatric surgeon James Lau Tai-kwan, died from SARS, even as his infected wife remained in quarantine.[11]

Amid this crisis atmosphere, what most galvanized Hong Kong's sense of doom that week was perhaps not the epidemic but the shocking suicide of one of the city's most iconic and beloved stars. On the evening of April 1, the singer-actor Leslie Cheung Kwok-wing—affectionately nicknamed Gor Gor (Big Brother) by locals—jumped to his death from a twenty-fourth-floor balcony of the Mandarin Oriental Hotel, a note in his pocket citing not SARS infection but clinical depression.[12] Overnight and within nine hours, six other people leaped from buildings in separate suicide attempts, five of them succeeding.[13] More would follow in subsequent weeks, with 134 suicides in all that month, a 35 percent increase from the previous months of that year and a 56 percent increase from the preceding five Aprils. While these deaths were attributed to a range of causes, from mental illness to unemployment to financial debt, the most noticeable spikes occurred in suicides by jumping from heights and among men in Cheung's age group, with several cases involving suicide notes that directly referenced him.[14] "A rich and depressed man like Cheung commits suicide," wrote one man. "Why not a poor and depressed person like me?"[15] This disturbing trend prompted intense scrutiny of the local media's role in reporting celebrity suicides. A group of University of Hong Kong faculty quickly called on journalists to refrain from overzealous coverage of Cheung's death and to focus instead "on the need to treasure life, mutual help and love," so as not to fuel public feelings of bleakness that would escalate the suicide epidemic.[16] Indeed, out of the entire outbreak period, that first week in April may have encapsulated the city's most concentrated sense of near extinction.

Yet, following the chronicle of Hong Kong that week also reveals the myriad ways Cheung's suicide unexpectedly reenlivened the city, in a perfect example of deextinction. If global memory of SARS-wrought Hong Kong tends to focus on eerie images of deserted urban landscapes, of empty restaurants and hollowed-out subways, in the days after Cheung's death, the streets were anything but barren. His fans networked by word of mouth and social media, so that by the night of April 5 over three hundred mourners had gathered outside the Mandarin Oriental in commemoration.[17] In addition to bouquets, they left face masks in front of the hotel, purportedly to protect Cheung's spirit from SARS in the afterlife.[18] On the night of his memorial service on April 7, nearly ten thousand people congregated outside the Hong Kong Funeral Home, packing two basketball courts across the street and braving the virus as much as a steady rain.[19] Some stayed overnight, and, by the next morning, with the rain unceasing, over a thousand mourners reappeared, lining the roads from the funeral parlor to the crematorium to see Cheung off on his final journey.[20] Archival footage of that week shows throngs dressed in black and seas of masked faces beneath a dense mosaic of umbrellas. When interviewed by local news, these fans talked not only about their admiration for Cheung's talent but also about his companionate place in their collective upbringing. Their language was plural, epochal: "His songs accompanied us as we grew up," said one woman to a reporter, as another woman beside her nodded vigorously. "They kept us company as we grew up in the eighties."[21] More than the loss of a brotherly idol, Cheung's demise seemed to mark the passing of a local world, the traumatic expiration of not just one generation's but the whole city's cultural bildungsroman. Yet, even in communal grief, the public was full of microactivities and far from inert with despondency.

For those in the entertainment industry, deextinction practices were harder to come by since the interlocking sense of epidemic catastrophe and cultural collapse was even more acute, not only because many knew Cheung personally, in a business notorious for its two degrees of separation, but also because they had been confronting the industry's decline for a decade by then. The film sector is a prime example. At its pinnacle in the early 1990s, Hong Kong released an average of 150 movies per year, surpassing the output of most national cinemas, including Western ones.[22] Local films consistently outgrossed foreign ones in the domestic market, stunningly "bucking the worldwide trend of Hollywood domination."[23] Hong Kong cinema ranked second in the world in terms of export, behind only the United States, dominating market shares in countries across East, Southeast, and South Asia.[24] Many awestruck observers of this phenomenon—whereby an Asian colonial city's indigenous culture industry achieved a magnitude of international commercial success that beat out even Hollywood's hegemony in regional markets—would echo David Bordwell in calling Hong Kong cinema "one of the success stories of film history."[25] However, beginning in 1993, a combination of factors drove this industry into a progressive slump. Contrary to expectations, the chief culprit was not the impending handover, not geopolitics, but neoliberal economics. In the nineties property boom, local developers tore down old-style cinema halls and built expensive high-tech multiplexes in their stead, which drove up ticket prices and in turn diminished movie attendance.[26] At the same time, overproduction of local flicks, made fast and cheap to meet transnational demand, meant that Hong Kong productions came to be equated with uneven quality. Demographic changes also fed audience fatigue, as what had seemed cool and novel to the eighties generation became tired formulas by the early nineties, when "everyone knew all the gimmicks."[27] Hence, local moviegoers increasingly turned to big-budget Hollywood imports for a fresher and more reliable viewing experience. In 1993 Steven Spielberg's *Jurassic Park* set record highs at the local box office, heralding a new period of Hollywood films eclipsing local ones.[28] These years also saw the rise of other film industries across East and Southeast Asia, drastically shrinking Hong Kong's shares in overseas markets. Finally, many locals never recovered from the 1997 Asian financial crisis, and, by 2002, the unemployment rate had soared to almost 8 percent while bankruptcy claims were at an all-time high.[29]

In this climate of financial gloom, the entertainment sector was in fact mostly hopeful about 1997, as an opportunity to integrate with the mainland economy and open up a much vaster market.[30] By 2003, though, not only had this much-anticipated market not materialized, but the Chinese government had also imposed ever-stricter protectionist quotas on Hong Kong films, even as these films were being rampantly pirated and shown openly in mainland theaters.[31] If there was fear of cultural encroachment from across the border at that juncture, it was evidently on the part of China as much as Hong Kong. With the further eruption of SARS that spring, the city's movie production all but ground to a halt. By the end of that first week in April, local cinema operators were reporting a 30–50 percent plummet in ticket sales, with numerous circuits cutting back daily screenings. Ironically, the small venues weathered the outbreak better than the large multiplex chains, as they had only two to three screens to manage and were not housed in shopping malls that were susceptible to mall closings.[32] Had theater outlets not corporatized but remained on a small-business model, the film sector might have fared the pandemic better.

In this context, the entertainment industry's attempt to rally itself and the populace for the film awards that week begs to be read in terms of prosociality and resilience. An air of melancholy hung over the ceremony, but, like the public in the wake of Cheung's death, local celebrities turned out en masse to demonstrate their communal spirit. Instead of the usual cocktail of awkward formalities and stiff banter, the master host that year—the actor-director-producer-emcee Eric Tsang Chi-wai, a household name known for his clownish persona, quick wit, gift of gab, and sometimes foulmouthed stumbles—delivered an unusually emotional and teary-eyed opening speech:

On the 19th of last month, when I received the nomination lists for this year's film awards, I was really excited, because I felt this might just be the most fun to watch year in the award's twenty-two-year history. All the nominated movies and actors are well-loved by everyone. But in the past two to three weeks, bad news has followed one after another. First, it was the Iraq War. Then, it was the viral outbreak here in Hong Kong. A few days ago, in our own showbiz circles, a very dear friend of ours left us. I suddenly felt like the world turned gray. I didn't want to do anything, touch anything, care about anything. I just wanted to back out completely.

So, a few days ago, I called the film awards' program director and told him I didn't want to host this ceremony. But in that instant, I saw on TV a frontline doctor who had just recovered from SARS turn to the camera and tell us that he plans to go back to work at the hospital. And when another medical professor, faced with an infected patient in the wards, asked the hundred-plus doctors gathered there to help him, not a single one said no. I knew then there's no retreat. Tonight's show *must* go on. Whether it was the 1991 East China flood, the Kunming earthquake, or Taiwan's 921 earthquake, Hong Kong show business has always been at the frontline of care for others, fundraising to help those in need. Today we have trouble at home—so all the more must we not lose our head and fall to pieces. I absolutely must step up and tell people: I love Hong Kong!

I hope everyone will understand that the scariest virus is not SARS but panic. I hope, through tonight, we can tell our friends around the world that, however they look upon us, we thank them for their care and concern, and we will do our best to clean up our house quickly, so that everyone can come back and be our guests. Today, through this annual ceremony, I hope to relay on behalf of our industry colleagues and fellow citizens our highest esteem and respect for Hong Kong's medical professionals. Thank you, thank you, and thank you again. Thank you for all your work; we feel proud because of you.[33]

Tsang's speech is revealing in the ways it casts Hong Kong's entertainment industry amid a citywide disaster: not as a purely commercial or frivolous institution or an elite and privileged tier of society removed from the rest of the city but as a sector with a sense of compassionate leadership and social responsibility, one that strives to emulate the courage and dedication of the medical professions. Tsang echoed health authorities when he reminded local viewers that "the scariest virus is not SARS but panic"; he modeled a voice of reason and empathy when he thanked frontline medical workers and destigmatized them as sources of contagion; and he assumed the role of not just industry but city spokesperson when he addressed international audiences and encouraged their future return, doing his bit to help the tourism economy. Above all, he portrayed himself and his colleagues as beholden to, devoted to, and deeply affectionate toward Hong Kong as a place and community. This industry self-image was also embodied in the many words of humble gratitude expressed toward the city's medical workers throughout the ceremony. Even when the tone occasionally lightened, what most strongly signaled the industry's joint message was the stars' very act of showing up. While there was an alleged drop in attendance by foreign invitees that year, including big-name mainland directors, local artists and filmmakers made a point of coming out rather than staying home, in a concerted display of mutual support for local viewers as much as each other.

In that act of mass assembly, the industry mirrored the public that week. Helen Siu and Jane Chan have argued that the outpouring of "respect and sadness" in Hong Kongers' public eulogies for medical workers that spring reflected not just "collective trauma" but "an agentive moment of repositioning through affirming civic practices."[34] Likewise, the mass eulogies for Cheung that April were not just rituals of mourning but agentive and prosocial civic practices that helped galvanize the city's distinct sense of self amid SARS. Not fortuitously, many stars who appeared at the award ceremony were also spotted at the various private services for Cheung in the following days. He was nominated in the best actor category that year, and, though not favored to win, his absence was surely keenly felt that night. In concluding his speech, Tsang, too, restored the spotlight on Cheung by paying tribute to "Gor Gor, our music king, our eternal movie emperor"—his words capturing an oddly imperial image of Hong Kong, even in its decline and crisis as an ex-colonial pandemic epicenter.

The Cantophone's Extinction/Deextinction Double Consciousness

This chapter extends the previous two's concerns by asking: What do pandemic ordinariness and prosociality look like at the site of not just a non-Western epicenter but one of ex-colonial semiautonomy, when the unexpected crisis of global disease unfolds over a protracted local crisis temporality of political domination and cultural besiegement? How do we read for its practices of pandemic resilience? In the year of SARS, Hong Kong's popular media industry was prolific in producing epidemic narratives, and, here too, sentimentality and humor in the stories of small people abound, as we will see below. But more than a sense of immediate crisis, what gets woven into the ordinariness of these works is something at once more sweeping and endemic, akin to a consciousness of slow apocalypse. This aesthetic affective form is not Whyte's model of crisis epistemology, with tenets of unprecedentedness and urgency that mask deeper historical and structural violences, but rather its inverse—an extinctionist temporality that stretches, embedding SARS within a longer local genealogy of colonial precarity whereby civilizational collapse seems all but overdue. This extinctionist ethos is certainly tied to the 1997 transfer of Hong Kong's sovereignty from Britain to China, and Ackbar Abbas has notably dubbed it a "culture and politics of disappearance."[35] As the local critic Li Cheuk-to put it at the time, 2003 brought to fruition the city's "apocalyptic anxieties" from 1997.[36] Indeed, this has become the dominant global narrative and memory of handover-era Hong Kong. Yet, crucially, extinctionism is only half the story.

Much less recognized is how Hong Kong's SARS texts are almost invariably shot through with a simultaneous exorbitant will to life and rejuvenation—what I call a subimperial extinction/deextinction double consciousness. If mainland Chinese culture is too often pigeonholed into what Xiaobing Tang terms the dissidence hypothesis, leading to a sorely truncated view of China that, as I have argued throughout the book, blots out a huge spectrum of social practices and expressions testifying to people's everyday microagency, so Hong Kong culture in general has too often been reductively read by global commentators within a narrow handover paradigm, what Jenny Lau calls an "elitist historiography" that fixates on the politics of 1997 as the de facto source of all meaning-making from the city.[37] Against such top-down hermeneutics, this chapter constructs, up from the ground of its popular media industry, the "local theories and nonce taxonomies" of Hong Kong's SARS encounter, to borrow Eve Sedgwick's phrase.[38] This intentionally weak theory, formulated out of local vernaculars as situated knowledges, is yet another modality by which I hope to decolonize Western pandemic epistemologies and do justice to local actions and affects. Where the handover-centric model sees only doom and gloom in Hong Kong's SARS articulations, I see above all their exuberant deextinctionist energy, their dogged practices of survival and renewal.

120   CHAPTER 3

I thus select for attention here three filmic projects that exemplify the local entertainment industry's de/extinctionist aesthetics: *Project 1:99* (*1:99 din jeng haang dung/1:99 dianying xingdong*), a compilation of eleven shorts sponsored by the Hong Kong government and directed by fifteen top local directors; *City of SARS* (*Fei din yan sang/Feidian rensheng*), a low-budget movie with three interlinked story lines featuring an ensemble cast of local stars, including a final segment starring Eric Tsang; and *Golden Chicken 2* (*Gam gai 2/Jin ji 2*), sequel to the award-winning raunchy comedy *Golden Chicken* from the year before, starring Sandra Ng Kwan-yu as a happy-go-lucky sex worker.[39] These films were all made and released in 2003, some shot during the outbreak period itself, others within weeks of the outbreak's end, thus representing the industry's near retrospective on the city's epidemic experiences. At first glance, they seem to possess value only as cultural documents of a minor archive vis-à-vis a global pandemic. None could be called high art, being quick productions made on relatively small budgets and tight timetables. Yet each brought together a host of local performers and/or filmmakers, mobilizing to the utmost the industry's star system and enclave networks to convey the sense of collective enterprise and communal perseverance. For their makers as much as their intended audiences—Hong Kongers weathering SARS and its aftermath—the films' raison d'être was the here and now. Not meant to be timeless texts for international spectators or even local viewers ten years hence, these films were closer to personal notes passed between classmates and neighbors, their messages crafted around a common present condition, their affects premised on insular bonds and intimate lingos. In their insider quality and invocation of a socius united in shared distress, they can be likened to chapter 2's digital SARS jokes that actively constructed an epidemic community rather than simply representing it.

What uniquely characterizes Hong Kong's SARS works, though, is a geocultural formation I call the Cantophone. As Lau contends, scholarship on Hong Kong culture often exhibits a handover reductionism, whereby "every contemporary film" is interpreted as always primarily fixated on "the 1997 issue," thus "eras[ing] the concrete details of cultural experiences and ... complex social and psychological realities of life in Hong Kong."[40] Hong Kong culture takes on critical worth for scholars abroad only if it fits into theoretical models of postcoloniality and subalternity articulated elsewhere, in global centers of discursive power. The dominance of this critical paradigm accounts, for example, for the international prominence of Hong Kong art-house cinema, often treated as an exclusive and almost transcendent art form because its sociopolitical contexts can be quickly explained away via 1997. By extension, visuality comes to be privileged as the system of signification that matters, obviating the need for remote viewers to know local languages and lingos.

Shifting from this framework, I elevate for analysis here precisely those filmic materials and components that would normally be dismissed or bracketed as inscrutably local: lowbrow genres of comedy and farce and their use of fleeting vernaculars and sounds. In fact, the rise of local cinema was never independent of a wider cultural sphere interlocking film with television and music. The fluidity and porousness between the various platforms of this multimedial ecosystem are also what lends local celebrities their aura of intimacy for the local public, a dynamic Leung Wing-Fai calls "multi-media stardom" (with Leslie Cheung being an eminent example).[41] Contemporary popular culture is rarely experienced with the visual severed from the aural, and, more often than not, sounds are intermeshed with images in a commingled sensory mediascape. This multimedial assemblage lies at the heart of what Po-King Choi terms "the indigenous culture of Hong Kong," which "furnishes the basis for a distinctive Hong Kong identity" from the late 1960s onward.[42] From the inception of this indigenous culture, sound—especially Cantonese sounds, in the full range of its accents—has been an indispensable component of local identifications. To downplay the language's vital role in the development of Hong Kong cultural identities is to risk amputating their historical and lived corporeality, rendering local sounds mere variants of a larger sinophone empire. And, during SARS, it was precisely Cantonese vernaculars that the entertainment industry marshaled, again and again, as localizing strategies to tell Hong Kong's epidemic stories and encode local epidemic memories. We cannot begin to analyze these works if we ignore Cantonese and its significance for Hong Kong cultural identity formation, and we would miss all the deextincting moves and nuances that each work weaves into its epidemic storytelling.

Since the handover, fears about the mainlandization of Hong Kong culture and the Mandarinization of Hong Kong education have continually stirred local outrage and fomented anxiety about the imminent "death of Cantonese," registered in such dystopian works as the 2015 indie film *Ten Years*.[43] In this context, I use the term *Cantophone* in order to put the accent not just on place but on language, and not just language but vernacular, and to amplify the phonic dimensions of local vernaculars—in speech and song, through soundtracks and soundscapes. Akin to Shu-mei Shih's concept of the

Sinophone, the Hong Kong Cantophone, too, defines itself in opposition to China's Mandarin culture by emphasizing linguistic difference rather than ethnic sameness, postcolonial hybridity rather than ethnonational solidarity. As a consciously deployed aesthetic, the Cantophone is highly assertive of its Cantonese sounds, not as one dialect within a universal Han Chinese but as an autonomous tongue with rich internal idioms irreducible to a master script. As such, the Cantophone fits well with Shih's characterization of the Sinophone as the aggregate "heterogeneity of Sinitic languages" produced "outside China and on the margins of China and Chineseness."[44] Like the Sinophone, too, the Cantophone is deeply tied to locality and often adamant about local branding, with the catchphrase "made in Hong Kong" connoting a separateness rather than contiguity with other regional Cantonese productions from southern China. Finally, the Cantophone, too, can manifest a strong "anticolonial intent against Chinese hegemony," even when it does not—and it typically does not—adopt an overt oppositional politics.[45]

What distinguishes the Cantophone, however, is its subimperial double consciousness—a sense not just of its post/colonial marginality but *also* of its cultural centrality in the Chinese world, especially during its so-called golden era. In its heyday, from the 1980s to mid-1990s, Hong Kong popular culture was a dominant force in shaping global Chineseness, with a sphere of influence spanning East and Southeast Asia, Australia, North America, and Europe. Its copious commercial exports included not just films, as noted above, but also pop music and television serials. For decades, Hong Kong television programs and Cantopop songs constituted defining forms of popular culture for Chinese communities across the world, functioning as powerful building blocks of imagined community in the diaspora.[46] Even into the early 2000s, Cantopop stars were often mobbed by fans when they held concerts in Taipei, Singapore, London, and Las Vegas.[47] This is a far cry from Shih's Sinophone as a "minor articulation" on the periphery of China and Chineseness.[48] Instead, the Cantophone exemplifies Kuan-Hsing Chen's concept of subempire: "a lower-level empire that depends on the larger structure of imperialism," subordinating itself to other capitalist world powers while targeting for expansion "politico-economically weaker countries."[49] For Chen, the archetypal subempire is 1990s Taiwan. Ding-Tzann Lii, though, views golden-era Hong Kong cinema as epitomizing a "colonized empire" and "marginal imperialism," insofar as its expansion into overseas markets led to the "underdevelopment" of other regional cinemas for decades, including in Taiwan and South Korea.[50] It is by virtue of the Cantophone's subimperial status that its cultural industry came to cultivate a dyadic image of Hong Kong as never simply a colonial underdog imperiled by annihilation and erasure but also a regional top dog, a source others look to for inspirational energy, a subjugated life that never quite dies but always has the capacity not just for survival but for dominion. Indeed, strife and crisis feed this self-image, so that extinction threats themselves become incorporated as essential fodder for sustaining deextinction narratives.

Still, unlike other subempires such as Taiwan and South Korea, Hong Kong lacks a sovereign state of its own to drive its capital accumulation and consolidate its expansionist energies. Its film industry, for one, "developed solely in response to market demands and in the absence of any protectionist government policy."[51] This dependence on transnational capital rendered it "susceptible to slumps and recessions in the regional economy, which are beyond [its] control."[52] As Abbas aptly puts it, Hong Kong cinema "has to be popular in order to be at all."[53] Without the stability and backing of a sovereign state, the city's popular media industry never had the luxury of conceiving of itself as something permanent, a subempire that would last. Hence, even at its height, it was fragile and contingent, a kind of subsistence subempire. If it attained astonishing market success and cultural influence during the boom period, this was in no small part due to feelings of insecurity about the city's future. As Law Kar and Frank Bren poignantly put it, local cultural producers labored with an acute sense of the clock ticking, as they "emptied their hearts and minds into their work to make the most of the time left."[54] These material conditions formed the sociohistorical backdrop to the Cantophone's extinctionist ethos and deextinctionist urgency.

Abbas has notably called this dynamic, this frenetic need to forge something that could properly be called a Hong Kong identity, the city's "politics and culture of disappearance": "The imminence of its disappearance," he contends, "was what precipitated an intense and unprecedented interest in Hong Kong culture. The anticipated end of Hong Kong as people knew it was the beginning of a profound concern with its historical and cultural specificity."[55] Along this argument, it was only when Hong Kongers faced the impending fate of being "reunified" with the mainland, of having their semiautonomy extinguished in a near future, that they for the first time threw themselves into the concerted project of identity construction. Abbas locates the start of this sensibility in 1982, with Margaret Thatcher's visit to China, and in 1984, with the signing of the Sino-British Joint Declaration that confirmed the 1997 handover date, and he sees it exemplified in Hong Kong's New Wave

124   CHAPTER 3

cinema.[56] Abbas's thesis, however, falls short on precisely what Lau insists on—"looking deeply into the history of local popular cinema"—and falls prey to the narrow reductionism of a 1997-centric reading.[57] If we look beyond art-house cinema and consider the wider Cantophone realm out of which its auteurs emerged, we can in fact trace the cultural matrix of disappearance to a decade earlier—to 1972, the year Cantonese cinema died for the first time.

The story is an uncannily familiar one: after flourishing for two decades post–World War II, when over a hundred and even two hundred films in the language were produced each year, Hong Kong's Cantonese cinema suffered a severe meltdown in the late 1960s. In 1970, only thirty-five Cantonese films were made; in 1971, only one; and in 1972, zero.[58] Back then as later, the reasons for collapse were several. It may be, back then as later, that the overproduction of low-budget works "reached saturation point" for the market.[59] Mandarin productions, while far fewer in number, tended to have much bigger budgets and "dazzling production values." Above all, even more so back then than later, "foreign sales drove local production," determining a movie's soundtrack as much as its genre and cast.[60] In that period, the choice between Mandarin and Cantonese was decided not by the place of production or the language spoken by the actors but by the studios and their target markets. Cantonese films had an audience of only eight to ten million worldwide, but Mandarin films, even with the mainland market closed during the Mao era, commanded an audience many times larger across Asia, with twenty million in Taiwan alone.[61] In the rivalry between big studios, resources ultimately shifted over to the production of more lucrative Mandarin films—even when the crews spoke mostly Cantonese.[62] "Hence the peculiar fact that each year Hong Kong made dozens of films in a tongue spoken by less than 5 percent of its population," observes Bordwell, with the "curious result . . . that Bruce Lee and other Cantonese-speaking stars were dubbed into Mandarin and their films subtitled for the local audiences."[63] The translocal funding structure for this original Hong Kong Cantonese cinema, and its embeddedness within a marketplace dominated by studio empires, throws into relief the city's historical peripheralness even for its own film industry. What's more, even the Cantonese used in this early cinema was not oriented to local lives and local issues, as it grew out of a regional agenda set by mainland emigrant filmmakers, most of whom were guided by a socialist vision.[64] This cinema's detachment from local viewers' concerns and tastes may be why it died so swiftly after the launch of local television broadcasting in 1967, which Stephen Teo calls its true "death-knell." Within a few years, the local station TVB, with its localized programming, supplanted Cantonese films as the "most popular entertainment medium for Cantonese-speaking audiences."[65] It is from this conjoined vanishing of a prelocal Canto-cinema and ascendence of localized Cantonese mass media that Hong Kong's Cantophone culture arose.

Given this history, the Hong Kong Cantophone can be said to always carry a trace of extinction consciousness. The memory of its birth is also one of its rebirth from a prior demise. This consciousness predates 1982 and 1984, and it postdates 1997 into 2003. Even at the height of its subimperial influence, the industry could anticipate a termination it had experienced before, in a not so distant past. It is within this history, too, that we can understand the city's deep and widespread bereavement over Leslie Cheung's death. Cheung's career was both a catalyst and a product of Hong Kong Cantophone culture, and, fatefully, his trajectory paralleled the latter's, in ascent as in decline. His struggling attempts to enter the Cantopop industry in the late seventies, followed by his explosive popularity as a local singer in the eighties and an internationally acclaimed actor in the nineties, not only coincided with but also epitomized for many the early toils, gradual entrenchment, and high glory days of the homegrown culture as a transnational phenomenon. His shocking suicide was a condensation point. So were the deaths of several other beloved local idols who departed in rapid succession during those two years—including the singer Law Man, singer-actress Anita Mui Yim-fong, and lyricist James Wong Jim, each of whom also brought out thousands and even tens of thousands of mourning fans. The colossal scale of these demonstrations of public grief suggests, paradoxically, the kind of sorrow experienced by an enclave of privileged insiders, as they watch their small and cherished dynasty crumbling, its founding royalties and iconic heirs dying off one by one, seemingly prematurely and yet also not. This sorrow persists despite everyone knowing all along that their dynasty's reign would not last, that it had a scheduled expiration date, and that that date had already passed.

Hannah Arendt wrote of postwar stateless peoples that their "first loss . . . was the loss of their homes, and this meant the loss of the entire social texture into which they were born and in which they established for themselves a distinct place in the world."[66] For Arendt, the loss of home was not the greatest calamity of the rightless, nor could post/colonial Hong Kongers be glibly equated with stateless refugees. Yet the historical predicament of Hong Kong has been such that its inhabitants continually face a similar loss of world. This loss occurs in situ, needing neither a global war nor a fascist regime nor the wholesale displacement of a people to be enacted. Instead,

126 CHAPTER 3

the city's experience of loss is the collateral damage of everyday geopolitics, the side effect of a legal transaction between adjacent and remote empires, executed through paperwork and handshakes rather than bombs and tanks. This loss of world unfolds in slow time, and slow death lacks the horrific grandeur of fast extinction. But, for those living under its shadow, the threat can be felt no less acutely. Following Rob Nixon, we might call this the "slow violence" of "long dyings": "a violence that occurs gradually and out of sight, a violence of delayed destruction that is dispersed across time and space, an attritional violence that is typically not viewed as violence at all."[67] And, following Lauren Berlant, we can see it as a form of collective "slow death": the "physical wearing out of a population in a way that points to its deterioration as a defining condition of its experience and historical existence," unfolding not in fast time but within "temporalities of the endemic."[68]

For Hong Kong, these articulations of slowly dying life within slowly toxifying environments are only too resonant. Like an endangered species, the cultural agents of this world have labored frenziedly to reproduce it and even briefly succeeded in propelling its creatures into the international limelight. SARS may have incited global fears of cataclysm and annihilation, but, in Hong Kong, another variety of slow extinction has been happening in plain sight, without the benefit of the name. But lest we overly romanticize this story, we must recall, too, that the ascendency of Hong Kong cinema had once "destroyed" other cultural forms such as Taiwanese cinema.[69] And where the local Cantonese cinema survived, what ultimately perished, in what Jeff Yang has called "a kind of mass-extinction event," was the earlier Mandarin film industry, in Taiwan as in Hong Kong.[70] Thus, at the affective core of the Cantophone is a double-edged quality—a double consciousness of both dominance and extinction, of being both top dog and underdog. This paradox is perhaps what gives rise to some of Hong Kong popular culture's signature bipolar styles: the manic tragicomedy, the self-serious yet self-parodic social satire melodrama, the exorbitant fantasy epic of rogues and small heroes, and that eccentric penchant for glamorized bad taste often analogized imperfectly to Western-style camp. Even in its crisis narratives, the Hong Kong Cantophone is never merely or wholly mournful but can possess a madcap energy, just as Ursula Heise recognizes that extinction narratives can assume more than "elegiac and tragic modes" and even take the path of comedy.[71]

Hong Kong's 2003 SARS films shore up these stylistic polarities in force. On the one hand, they marshal a set of tropes that are distinctively Hong

PANDEMIC RESILIENCE   127

Kong in their imagining of extinction: suicide is a recurrent motif, as are gallows humor, unemployment, bankruptcy, spousal abandonment, amnesia, and the life-or-death gamble. Disease and sickness actually occupy minor roles in these epidemic narratives, functioning as circumstantial backdrops or plot triggers rather than ends in themselves. On the other, tightly conjoined with these motifs are a host of companion deextinction tropes: the underdog comeback, the reversal of fortune, the eleventh-hour rescue, the overdue miracle. Just as extinction is envisaged as nonfinal, so is deextinction posited as provisional: there is no theology of eternal triumph here except hyperbolically self-ironic ones. More often than not, the implied metaphysics is one of cyclical fortune and ceaseless return, and the attendant ethos is not one of victorious overcoming but of continual resilience.

On a formal level, the SARS films enact this resilience through an excess of Cantophoneness, an intensified claiming of a unique Hong Kong identity through reiterations of its signature cultural artifacts. Genre recycling, intertextual self-citation, archival footage replay, sonic memory retrieval—these are some of the industry's staple methods for selectively rebreeding its past productions and editing its own genomic materials for adaptation in a changing habitat. Inside jokes, inside allusions, and insider networks proliferate. It is as if, in the wake of the virus crossing the border from China, the films could compensatorily seal off their borders of spectatorship or comprehension. By virtue of being traveling media, they are still available to transnational and diasporic audiences for consumption, but the Cantophone community they interpellate, however translocal, is imagined as existentially tethered to local life and survival. Their hodgepodge picaresque plotlines, the almost inhuman vitality of their protagonists, the proliferation of local references, the thickening of an interior intertextuality, the accentuating of Cantonese slang and Cantopop songs, and the myriad layers of what can easily be mistaken for trivial nostalgia but are in fact local memory cues—these are all gestures of a besieged industry, playing out its part as guardian of a collapsing subempire for an exclusive enclave as it inoculates itself against ongoing attrition. The Cantophone, in all its multimedial bits and pieces, serves as the crux vehicle for not just memorializing but revivifying this cultural world. In relation to SARS, this Cantophone self-resuscitation may strike outside observers as the wretched dying gasp of a narcissistic industry. But to those who are clued into their purpose and methods, their anguish and longing, these films are nothing short of dreams of collective deextinction. In our pandemic times, if we are to search for a model of communal resiliency, what better place to find it than in a city so experienced in dreaming crisis comebacks?

Local Luck and Local Laughs in *Project 1:99*

Deextinction themes of Hong Kongers' inveterate capacity for communal can-do-ness and lucky survival pervade *Project 1:99*, underpinning its creators' very memory of the project's origins. As the director Gordon Chan Ka-seung recounts, "When SARS came, we [of the Hong Kong Film Directors' Guild] all knew we needed to do something. That was such a depressing moment for Hong Kong. Leslie passed away, SARS came. So it was like the end of the world." *Project 1:99* thus has its psychic roots in that first week of April 2003, and, characteristically for this industry, apocalyptic prospects only spurred productivity. "Tsui Hark and I and Peter Chan were the initiators for this project," Chan recalls. "We went to the government, luckily we got the money and we started shooting.... We are a part of Hong Kong. Every time, when something happens we know we need to come up with something."[72] Peter Chan Ho-sun echoes this sentiment: "I think the 1:99 project was something we needed to do as part of the Hong Kong community ... people will look at these films and recognize something of their own experiences in what we have produced or be inspired by their messages."[73] John Shum Kin-fun, actor-producer and political activist, also helped secure government funding for the project. "Show-business people might seem egotistical in some ways," he comments, "but when it comes to something like [SARS] they are very conscious of their responsibilities to society. In Hong Kong especially they are very generous." And, he adds, very savvy: "We understand the role of the media much better than the government. We can mobilize very fast to respond to the needs of a situation. We have done it several times now and we have the manual ready."[74] At these filmmakers' urging, the Television and Entertainment Licensing Authority agreed to provide HK$500,000 to cover production costs, and, within the month, a dozen major directors signed on.[75] The idea was to compile an anthology of shorts of one to two minutes each, all focusing on some aspect of Hong Kong life amid SARS. Wong Kar-wai, who originally intended to shoot his piece in the city's first infected hospital but was unable to complete shooting on time, was nonetheless credited with the project's title: "1:99" refers to the ratio of bleach to water for mixing a disinfectant (so went local lore), so the slogan was meant to arouse a feeling, as Peter Chan puts it, of "doing things for yourself . . . getting on with life."[76]

The eventual roster of filmmakers and performers was a veritable who's who of the local entertainment industry, spanning famous directors and megastars with international profiles to television veterans and Cantopop idols across several generations. Besides Gordon Chan, Peter Chan, and Tsui Hark, the contributing directors were Fruit Chan Gor, Teddy Chan Tak-sum, Mabel Cheung Yuen-ting, Stephen Chow Sing-chi, Dante Lam Chiu-yin, Andrew Lau Wai-keung, Alex Law Kai-yui, Joe Ma Wai-ho, Alan Mak Siu-fai, Johnnie To Kei-fung, Brian Tse Lap-man, and Wai Kar-fai. Child actors and new performers were also given parts, some with starring roles. Many participants, including high-salaried actors and filmmakers, reputedly worked without pay, out of a public-minded spirit to boost Hong Kongers' morale. Shooting began in May, when SARS was still ongoing but starting to abate in the city, and wrapped up by July. The shorts were then submitted to the Hong Kong government for distribution to local television stations, airing for the first time on TVB in August.

As Gordon Chan notes, one special emphasis of *Project 1:99* was on comedy, to "do a lot of comedy."[77] Like the digital SARS jokes in chapter 2, this turn to humor was not a matter of pandemic denial or schadenfreude, nor was it disaster capitalism's crass exploitation of a lucrative local film genre.[78] As with small humor, the comedy of these SARS shorts puts the accent on the ordinary, the prosocial, the playful. But more pointedly for Hong Kong, the comedy film—especially social comedy that situates slapstick entertainment within local societal issues—is intimately tied to the history of Cantophone deextinction. When Hong Kong's Cantonese cinema died for the first time in 1972, what revived it were two social comedy films: *The House of 72 Tenants* in 1973, directed by Chor Yuen, and *Games Gamblers Play* in 1974, directed by Michael Hui Koon-man. If *The House of 72 Tenants* was "an unexpected box office success," *Games Gamblers Play* was a super "blockbuster . . . hitting number one in the box office and essentially inventing the Canto-comedy genre."[79] Cantonese social comedy hence carries a very specific historical residue for Hong Kong's popular media industry, bearing the trace of an ur-genre for underdog comebacks and local culture's resilience. Indeed, all the SARS films in this chapter owe much to this lineage. So, while the shorts in *Project 1:99* span numerous genres—from historical documentary to speculative dystopia, animal advocacy to intergenerational family drama, animated

130 CHAPTER 3

children's fable to motivational music video—comedy stands out as a recurrent device. Of the eleven shorts, five make substantial use of humor that has clear roots in Cantonese social comedy. Their points of reference are insistently local, evincing the deliberateness with which the directors reactivated indigenous comic traditions and practices. Their message—that these are Hong Kong productions made *by* Hong Kongers *for* Hong Kongers—was crafted with precision and care.

For instance, Tsui Hark's "Believe It or Not" is a video game action cartoon that draws on the characters of *Old Master Q*, Hong Kong's longest-running comic strip, created in 1962 by the local *manhua* artist Alfonso Wong under the pen name Wong Chak. This comic is "well-known for [its] witty and lampooning portrayals on a broad range of topics—from current affairs to the minutiae of daily life in Hong Kong."[80] In the short, Miss Chan, Old Master Q's love interest, is stranded at sea on a raft and beleaguered by SARS sharks. With the help of his sidekicks Big Potato and Mr. Chin, Old Master Q rescues Miss Chan by catapulting from a nearby island's coconut tree and kungfu blitzing the sharks with coconut cannonballs. In contrast to the militarized rhetoric deployed by both global health discourses and the mainland government during SARS, metaphors of epidemic isolation, besiegement, and defense get routed here through the gentle humor of an indigenous comics and its feel-good scenario of buddy teamwork and last-minute romantic rescue. "We all grew up with this comic strip, which has been running for forty years," said Nansum Shi, Tsui's wife and collaborator, during the short's production. "[Wong Chak's] stories are about sticking together in times of crisis," so the short's "essential theme is . . . when this city unites, it wins."[81] This language of winning suggests not warfare but games and gamblers, a motif that runs through all the comedies in *Project 1:99*.

Gordon Chan and Dante Lam's "Waiting for Luck" offers another example of de/extinction aesthetics. The short stars Dayo Wong Tze-wah, Hong Kong's premier stand-up comedian of the post-1997 generation, famous for his political satire routines that are dense with local references and Cantonese witticisms. Here, Wong plays an out-of-work and presumably homeless man, sitting idly at the harbor and staring dejectedly out at the water. Suddenly, a chic black-suited woman (played by Gigi Leung Wing-kei) materializes beside him and whisks him away to a computer-generated white room à la *The Matrix*. But instead of being seduced into a too-good-to-be-true simulated life complete with convertible sports car and starlet girlfriend (played by Gigi Lai Chi), he opts to live by his own honest labor and ends up selling discounted face masks at street intersections. In the final frame, he wears a traffic cop's cross straps and holds an upright broom by his side, a pose that mimics the Cantonese martial arts folk hero Beggar So. The short thus promotes Hong Kong self-reliance amid SARS and anchors it in Cantonese folk ethics and humor, suggesting that, with a spirit of genial and resourceful diligence, good fortune will come just when one thinks luck has run out.

The other three comedic shorts directly take up themes of games and lucky wins, with two reenacting the 1970s milieu to deextinct the decade when the city's Cantophone humor culture flourished. Joe Ma's "Who's Miss Hong Kong?" whimsically dramatizes a 1970s-era Miss Hong Kong Pageant in which a stuffed pillow in the shape of the territory is crowned the year's beauty queen. The other contestants (played by eleven Hong Kong idol actresses and singers) all squeal with delight and cheer the pillow on, signaling a non-zero sum game where Hong Kong's win embodies everyone's win. This short's industry self-parody also includes period impersonations of two iconic figures, Ivan Ho Sau-sun (played by Eason Chan Yik-shun) and Lydia Shum Din-ha, endearingly known to locals as Fei Fei ("Fat Fat") (played by a cross-dressing Bowie Wu Fung), hosts of the by-then-defunct television variety show *Enjoy Yourself Tonight*, one of the longest running live broadcast shows in the world and at one time compared to America's *Saturday Night Live*. Both Ho and Shum, not fortuitously, were comic actors and part of the original cast of *The House of 72 Tenants*.

With greater emphasis on local sounds, Johnnie To and Wai Kar-fai's "Rhapsody" revives not just 1970s costumes and hairstyles but also the foundational music of Sam Hui Koon-kit, often hailed as the Father of Cantopop. The youngest brother and frequent collaborator of Michael Hui, Sam also costarred, alongside Michael, in all of the latter's films in that era, including *Games Gamblers Play*. While Michael wrote the scripts and directed, Sam composed and sang the theme songs. Both are credited with forging the cultural zeitgeist of the 1970s working class, Michael for capturing "the everyday person who is caught in the reality of a fast-paced society . . . in comic forms," Sam for giving voice, in a modern folk musical style fashioned out of Hong Kong vernacular, to "small-time city-dwellers . . . their energy and vigor, their optimism, but also that bit of helplessness behind their drive to live as if their lives are on the line."[82] In "Rhapsody," the immensely popular actor Andy Lau Tak-wah plays the part of a *daa gung zai*, a working-class guy, standing in a line of jobseekers and jocularly belting out Sam Hui's "The Private Eyes" ("Bun gan baat loeng"/"Banjinbaliang"). This iconic theme song to the 1976 movie of the same name, written and directed by Michael and starring both brothers, is an upbeat, witty, and slang-filled anthem to Hong Kong's working-class men yoked to a lifetime of wage slavery. The short ends with Lau joining a chorus of other stars in the more heartwarming Sam Hui aria "Gifting You This Song" ("Ze jat kuk sung kap nei"/"Zhe yi qu song gei ni"), about fellowship and hope amid loneliness and hardship. The quick takeaway is that Hong Kongers would recover from SARS, even those hard hit by the epidemic, just as the city's downtrodden have been able to survive for decades—accompanied, comforted, and cheered throughout by the tunes of native Cantopop. As Johnnie To remarked during the making of the short: "I want Hong Kong people to remember the feelings we had [from the 1970s]. Times were very tough but just around the corner was a golden period for Hong Kong. We will get there again, we just have to work hard and stick together."[83] By assembling a contemporary cohort of readily recognizable local celebrities (represented, besides Andy Lau, by Sammi Cheng Sau-man, Lam Suet, Sean Lau Ching-wan, and Chapman To Man-chat), the short signaled to its 2003 public not just a present solidarity but a historical continuity with the Hui brothers' comic world, of small people grinding along with self-deprecating wit and resilient humor.

In the longer three-minute version of "Rhapsody," in two middle scenes deleted from the short's official release, the gambling trope takes center stage. The cast is shown exuberantly playing mahjong while singing a third Sam Hui song, "Legend of Mahjong Playing Heroes" ("Da zoek jing hung zyun"/"Da que yingxiong zhuan"), the title of which plays on the martial arts novelist Jin Yong's *Legend of the Condor Heroes*, adding another layer of local intertextual humor. The emphasis of this mahjong playing is clearly less on gambling to win than gambling to socialize—to generate what Desmond Lam calls "social heat," the "liveliness, warmth, and noisiness of social gathering" reminiscent of a "Chinese celebrative event."[84] And, sure enough, this scene is followed by another in which Sean Lau sings a fourth Sam Hui song, the New Year jingle "Here Comes the God of Wealth" ("Coi san dou"/"Caishen dao"). As with many Hong Kong gambling-themed movies, there is an implication that a person's reversal of fortune can be mysteriously routed through the gambling table, and that gamblers are united by a faith in some folk deity or cosmic force that ensures the continual circulation of fortune. But more than mere superstition, the short invokes the god of wealth via mahjong as a highly localizing gesture, a rallying cry for Hong Kongers to remember amid the epidemic those everyday folk beliefs and communal rituals, that element of luck and magic, that stitch together the fabric of the city's social life.

Within *Project 1:99*, Stephen Chow's "Hong Kong Will Sure Win" is perhaps the most direct heir to Michael Hui's comic cinema. This short opens with a middle-aged woman (played by Yuen Qiu) lying in a hospital bed and video chatting with her daughter (played by Jenny Yip). The mood is somber, the mother's face is wan, her voice weak, and the daughter looks close to tears. The camera then cuts to the father (played by David Hung Wai-to), who takes off his glasses and massages his eyes tiredly with the back of his hand. "I don't worry about your dad," murmurs the mother. "I worry most about your older brother." The camera cuts to the brother (played by Wu Fan), who is seen coughing violently into his mask, then taking a sip of water only to spew it back out as he hacks away. "Mom," the daughter wails, "I really can't do this without you here!" "What's there to be afraid of?" answers the mother, her voice a bit stronger. "We won't lose." At this titular phrase, as if by magical incantation, the mood reverses. The daughter yells, "Okay, you said so!" as the camera pans out to reveal a family living room and an ongoing mahjong game. The daughter discards a tile, at which her brother gleefully barks, "Pong!" and guffaws at his winning hand. "I told you I didn't know how to play!" whines the daughter, as the mahjong players disband for the night. "Jesus, your brother threw out a six of circles," the mother says in self-defense over the video screen. "How did I know he'd be so sneaky as to bait you for a three of circles?"

The building up of tragic suspense and its swift deflation, the surprising last-minute overturning of atmosphere and plot, the self-ironic spoof on inflated emotions and rhetoric quickly undercut by Cantonese colloquial dialogue for anticlimactic bathos—these are all signature Stephen Chow directorial techniques. In Hong Kong's gambling films, the gambling motif often juxtaposes seemingly opposite categories: not just victory and loss but also expertise and amateurishness, luck and calculation, usurpation and restoration, extinction and resurrection. Fittingly, Chow makes this genre central to his staging of SARS, constellating seemingly oppositional paradigms and affects: crisis and ordinariness, epidemic catastrophe and daily familial life, debilitation and activity, illness and play, tragedy and camp. His short spatializes these juxtapositions by alternating between hospital room and living room, sickbed and mahjong table. But rather than blurring the line between these spaces to intimate the expansion of a state of exception, the weight here falls on the persistence of the mundane, the playful, the droll. If there is expansion, it is decidedly on the side of nonexceptional local life infiltrating and engulfing the zone of global disease emergency. In this magic theater, comedy and life are reciprocally animating; there is an inveterate faith in the power of humor and play to reawaken even the dead. The short's message toys with a classic local self-image: that Hong Kongers will come back from the grave just to play a game of mahjong.

Games Gamblers Play arguably inaugurated this comedic self-image for contemporary Hong Kong cinema. Hui's political satire, though, was overtly Marxist, as he tied gambling not to middle-class leisure and domestic play but to the capitalist colony's entrapment of its underclass men, with apparatuses of gambling promising fast affluence but actually functioning to exploit and contain these men's excess energy and desires. Yet what the movie offered pre–golden era Hong Kong audiences was not just an intellectual critique from up high but a set of cultural aesthetics from below, a popular cinema and music style accessible to and derived from the vernaculars of the working masses, epitomized by Sam Hui's title theme song. To outsiders and in translation, this song's chorus may sound trite, but its distinct power lies in its groundbreaking use of idiomatic gutter Cantonese to convey a gut-level sentiment to and for local speakers:

> Life is like gambling: [*jan sang jyu dou bok*]
> there's no telling about winning or losing. [*jeng syu dou mou si ding*]
> If you win, you only get a good laugh, [*jeng zo dak caan siu*]
> but if you lose everything, you don't have to get worked up either!
> [*syu gwong m sai hing*][85]

Chow's oeuvre at large builds on the Huis' prototype. His films also invariably feature a little-guy protagonist, also often played by himself, with the dramatic tension shaped by this character's rise and fall in fortune as he learns moral lessons along the way. Beyond gamblers and cheaters, thieves and petty criminals, his films are frequently populated by beggars and refugees as well as fallen gods and masters, not just the rascals and nobodies of the post/colony but also its moral sinners in need of karmic redemption. Especially salient in his films is a fascination with the self-debasement of a rock-bottom underdog figure: what lengths he would go to in order to survive, how much of his conscience he would compromise in order to claw his way out of the pits, and how much dignity he would cede to those in power until he finally draws the line and strikes back. Chow's films often wallow in the spectacle of public humiliation as well as the reckoning of private shame, both of which constitute the psychic and emotional price of living the life of the earth's unresigned wretched. Beneath their wounded masculinity is an undercurrent of male aggression and rage that finds an outlet in the frenzy of pastiche and camp. This comic vitality prevents his protagonists from devolving into permanent depression and collapse, but it also prevents them from mounting into the righteous anger of revolutionary politics or fully transcending into spiritual bliss. If global critics habitually label his style *mo lei tau*, or "brainless nonsense," Chow himself professed early on not to understand the meaning of this term. In a 1993 TVB talk show interview with Wong Jim, Chow pointedly embedded his comic mode within a longer and more eclectic local lineage, one extending from the Cantonese opera performer and pioneer TVB actor Leung Sing-bor to Wong Jim himself, who was not just a prolific Cantopop lyricist but a widely respected comedic host. And Michael Hui, Chow remarked, was certainly someone he studied and emulated, as a "creative target and partner."[86] It is also within this descent line of Cantonese social comedy that we can situate the irreverent approach to SARS taken by both *City of SARS* and *Golden Chicken 2*.

Self-Extinction Farce in *City of SARS*

City of SARS was Hong Kong's first full-length feature on SARS, its very existence exemplifying "Hong Kong's resilience": the movie was shot in just fifteen days during May 2003, on a tiny budget of HK$5 million. As the Hong Kong–based journalist Tom Hilditch put it at the time, "The city is not just beating SARS but turning it into entertainment," going from "panic to popcorn in 90 days."[87] Despite its low production value, the production team did not regard the film as a mere commercial flick. The scriptwriter Edmond Wong Chi-woon confessed that he wrote and rewrote the script as he went along, its ending as uncertain to him as the epidemic's outcome for the city. Rather than the formulaic Hollywood virus movie, this, he said, was more akin to "a war movie crossed with reality TV," but one fraught with "a tremendous sense of responsibility."[88]

Unlike *Project 1:99*, *City of SARS* consists of a crew and cast Hilditch calls "mostly B-list," and its director, Steve Cheng Wai-man, is associated mainly with lowbrow genre flicks.[89] Yet, for local audiences that summer, easy viewing fit the bill. The actors were all familiar faces in their own right from local television, hence all the more down-to-earth and relatable as fellow citizens weathering the same predicament. The three-part anthology

136   CHAPTER 3

format catered to a range of tastes, with each segment marshaling conventions from popular television serials: hospital medical drama in the first, adolescent romance in the second, and social comedy in the third. The generic plotlines and stock characters did not challenge audiences' values and beliefs but inspired a comforting sense of genre familiarity amid SARS. By multiplying recognizable actors and tropes drawn from local entertainment, the movie established a pandemic ordinariness effect very specific to Hong Kong in that moment. And in the tradition of local social comedy films, the last segment revels in the incongruous yoking of an epidemic crisis to a cinema of bad taste, packing to the hilt puerile, over-the-top, scatological, and sick gallows humor, in a protracted SARS extinction farce.

At the segment's start, Hung—played by Eric Tsang—is a former street peddler turned lottery winner turned small-business magnate who now owns a chain of restaurants, karaoke clubs, movie theaters, and travel agencies. He is a caricature of the opportunistic and vulgar small-time bossman, and, when SARS hits the city, he loses no time in announcing to his business partners and lackeys that he will profit from the virus by opening a funeral home, as he chortles away maniacally at his own ingenuity. Techniques of slapstick and vaudeville heighten the satire of disaster capitalism: actors assume cartoonishly exaggerated facial expressions and body postures to signal their character types, fast-paced cheeky dialogues magnify moral foibles, and skewed camera angles and disjointedly upbeat background music convey the sense of a madcap circus world. In one scene, Hung gets a phone call from a distant aunt (the mother of the teenage protagonist in the middle segment), and, when she tells him her son has been taken ill with SARS, he replies with sincere gusto: "Many congratulations to you then! One less pair of chopsticks and one fewer mouth to feed. You know how expensive college is; now you get to save that expense. Besides, it's a popular trend these days: when someone in the family gets SARS, the whole family benefits because the government pays you compensation money." Hung speaks according to the logic of the marketplace, and, to him, SARS has its ready translation in the language of Hong Kong dollars.

As the outbreak intensifies and people begin to avoid public spaces, Hung's various businesses, all part of the city's entertainment and service industries, are dealt a devastating blow and he sinks into exorbitant debt. By his assistant's calculations, even if he sells all his assets, he would still owe the banks and loan sharks $15 million. This is the point at which the story combines social satire with family melodrama, as brotherly love comes to the fore. Though mercenary and unscrupulous, Hung is far from heartless. He is devoted to his younger sister (played by Sharon Chan Man-chi), the only family he has left and whom he has raised like his own child. To shield her from the consequences of his financial ruin, Hung decides to commit suicide instead of declaring bankruptcy, hoping she can live off the payout from his life insurance policy. From poor peddler to prosperous businessman to desperate debtor, Hung perfectly fits the mold of the comic little guy and fallen antihero, having risen in life through the random chance of a lottery ticket and now plummeting again in fortune due to the collateral effects of a global pandemic. In this vein, his suicide attempts take on the quality of a series of gambles, contingent on the mysterious and impish workings of fate. However zealously he throws himself into self-destruction, he is repeatedly thwarted, not by anyone's intentional interference but by sheer bad/good luck. Though wrapped in morbid humor, this theme of unattainable extinction translates to a deextinctionist fantasy that Hong Kongers will never be entirely wiped out, not even in a pandemic, and not even if they actively work toward it.

First, Hung directs his assistant (played by Jerry Lamb Hiu-fung) to compile a list of reliable suicide methods. His assistant complies with macabre glee, consulting a how-to manual and ranking each method on a five-point scale of success rate and degree of suffering, reveling in the gruesome details of each death as he describes them to Hung. Despite these meticulous computations, Hung encounters snags at every step. His first attempt is to jump off a high-rise (with silent echoes of Leslie Cheung's death). "According to this book," the assistant informs him, as they stand on the rooftop of a skyscraper, "this approach to suicide has four points for fatality and only one point for pain. It's one of those that come highly recommended. . . . And Boss, you've chosen the right venue. The most important factors are that you're at least twenty meters up with nothing around you, that the ground surface is hard, and that there're no trees, cars, or people in the way. Why? Because if you land on someone, you'd have to pay them compensation, and then all your insurance money will go not to your sister but to them." When Hung asks about the best body position to take, the assistant answers cheerfully, "Boss, the safest bet is to land head first. Then your head will explode and you won't see a thing. But if you land feet first, your leg bones will jut up through your body, and that will be quite ugly and disgusting." As Hung approaches the building's edge and prepares to jump, the assistant hurriedly reminds Hung that he has not been paid his final wages. Hung takes a check out of his suit jacket pocket and hands it to the assistant, noting that he has included a bonus. "Can you do me one more favor and push me over?" Hung asks glumly, to which the assistant yelps a quick "Sure!" and eagerly shoves Hung with one hand while turning away grinning at his check. The camera then swerves to show Hung landing with a thud on a platform a few feet below. "Damn you!" he screams. "I wasn't even done talking and you already pushed me! Get down here now and help me up!"

Hung's next attempt involves carbon monoxide poisoning by charcoal burning. "According to my research," resumes the unflappable assistant, "the pain level here is only three. And as long as you set everything up just right, and no one interrupts you, and you don't fail, your success rate is pretty high too." In ritual preparation, Hung paints his cheeks and lips bright red. The camera's close-up of his face draws attention to his paradoxical embodiment of the cadaver clown, suspended between laughter and death. But then his assistant returns with news that all the stores are sold out of charcoal because it happens to be Easter, a popular day for barbeques in the suburbs. "No need to be disappointed, though," he reassures Hung jovially. "Surveys show that apparently 85 percent of coal-burning suicide attempts fail. Due to oxygen deprivation in the brain, people end up as human vegetables in the hospital, needing care from others. That'd affect your sister. What's more, if you lie there all day, the flesh on your back would start to decay and bleed and get infected with maggots, which would affect the hospital workers. The corners of your mouth would rot, and since you won't be brushing your teeth, they would stink. If your girlfriend doesn't visit or look after you, you'd be harming yourself too. And another thing: since you won't be able to relieve yourself, when you piss and shit, I'd have to buy you diapers, and that would affect me . . ." The dark comedy of this scene is reminiscent of the class critique in Michael Hui's films but delivered in Stephen Chow's trademark style of extravagantly coldhearted humor. The assistant's suicide data, though callously and garishly narrated, in fact spotlight the endemic problem of economic suicide in nonepidemic times. So, while not a social protest film by any stretch, this story line situates Hung's SARS-era predicament within a socioeconomic and psychological precarity faced by many superficially secure middle-class Hong Kongers.

Having exhausted the common avenues for suicide, the assistant finally suggests to Hung that he try contracting SARS. This timely method, the assistant argues, has the additional advantage of procuring government reparation money for Hung's sister, and it can even propel Hung into media stardom. Exhilarated by the idea, Hung launches into a quest for contagion. In the elevator of his apartment building, he takes his first stab at self-infection. The elevator is packed with masked residents, so Hung enthusiastically offers to punch the floor buttons for everyone. He rips off the plastic cover from the keypad and rubs a bare hand over the panel several times. "What, scared?" he asks the other passengers merrily. "Oy! We're Hong Kongers. We have to have confidence in Hong Kong. See—" He smears his contaminated fingers across his eyes, nose, and mouth. "—I'm fine! No problem!" He then makes a monster face, spreading both hands up in a mock growl, playfully threatening a violent sneeze as he pivots to face the recoiling crowd around him. In SARS iconography, the elevator is often depicted as a zone of heightened epidemic danger, a spatial synecdoche for the overpopulated global city and an urban microcosm for contagion. This scene effectively recodes the fear-charged space of the urban elevator by turning it into a site of farcical laughter, the comic hyperbole for one man's death-seeking mission.

The next plot sequence resignifies an even more iconic space of infectious disease peril: the SARS hospital. Departing from the biopolitical and sentimental paradigms in Hu Fayun's and Chen Baozhen's novels (and in the movie's own first segment), the last segment here saturates the SARS hospital with a frivolous gallows humor. Watching the news on television, Hung learns that another four local frontline medical workers have been diagnosed with SARS, suspected to have contracted the virus through close contact with infected patients. Hung's face lights up as he devises his next plan for self-infection. He marches into a SARS hospital but is stopped in the hallway by two staff members garbed in protective gear. When asked to name the patient he is visiting, he rattles off a string of random names before offering, with exasperation, that of superstar Andy Lau. The staff escort him out and threaten to call security. Outside, Hung makes several calls on his cell phone, hoping to find an acquaintance with a SARS-infected relative but is hung up on by everyone. Remembering the aunt who had called him earlier, he quickly dials her number to gather intel on his cousin. Thus armed, Hung smugly marches back into the hospital. He is stopped again by the staff, but, this time, they inform him that his cousin is in SARS isolation and cannot receive any visitors except medical personnel. "To be quite honest, I, too, studied medicine," he improvises. "I'm a veterinarian!" He is escorted out again. On his third try, Hung disguises himself as a physician, donning a face shield and lab coat, and, this time, he successfully infiltrates a private sickroom in the isolation ward. He vigorously inhales what he imagines to be tainted air and, just for good measure, sucks from the mouth of a bedridden patient. A nurse surprises him from behind and tells him that the patient has just died, that they are in the middle of wrapping up the body. At this, Hung faints dramatically, cartoon-style, as the film relishes its own over-the-top silliness. SARS and illness, death and suicide are stripped of all gravitas, all aura of the sacred, as the dead and the living are literally made to kiss. Extinctionist farce turns the SARS hospital into a stage for the little-guy's self-martyring antics.

Bad body fluid humor as a device for overturning contagion fears is mustered with even more carnival energy in Hung's final suicide attempt. Still not feeling sick, he is driven to extreme desperation, and, in the tradition of Stephen Chow's rock-bottom underdog antiheroes, he literally sinks into the gutters to achieve his goal. At a chance remark by his sister, Hung decides to contract SARS by swallowing contaminated sewage from the Amoy Gardens housing complex. While it was common knowledge at the time that SARS was transmitted through respiratory droplets, the Amoy Gardens outbreak initially presented an epidemiological mystery, as there were no clearly identifiable transmission vectors. Eventually, it was discovered that virus-laden feces had been aerosolized into the bathrooms of individual apartment units through an obsolete drainage system, exacerbated by a cracked sewer vent pipe and "poor hygiene and pest infestations."[90] By pedagogically including some of these epidemiological facts, the film demonstrates its sense of social responsibility in educating the public and demystifying that outbreak. Moreover, by spotlighting the substandard environment of this one lower-middle-income housing complex, the film registers the socioeconomic inequalities within everyday public health. In this scene, as Hung approaches the light well of one of the evacuated blocks, the camera makes a point of pausing on the corroded sewage pipes, leaky building walls, and garbage-strewn floor. Instead of showcasing Amoy Gardens as the terrifying site of invisible but lethal viral particles, the camera focuses on surfaces, on a plainly and grossly visible view of a housing estate in disrepair and neglect, alluding to the precarity of Hong Kongers who live in these housing projects. Though not among the city's most poor and squalid, this lower-middle population is nonetheless made vulnerable to environmental hazards from the shoddy infrastructure of their residences, and they can be uprooted en masse and expelled at one stroke if they become a possible source of contagion. Hung metaphorically descends into this class when he squats down to scoop up a cupful of dirty water from the ground. His readiness to consume this sewage reminds us that he came from the social gutters to begin with, in the film's subtle nod to the cycle of fortune/misfortune guiding his life and other little guys like him. It is in this near final moment of gritty resolve that Hung's sister and her boyfriend (played by Chin Kar-lok) arrive on the scene and rush to his side, but not before Hung hastily gulps down the drainage water.

A half-fairytale ending is engineered when the sister's boyfriend reveals that he is actually the heir to a now booming face mask and medical equipment factory and can cover Hung's debts. Financial doom is averted, and Hung bestows his blessings on the young couple. Yet in this very instant, he starts to feel feverish. In the ambiguous coda, Hung is shown on local news as Hong Kong's last SARS patient. He has successfully infected himself after all, but, having also ingested large doses of herbal medicine, fed to him by his ever-conscientious sister, he fluctuates between recovery and relapse, hospitalized until the end. Hung's indeterminate fate reflects the epidemic's uncertain future during the film's actual shooting, and, as a result, *City of SARS* as a whole ends on an ambivalent note of completed disaster but ongoing affliction, suspended between normality and crisis. Unlike Hollywood pandemic movies such as Steven Soderbergh's much-cited *Contagion*, there is neither worldwide collapse nor a world-saving antidote. Rather than the gambler being punished with horrendous viral death for fraternizing with Asian bodies à la Gwyneth Paltrow's character in that film, Hung continues to hang on. His every suicide attempt has been like a toss of the dice or a pull of the slot machine, and his every gamble for death begins from and returns to zero, with no ultimate accumulation or loss of fortune. If there is no decisive resurrection, there is no permanent extinction either.

It would take another few months, until after SARS had been declared over globally, before Hong Kong's entertainment industry would return to this template of extinction farce in another full-length feature. This time, the telos toward deextinction will be much more assured, and much more overtly self-referential and allegorical.

Deextincting the Golden Age
in *Golden Chicken 1* and *2*

Promoting *Golden Chicken 2* for its Christmas release, the screenwriter James Yuen Sai-sang recalled at year's end: "2003 had a lot of things happen that nobody expected. We Hong Kongers felt this year deserves something that would tell the stories of Hong Kong." Chapman To, who had parts in both the original *Golden Chicken* and its sequel, called 2003 "a year worth recording." Peter Chan, the films' producer, likewise told prospective audiences, "I think this year is one you'd be most unlikely to forget. I wanted to capture those feelings, those sensations. . . . If Hong Kongers understand this movie, we'll be happy." Sandra Ng, the lead in both films, echoed these sentiments, describing 2003 as much as *Golden Chicken 2* as *"fung wui lou zyun,"* full of twists and turns where every winding of the road brings new surprises. "I really want to experience this year again," she said.[91] To narrate local stories, to document a momentous year, to preserve its sensory memories for fellow citizens, and to make relivable that which had just passed in all its bittersweetness and silly joy—these were the impulses that animated the last SARS film of 2003 Hong Kong.

Unlike the anthology format of *Project 1:99* and *City of SARS*, *Golden Chicken 2* centers on one main character: Kum Yu, nicknamed Ah Kum, a prostitute with the proverbial heart of gold and a larger-than-life ebullient spirit. On the surface, a bawdy comedy about a sex worker with an upbeat personality may seem a tasteless choice for allegorizing Hong Kong as the global epicenter of a pandemic. But Ng had played Kum in *Golden Chicken* the year before and won a Golden Horse Award for Best Actress for the role, and the movie had been a surprise hit at the home box office. Peter Chan calls it "something that truly belongs to Hong Kong," a film focused on the city's contemporary past and a genre that he "had not seen in a long time."[92] Kum's persona, moreover, resonated strongly with a Cantophone sensibility, so it seemed a fitting vehicle to reprise for telling local stories around SARS. As one online reviewer aptly puts it, "Ah Kum is an all too ordinary nobody," a small-timer always struggling against the odds and yet always managing to stay afloat.[93] "Ah Kum is not pretty, she's an underdog, and Kwan-yu is most fun to watch when she plays underdogs," remarks Chan in the promotional featurette. Aside from being an acclaimed director and producer, Chan is also well-known to locals as Ng's real-life longtime partner, in one of the many insider relationships of the two films. "Ah Kum is a very optimistic and happy-go-lucky person, the type that, as the saying goes, 'if the sky falls down she'll use it as a coverlet.' So, along the way, she doesn't know to be afraid, doesn't know what it means to fail."[94] And when she does fail, she is not afraid to start over again, and again, and again. By the early 2000s, Ng had played dozens of comparable stock characters in supporting roles, and she projected the same temperament off-screen, so it was well-trodden and comfortingly familiar acting ground both for her and for local viewers.

PANDEMIC RESILIENCE   **143**

If Hong Kong has an iconic little guy in female form, a second-tier actress who embodies the image of being all too mediocre, lacking the grand pathos of tragedy yet seeming eternally resilient and never truly beaten down, Ng was it. During a citywide crisis, Ng qua Kum served only too well as a beacon for local viewers. Even Kum Yu's name is meant to be a near homonym of Ng's (Kwan-yu), and Ng's Golden Horse win for the role the year before only boosted her patina of underdog triumph.

Even more than *Project 1:99* and *City of SARS*, the 2002–3 *Golden Chicken* franchise taps into the social comedy genre that reanimated Cantonese cinema. Like Michael Hui's films, the two *Golden Chicken*s zero in on Kum as an underclass protagonist caught in the whirlwind of social change, from late-1970s to early-2000s Hong Kong, in effect giving the genre an afterlife into the present. Unlike New Wave cinema's social realism—which prompts audiences to suspend disbelief and ignore the star quality of celebrities playing ordinary people—local social comedies tend to invert the hyperreal principle, so that simulacra reaffirm rather than dislodge the sense of a shared communal reality. With both *Golden Chicken*s, where the veil between script and life, diegetic milieu and extradiegetic present, remains teasingly thin by design, audiences are interpellated as accomplices in a shared fictional romp. The sequel pointedly borrows this local style to reconstruct the density of just-lived epidemic life, even if the stylistic choice may strike remote viewers as inappropriate or trashy.

To be sure, neither *Golden Chicken* is radically progressive in its gender and class politics. As Vivian Lee rightly points out, the films contain "an underlying elitist romanticism in the portrayal of the lower class . . . [and] Kum's image as a 'happy prostitute' glosses over the harsher realities not only of women in her profession but also the social class she comes to represent."[95] Indeed, the films are not centrally concerned with gender oppression per se, leveraging Kum as an allegory of mostly male abjection, evincing a sexism that runs deep in the Hong Kong entertainment industry. While the plotlines do not entirely ignore the exploitative economy around women's bodies, the impetus is not to agitate for social reform but to give a nonexceptionalized portrait of female sex work, as no more and no less degrading or undignified than other modalities of underclass life in the city. But by the same token, the films meaningfully expand the cinematic genre codes available for narrativizing female sex work by eschewing moralizing formulas. Kum is a woman in her forties and a career prostitute who enjoys her work, treating it as well as herself with professional respect. Her character thus facilitates what some local grassroots groups have long been advocating for: dismantling societal stereotypes around the sex industry, destigmatizing sex work, and cultivating greater understanding about sex workers' diverse experiences. "For many people, sex workers are always either single, poor mothers or women from the mainland who have divorced their Hong Kong partners because of marriage problems. Of course, these cases do exist—but they are not the only ones," comments the director of one advocacy group. "We have women who do sex work because they enjoy it, or because they think it's a way of contributing to society. It's not necessarily either a situation of dependence versus full agency. There is a broader spectrum than that."[96]

The *Golden Chicken* films highlight exactly this sense of professional ownership and agency. Kum is not cloaked in self-sacrificing tragedy or victimhood; she is an agent of humor, someone who sets the terms of laughter and sustains its energy, not the mere target or excluded object of it. This is a key departure from the social comedies of the Hui brothers and of Stephen Chow, where the central drama and tragicomic gravitas almost always revolve around male buddies or else a rogue hero wallowing in his own self-debasement, while women orbit them as ornamental objects of lust and conquest. Within this tradition, Kum presents a significant regendering: she is a sex worker who works for her own ends, not to support an impoverished family or love interest, not to satiate vanity or greed but simply because it is her job and it gives her a decent livelihood and a modicum of pleasure. Her story does not need to be legitimized by heterosexual romance, familial redemption, or an ultimate return to the folds of patriarchal kinship. Instead, she constitutes her own telos.

What the films reflect at their core, though, is the local popular media industry's posthandover grappling with the dissolution of its subempire. As Vivian Lee notes, the "elitist projection of the local" onto Kum as underclass "hero and emblem" can be attributed to the privileged status of the films' production crew, which "consists of members of the cultural elite who left the territory in the late 1990s and relocated back to Hong Kong afterwards to continue filmmaking." Both *Golden Chicken*s, therefore, "bear the imprint of the disillusionment and cynicism of the elite towards the new political realities of the excolony."[97] Most salient in this regard is Peter Chan. Right before the handover, Chan left Hong Kong and worked in Hollywood for three years, but he returned in 2000 to found Applause Pictures, a company dedicated to producing "pan-Asian films" with collaborations across Hong Kong, Thailand, Singapore, South Korea, and Japan.[98] He initially resisted tailoring his films to a strictly mainland market, but, like many other Hong Kong directors since the mid-2000s, he has increasingly "shifted his attention to projects with mainland appeal" and eventually advised other filmmakers to forego aesthetic localism.[99] His short for *Project 1:99*, "Memories of Spring 2003," already registers these ambivalences, depicting SARS-stricken Hong Kong as a surreal city in what John Nguyet Erni calls "double take," split between a haunting emptiness and disappearance, on the one hand, and the displacement effect of "urban deterritorialization" and "delta-fication," on the other.[100] In retrospect, the two *Golden Chicken*s represent a kind of last hurrah to thick localism in Chan's oeuvre, with SARS as his farewell event. All the more so then do the films illuminate what SARS brought to a head: the Hong Kong Cantophone's subimperial extinction consciousness.

Yet it is exactly from this extinctionism that a proliferation of deextinction tales and tropes emerged, encapsulating a hopefulness about the filmic medium's potential to remember and thereby reanimate the Cantophone world. To grasp this aspect of *Golden Chicken 2* in relation to SARS, we must focus on both films' formal elements—their idioms and vernaculars, intertextual quotations and allusions, and recyclings of local popular culture's images and sounds. Linda Lai calls this practice "enigmatization": "the selection and reorganization of existing images from popular culture in order to distinctly select the local audience as a privileged hermeneutic community, thus facilitating a state of internal dialogue, distinguishing those within from the 'outsiders' by marking who partakes in a shared history of popular culture."[101] With the onset of SARS, enigmatization went into overdrive. The first *Golden Chicken* had already been an apotheosis of the enigmatization aesthetic: marshaling copious markers of local history and popular culture, it had aimed precisely to reconstitute, sustain, and prolong a unique sense of Hong Kong identity for local audiences as they wrestled with this cultural world's disintegration. The first film's parable of Hong Kong's continued survival and limitless adaptability—through Kum as a special species with absolutely dogged staying power—became profoundly resonant during SARS. *Golden Chicken 2* thus returned with an intensified enigmatization, as the tools of its predecessor got revived and amplified. But to make this vision legible, we must first learn to read its enigmas.

Localism and Vernacular

Very much a bildungsroman, the first *Golden Chicken* covers a quarter century of Kum's life, from fifteen to forty, as she matures in tandem with Hong Kong. Like its sequel, the film is an exemplary Cantophone work, chock-full of local slang and period references, with much of the script relying on Hong Kong Cantonese idioms for its operative vocabulary, puns, and metaphors. The crew also took pains to replicate the decorative details, costume changes, and media environment of each era. Toward the film's opening, Kum is presented in flashback as a lower-class teenager in late-1970s Hong Kong, when she first entered the sex trade as a "fishball girl" (*jyu daan mui*) in one of the so-called neighborhood "fishball stalls" (*jyu daan dong*), dimly lit dives where male customers groped underage girls in semidarkness while being given handjobs by them, the girls' hand motion mimicking the kneading of fishballs from dough. This terminology is distinctively Hong Kong. Kum Yu's very name, pronounced *gam jyu* in Cantonese, puns on "goldfish" (*gam jyu*), and this dialect-specific pun conjures up for locals the phrase "goldfish guy" (*gam jyu lou*), a uniquely homegrown term for pedophiles that has no equivalent in other Chinese dialects, derived from a notorious 1968 case in which a local serial child molester baited young girls with promises of taking them to look at goldfish.[102] Right from the outset, then, the film underscores the locatedness of Kum's story, the tight knotting of person to place, and the linguistic nonsubstitutability of Cantonese in memorializing local life—in short, all the nontransportable elements of Kum's existence and milieu.

At this early point, Kum was still in pigtails and wore nerdy oversized glasses, shuttling from school to work every day in her sailor-dress school uniform. She was the happy-go-lucky type, delighted to earn a few bucks and completely unperturbed by the sordid nature of her work. When she began to lose her eyesight from the fishball shop's poor lighting, she switched jobs and became a nightclub "dance girl" (*mou neoi*), euphemistically called a "miss" (*siu ze*). She was eighteen and the year was 1980. "This was the golden era of Hong Kong," Chan explains in the movie's featurette. "When Hong Kong's economy was at its zenith, a beautiful nightclub miss could make over $100,000 a month. Under these circumstances, even a Plain Jane like Ah Kum could rely on her goofy antics and take little shortcuts, like faking kungfu moves for clients' amusement, to make about $60,000 to $70,000 a month. In that time of splendor, even if you were just a second-liner, you could still make a lot of money."[103] These nightclubs are obsolete now, but, in their heyday in the eighties, they were the favorite playground of the city's nouveaux riches. Patrons willing to pay were fawned over by armfuls of young women and treated like royalty, "driven to their private booth in golf carts kitted out as gold Rolls-Royces."[104] Kum landed at one of the ritziest of these establishments, Club BBoss, once "a Tsim Sha Tsui landmark, a 70,000 sq. ft. nightclub-cum-amusement park for men that boasted bright lights, lavish floor shows and more than 1000 perfectly coiffed hostesses."[105] It was a competitive time for the women who worked there. Topline misses— "with the faces of angels and the bodies of devils," as Kum says dryly in voiceover—were frequently fought over and "contracted," or *baau* in local slang, as the exclusive goods of wealthy men. Ambitious misses could make extra cash on the side by cajoling clients into paying for luxury merchandise that "they had their eye on," or *tai zung* in local slang. Kum, with neither extraordinary looks nor smarts, nonetheless assimilated quickly and found her niche. The pigtails and pink scrunchies gave way to a fashionable bob perm, the plastic glasses and school uniform to a glittery gold dress with cleavage. She had no patron to *baau* her, no customer to fight over her, not even a seat at the booth to accommodate her, but, even so, she could resort to performing Jackie Chan–style drunken fist—his *Drunken Master* had been a huge local hit a few years back and played on the club's screens, in one of the movie's many enigmatization gestures—to keep clients entertained and create at least a standing spot for herself in the private room.

In one telling scene, Kimmy (played by Tiffany Lee Lung-yee), the club's premier miss, rode on a ballroom golf cart with a client and counted her wad of cash after successfully coaxing him into buying her "a little handbag." Meanwhile, Kum ran alongside behind the cart, out of breath but characteristically jovial, declaring that she, too, "had her eye on a red-white-blue bag." These cheap but utilitarian nylon canvas bags used to be ubiquitous as border-crossing luggage among Hong Kong's working-class poor in the eighties, after the mainland opened its border, so Kum's reference was a period- as well as place-specific joke, one that insinuated her own worth as inexpensive but hardy ware. Delivered with her usual broad smile and a self-deprecating drollness that did not embarrass or guilt-trip, Kum's facetious line subtly signaled to the client that she knew her place at the bottom of the nightclub hierarchy and would gladly settle for whatever scraps he was generous enough to throw her way. For this little burst of humor, and for her tactful and unrelenting effort, she was rewarded with a few bills, which she gratefully lapped up. In this atmosphere of extravagant high life, so long as she never deemed it beneath her dignity to play the clown, to run after the pack, to stoop and pick up spare change tossed over the shoulder, Kum could make a decent living—*wan dou sik* in local slang, a mantra she chanted to herself as she gleefully jumped up and down on her first "big bed" (queen-size) in her first "big house" (a one-bedroom flat of her own). Her income came from these petty survival techniques and this tenacious work ethic as much as actual sexual labor, for in this high-rolling milieu, the economy of sex trickled down to her only with the stingiest of patrons. In this manner, she weathered economic and political storms, as footage of the 1987 stock market crash and the 1989 Tiananmen movement flashes across the screen and in the backdrop.

The sociopolitical world that enabled this arrangement was uprooted in the early nineties, and, again, Kum's fortune was interwoven with Hong Kong's, refracted through the lives of the local misses. "The nineties had three important inventions that affected us in a huge way," Kum narrates in voiceover. "The first was the mobile phone. The second was karaoke. The third 'invention,' which had the biggest impact of all on us, was those girls who migrated from the north, who came to be known as 'that piece of northern chick' [*gor gin bak gu*]." In common Chinese slang, "chicken" (*gai*) is a colloquialism for prostitutes, as alluded to by the movie's title, but the largely derogatory term "northern chick" (*bak gu*) is a uniquely Hong Kong Cantonese invention, coined when thousands of mainland women flooded the city's nightclubs and sex market in the wake of Deng Xiaoping's 1992 southern tour. This moniker derives from a series of puns: "northern girls" (*bak fong gu noeng*) who join the sex trade and become "chickens" are named after the culinary dish "northern mushroom chicken" (*bak gu gai*) and shortened to *bak gu*, with *gu* equivocating on "mushroom" and "girl," the lewd implication being that both are edible commodities.[106] By this point in the film's timeline, some Hong Kong misses had managed to marry their patrons and immigrate abroad, but the ones who remained behind, even former top-tier girls such as Kimmy, found themselves increasingly sidelined by the newcomers. "Bad accents, big boobs, wrong makeup, and wrong style, but also hardworking in the extreme, and willing to do anything for money—these were the trademarks of the *bak gu*," Kum explains in voiceover, documenting this history from an industry insider's perspective. While the other local misses at Club BBoss strongly resented and at times publicly insulted their mainland colleagues, Kum alone tried to mediate. She silently recognized that, to some

PANDEMIC RESILIENCE   **149**

extent, she herself was a version of what the northern girls represented now, tolerated only because she was an underdog native rather than an underdog migrant. The key difference was that she had never been considered attractive or ruthless enough to be a true rival to the other women. So, even as she herself was gradually pushed out of the club by the northerners, she conceded empathetically with a sigh: "All of us just wanted to *wan sik*. How could one blame them? We Hong Kongers are so prim and delicate. How could we possibly go up against those *bak gu*?"

Through Kum's voice, the film captures a two-sided perception: at once sympathetically staging the plight of local female sex workers, whose livelihood lay at the mercy of geopolitics and translocal capital as much as masculine privilege, while also highlighting these women's sense of urban entitlement and prejudice against rural migrants. In this respect, the local nightclub misses also epitomized Hong Kong's subimperial attitude during the boom era. They saw their work as not just selling raw sex but maintaining a privileged bubble world of glamor, opulence, and refinement, and they saw themselves as cultured gatekeepers rather than oppressed subalterns. The line between the two might be thin, but self-image mattered, and it mattered all the more for the Hong Kong misses in the face of their more desperately wealth-seeking mainland counterparts. Even Kum, a hanger-on in this industry, realized that, in comparison to the *bak gu*, she had been "*san gui yuk gwai*," a precious princess and pampered regional elite, despite the shabbiness and squalor of her lowly place in this golden milieu. At twenty-nine, she was feeling old, too old to compete with the migrant women, yet not savvy enough to get promoted to a "mamasan" like her friend Madam (played by Kristal Tin Yui-nei). So she decided to switch jobs again and was hired as a "bone girl" (*gwat neoi*), after the local slang term for massage (*dap gwat*), at a massage parlor cum illegal sex den. Incidentally, the Cantonese word *dap*, denoting a gentle fist-hitting motion, has no pronunciation equivalent in Mandarin, evoking yet another instance of the uniquely Cantophone within the film's soundscape.

One scene in this next segment showcases again how local language evolved in response to the changing times, as Hong Kongers in Kum's ever-less-glitzy underworld industry strove to preserve a semblance of subimperial classiness in the early nineties. At the massage parlor, when one customer complained about the long wait in the "airport waiting room," Dragon (played by Chapman To), the former nightclub manager turned massage parlor supervisor, answered good-naturedly, "Well, the plane's *delayed* [in

150   CHAPTER 3

English]. How about this? In a bit, I'll *upgrade* [in English] you to a first-class private cabin." To another waiting customer, a bathrobed obese man sipping from a beer mug, he crooned, "Today I found a Skymaster Boeing 747 for your delectation." When the customer growled, "For real? Don't let me find out later that it's old and ugly," Dragon replied, "No way! We're a new airport, so of course everything's young and enormous." The customer then said enthusiastically, "I want to eat your flight set dinner, and I want it both cold and hot!" To which Dragon laughed with understanding: "'Ice fire' [in English]? Sure, just get yourself ready for the docking bay." Small scenes like this one suffuse the film. Eschewing exegesis, the script allows the audience to soak up the argot-rich dialogue in context. "Skymaster" (*hung zung baa wong*) and "Boeing" (*bo jam*) play on local slang for "big-breasted" (*bo baa*); the word used for "young" (*nyun*) is a vulgar way to refer to the tenderness of youthful female flesh; and "eating" (*sik*) is a long-standing code word for sex. In the airport conceit of this business, lower-class men could pretend to be high-flying jetsetters and fallen pimps could indulge this image of lavish consumption. Through Kum, viewers learn, too, that masturbation had a range of trade expressions, from "hitting the airplane" (*daa fei gei*) to "butchering a snake" (*tong se*) to "releasing fire" (*ceot fo*). This industry jargon intermingles with Cantonese-specific idioms such as *taan* for "enjoy," from the phrase *taan sai gaai* or "enjoying the world," whose denotation has no equivalence in Mandarin, where the written character means simply to sigh or exclaim. Even the peppering of one's speech with English words—such as "ice fire," for the American slang phrase "fire and ice" for temperature sex play—is a pointedly Hong Kongizing gesture, alluding to locals' habit of randomly dropping English words, sometimes gratuitously and incorrectly, into conversation in order to signal the speaker's post/colonial cosmopolitanism, linguistic hybridity, and creative panache, all wrapped in a tacky showiness.

The film's extended chronicle of Kum's life continually emphasizes these inseparable links between lived local history and a living, changing vernacular. "Chicken" may be general lingo for prostitutes across Chinese dialects, but the vicissitudes of Kum's story accentuate the inadequacy of that one word to encapsulate the myriad permutations of local sex work throughout the decades, much less the insider lexicons that gave these social microcosms meaning and texture, in all their flamboyance and seediness. From a "fishball girl" to a "nightclub miss" to a "bone girl," Kum's occupation as a "chicken" has many avatars. Taken together, her jobs mirror the highs and lows of Hong Kong, calling attention to the rise and fall of the city's various lifeworlds.

PANDEMIC RESILIENCE **151**

Once-pervasive formations such as the fishball shops and the dancehall night-clubs are all but extinct today, but their memory imprints live on in the film. Each phase of Kum's working life is rendered with so much nuance, each milieu and its sounds and sights reconstituted with so much specificity, that the thickness of lived experience seems impossible to transplant to another locale, another language.

Toward the movie's end, Kum's status changed again. After injuring her finger at the massage parlor and after her doctor friend accidentally botched the medical procedure, Kum had to quit the *dap gwat* business. Meanwhile, 1997 passed quietly in the background, with both the handover and the Asian financial crisis, and Kum was able to survive these watershed macro events unscathed. What devastated her personal savings at one stroke, though, was something that made only local headlines: the news in 2001 that the company Pacific Century CyberWorks owed billions in negative assets, leading to a plummet in its stock market price. The company's CEO, Richard Li Tzar-kai, was once touted as an entrepreneurial wunderkind during the dot-com bubble, a fitting heir to his "Superman" tycoon father Li Ka-shing, at the time the richest man not just in Hong Kong but in all of Asia. Richard Li was known for using flashy moves such as giant corporate takeovers to enhance his image as an audacious capitalist equal to his father, but the crashing of PCCW was so dramatic and so unexpected that it bankrupted many local small-time investors. It also brought to public light that the Hong Kong Stock Exchange had secretly altered its rules to accommodate the company and give Li favored treatment.[107] In spotlighting this incident as the concrete cause of Kum's bankruptcy, the film keeps its class critique squarely trained on the local oligarchy, insisting on the responsibility of home-based actors rather than remote ideologies or global forces in bloating local dreams and shattering local lives. In a brief vignette, the film integrates footage of an older woman confronting PCCW's board of shareholders during a news confer-ence, yelling at them accusingly: "Who knows how many hundred millions you guys have made in profit already? But the ones you swallow up are all the little shareholders like me. Do you think that's right?" In the next clip, Rich-ard Li is shown stuttering incoherently to the press, and Kum, as if captured in archival footage, angrily shouted at him and demanded her money back, as security guards dragged her away. By reduplicating just a few news media fragments and inserting them into Kum's plotline, the film cues local viewers in to a memory of the recent past, an episode that would carry very little reso-nance for nonlocal viewers. This is an exemplary moment of enigmatization, in which the film selects for historical materials "integral to the collective memory of the local people of Hong Kong but [that] are basically unknown to the 'outsider.'"[108] Without careful attention to this Hong Kong story, a viewer can easily impute Kum's misfortune to the wrong global history.

Despite her hitting rock bottom at this point, or *puk gaai* as she puts it in gutter Cantonese in voiceover, Kum was ultimately resurrected from the brink of extinction. Forced out of her nice flat into a rundown apartment, with all her belongings except her bed, now sawed in half, confiscated by the bankruptcy company, Kum glumly wandered the streets. In the long line of employment seekers outside the labor department office, she ran into a former customer, a bucktoothed math teacher who went by Professor Chan (played by Tony Leung Ka-fai). At her invitation, he followed her home, and, for old times' sake, they had sex. But afterward, the two haggled over the fee. "Back in the day," Kum grumbled, "when I was at the top of my game, I didn't even need to sleep with a client and still could earn a few thousand dollars." To this, Chan quickly retorted, in one of the film's most explicit thesis moments, "Back then?! Back then, I exerted 50 percent effort and got full payment! Back then I was referred to as Professor Chan, but now there's no one to call me even Teacher Chan! 'Back then' has been flushed down the toilet. Nowadays, there's no reaping without sowing, only working more to get more. Have you heard of the saying: work is hard, but it's still better than being idle? Wake up, Double Seven." Chan's rousing lecture here is replete with Cantophonisms. His made-up proverb, "work is hard, but it's still better than being idle" (*gung zok gaan naan, zung hou gwo jau jau haan haan*), plays on Cantonese slang and rhyme. More wittily, his phrase for "back then" (*gau si*) is an exact pun in Cantonese on "piece of shit" (*gau si*), paving the way for his toilet metaphor. Even his pet name for Kum, "Double Seven" (*maa cat*), recalls a bygone era of local vernacular practice when workers with on-call jobs would commonly refer to each other by their pager numbers, before mobile phones replaced beepers in the late nineties. None of these linguistic elements would work in other dialects or in other sinophone cities with a different vernacular history. They are pointedly summoned in this scene not just for communicative flavor but for their embodiment of an in-group local identity and memory, a sense of Hong Kong Cantophone community and history—even as, and precisely because, this identity faces increasing internal displacement in the posthandover period.

At heart, Chan's lesson was this: in the old days, Hong Kongers, even bottom-feeders like Kum and himself, were regional top dogs, reaping the overflowing fortunes of the city's miracle economy. But in the new millennium, they could no longer bank on subimperial privilege or consumer decadence, cheap tricks or easy money, for a living. Chan advised Kum to relinquish the past and start over. Through this speech, the film encourages locals to let go of a fixation on Hong Kong's golden age and find a way to move on in the new epoch. This does not necessarily entail forgetting one's previous life, just creative entrepreneurship with the skills and resources one already possesses. When Kum scoffed that she could reboot her career by selling pineapples out of her apartment, Chan solemnly proposed an alternative business model that would become Kum's new livelihood into the sequel: a one-woman brothel, popularly dubbed "one building one phoenix" (*jat lau jat fung*), with "one building" (*jat lau*) punning on another Cantonese slang phrase for "top-rate" (*jat lau*). According to Hong Kong crime ordinances, prostitution is not illegal per se, so long as a sexual transaction is not "organized," whether by human trafficking, sexual coercion, pimping, or public solicitation. In turn, a "vice establishment" is defined as a venue of sexual service with two or more employees, so "a lone sex worker who sells her body for money inside an apartment (one-woman brothel) is not technically committing any . . . offences."[109] When the city's nightclubs and dancehalls began to close in the late nineties during the posthandover crackdown, these one-woman operations sprang up to fill the market gap, offering low-cost and no-frills sex for low-income clients as well as flexible self-employment, with no middleman or mamasan cuts, for female sex workers. Here as elsewhere, the film does not explicate this terminology or elaborate on the legal context, taking for granted a baseline social knowledge among its audience. In the next scene, Kum is shown busily advertising her new business around town, paying for her photos and videos to be posted on prostitution websites and putting up flyers around her neighborhood. Thus commenced her final "chicken" avatar, at the age of forty, as a "phoenix sister" (*fung ze*)—the very point at which *Golden Chicken 2* would pick up when SARS broke out a few months later, in real time.

In the making-of featurette to *Golden Chicken*, both the director and producer tackle the question of Kum as an allegory for Hong Kong. Instead of allotting her the auxiliary role of vehicle to the city as tenor, they readily see her as a paragon and archetype—and her tale as a moral parable of subempire's deextinction. The two men's remarks emphasize the degree to which Kum's character is conceived as an aspirational model of species survival for posthandover Hong Kongers, a figure who refuses to disappear or go extinct,

154   CHAPTER 3

despite the repeated wrecking of her habitats and lifeworlds. From one job to the next, even as each incarnation's ecosystem fades away, Kum always manages to crawl out from under the rubble and rise again from the ashes. "By the end of the movie," Peter Chan notes, "that's when you have to consider genuine ability (*sat lik*). It's about today, now. In this day and age, the old attitude is not enough. The movie's not saying that the old attitude is bad, just that it's not enough. . . . We can't forever rely on the old methods of the past." The director Samson Chiu Leung-chun explains in similar terms: "The spirit of the golden chicken is this: the person who thinks of ways to change with the times will be happier than the person who feels forced to do so." As Chan sums up, "When you've done your 100%, your very utmost, then you're truly a 'golden chicken.' Or, if you're not a prostitute, then you're a golden human. Or a golden Hong Konger."[110]

For the filmmakers, that Kum never thinks it beneath her to compensate for her shortcomings with extra effort and a huge dose of clownishness, that she can pick herself back up after losing all her gains in adult life and start over in a tabooed profession in midlife, undefeated and full of zest, epitomizes this "golden chicken spirit." Her relentless tenacity and underdog resilience, her capacity to rebound from blows and calamities despite continual indignities, and her willingness to adapt to new epochs and transmute herself with cheerfulness rather than dread or resentment, these qualities constitute the film's pedagogical ideals for a populace that has weathered the same local history and confronted an overlapping local present. Kum's narrative is offered as a lesson to those subimperial postcolonials who think themselves too good for compromise, too weary for self-transformation, or too jaded for exertion. This moral tale evokes a cultural consciousness of disappearance along Abbas's argument, but, much more than that, Kum is meant to be a paragon of revitalization through dogged persistence. She may appear sui generis in the film, but, for the filmmakers, she models a broader esprit de corps.

One short scene toward the film's end exemplifies this sheer life force, with a return to the trope of indigenous luck practices. Having set up her new apartment as a one-woman brothel, Kum decided to celebrate opening day by blessing her business, modestly but like any other respectable venture, by setting off a token string of firecrackers in the hallway for good luck. In that instant, a neighbor, happening to walk by, yelled out sneeringly at her, channeling the voice of state authorities and the moral public, "Aunty, what are you doing? Lighting firecrackers? There's a fine! Don't mess around!" Kum thumbed her nose at the young man's retreating back, paused for a few seconds in thought, then mimed the action of lighting the firecrackers anyway. As she imitated the sounds of exploding firecrackers under her breath and hopped wildly around the corridor, as if she herself had been turned into a blazing sparkler, she mouthed defiantly after the by-then long-gone neighbor, "*Ceoi ah! Ceoi ah! Ceoi ah!*," a slang expression of annoyance that roughly translates to "blow me!" Fittingly for a film that permeates its telling of local history with Cantophone sounds, Kum's "golden chicken spirit" ends with a distinctly local curse, even if unheard by the other.

From Underdog Allegory to Underclass Assemblages

So far, I have discussed the ways *Golden Chicken* mobilizes and proliferates references to the local, particularly through language and vernacular, to reconstruct its vision of Hong Kong history and social life as nontransportable and inimitably Cantophone. These gestures paradoxically shore up both a consciousness of extinction, of local life's passing, and a fantasy of deextinction, of this life's regeneration—not least through the filmic medium itself and the collective acts of audience recognition and remembrance it mediates. By 2003 a repertoire of interlinked de/extinction motifs had become well-established in local popular media culture. Below, I analyze some of these motifs that run through both *Golden Chicken*s: bankruptcy, unemployment, suicide, spousal abandonment, amnesia, mental illness, and, finally, golden-era Cantopop. By observing how de/extinction concerns predate and persist beyond SARS, we can also see how *Golden Chicken 2* nonexceptionalizes epidemic outbreak, rendering it not an event of epic rupture but one episode within an ongoing local crucible. In this respect, the film presents a postcolonial overturning of the pandemic crisis paradigm, provincializing supposedly global urgencies within enduring small local dramas.

Golden Chicken 2, and 2003, begin with auspicious tidings for Kum, as she and a group of her fellow sex workers visit a temple on Chinese New Year to seek blessings for the coming year. In a rapid enigmatizing opening sequence comprehensible to those cued in to recent local history, two temple attendants are shown secretly rearranging several tubes of divination sticks. In the chaos of the jostling crowds, Kum by chance picks up one of the rigged containers. She proceeds to pray and draw first stick #4, which she puts back because of the number's unlucky rhyme with "death," and then #10, which the oracle deciphers as a *soeng soeng cim*, a "very best fortune," one that promises marriage in the new year. As an elated Kum and her high-

156 CHAPTER 3

spirited companions get ready to leave, they run into a throng of journalists photographing a VIP outside the temple. Kum recognizes this off-screen personage as a local government official, but, forgetting his name, she identifies him to the younger women as the husband of Wu Wai-zung, or Sibelle Hu, an old-time Taiwanese actress.

The film then cuts to a series of recycled news footage in which a portly man is shown at this same temple drawing stick #83, which bodes "bad luck in everything" for the whole year. This footage is left largely unexplained, in yet another enigmatizing gesture to local life and memory. Audiences are expected to know the annual *kau chim* ritual, whereby a member of the Hong Kong government represents the city in praying for its prosperity every Chinese New Year at Sha Tin's Che Kung Temple, and they are expected to remember this embarrassing episode of Patrick Ho Chi-ping's disastrous divination earlier that year. This newly appointed secretary of home affairs was a former ophthalmologist, and local tabloids rumored that he turned politician only after performing eye surgery on several mainland state leaders.[111] Blaming Ho for SARS's spread into Hong Kong, Kum fumes in voiceover: "Bad luck for this fat dude, since I took the best fortune stick. It would've been fine had he just prayed for himself. Why the heck did he have to go and pray for all of us Hong Kongers?" Kum's unstated complaint here, that she would have made a better proxy for the local citizenry, underscores the gulf between Ho and herself. He may be a puppet emissary of the state, but she is an utter nonentity and mere spectator to her own hometown's providence. She may have her small-time fortune, but it does not trump Ho's big-man misfortune, nor does it immunize her or the populace against the fallout suffering of his divination reading. The situational irony the audience is privy to is concealed from Kum herself, who never realizes that she took the rigged tube of lucky sticks while Ho was thereby left with a tube packed with rejected omens.

From the outset, then, *Golden Chicken 2* spotlights the power inequality between different Hong Kongers' ability to claim representative Hong Kongness. The government *kau chim* ritual is satirized as a product of secular corruption reaching into the inner temple space, and local officials are mocked as incompetently executing even pro forma spectacles. Yet the film does not discount but actually underscores the potency of local divinations and small-time prayers. By teasingly embedding the local genesis of SARS in stealth maneuvers and chance switcheroos, this opening sequence pits the film against both official state scripts and global narratives of the pandemic, marking itself as a sublocal countermemory. Postcolonial underclasses are not simply at the mercy of macro power plays, the film suggests, and the most unexpected minor actors and inadvertent fumbles can snowball into astonishing outcomes. In this pandemic counternarrative, Kum, too, may emerge as not just an accidental victim but a fortuitous beneficiary, with her "very best fortune" augury.

As mentioned earlier, the 1973 social comedy *The House of 72 Tenants* brought Cantonese cinema out of its industry demise, and, here, we can see *Golden Chicken 2*'s subtle debts to it.[112] The sole Cantonese title to be released that year, this Shaw Brothers production was itself a remake of a 1963 mainland film of the same name set in Guangzhou. Updated and localized, the Hong Kong remake drew its huge cast almost entirely from TVB artists, thus establishing the new paradigm of a direct talent conduit between local television and film.[113] It was an unexpected hit, breaking even box office records set by the kungfu blockbusters of Bruce Lee, who had died two months prior.[114] One of the film's most appealing qualities was its use of the ensemble cast to dramatize an underclass assemblage's everyday survival antics in an urban slum. Its unabashedly feel-good premise celebrated not just commoners' endurance but their quirks and triumphs in 1970s Hong Kong, "a time of socio-economic transition" when "the territory was mired in social problems brought about by its rise as a manufacturing centre exploiting cheap labour."[115] The film's crowded tenement setting prominently called attention to the housing crisis of the period, and its central plot of a lower-class community banding together against a ruthlessly exploitative landlady and her husband emphasized the priority of place, of locality and neighborhood, in defining Hong Kongers' contemporary social identity, in a region increasingly marked by waves of migration. The film hence performed what Arjun Appadurai calls a "production of locality under the conditions of contemporary urban life."[116] Perhaps most significant for the film's legacy was that, though the characters were supposed to hail from diverse mainland backgrounds, from Shanghai to Shandong, and though many of the actors themselves were migrants from China and Taiwan rather than Hong Kong natives, everyone was scripted to speak in Cantonese, however accented. In this new Cantophone mediascape, Hong Kong was depicted as "a Cantonese society able to assimilate Chinese people from different regions."[117] The film's picaresque quality, with its "series of vaudeville-like bits," "endless parade of characters," "episodic treatment of the plot," and Cantonese colloquial humor that "didn't translate" all worked to construct an enclave-oriented panorama of the local underclasses.[118] This was the beginning of Hong Kong's Cantophone multimedial culture and its inverted hyperreal, where familiar faces on the small screen could be expected to appear on the big screen and vice versa, and local celebrities playing slum dwellers or refugees could reinforce rather than undercut the aura of a shared material reality.

*Golden Chicken*s recuperated all these elements. Aside from the emphasis on locality and the liberal use of Cantonese humor and untranslated vernacular, both films deployed star-studded casts playing mostly underclass figures, in a vaudeville-like episodic parade. While centered on Kum, the films utilize her profession as a narrative device to constellate a roster of key side characters: less affluent men who cannot afford topline dancehall misses during the golden era or higher-priced call girls and society mistresses later on, men who frequent massage parlors or one-woman brothels for cheap thrills, and indigent men down on their luck and out of work, sometimes becoming desperate criminals on varying scales. The suggestion is that Kum, as a second-rate "chicken" through all her avatars, can open a time-capsule window into wider segments of the lower-class fringe, mainly but not exclusively male, that would otherwise remain invisible to cameras trained on more reputable and palatable spaces of the city. These are some of the people at the bottom rungs of Hong Kong society in the quarter century leading up to SARS. They are united, in an essential way, by their inability to immigrate, stuck as they are, like Kum, by their changing fortunes in a local slave-wage economy, or else by a lack of savings and education that would allow them to start over and thrive abroad. As Peter Chan describes the prehandover era, "People who could emigrate would do so. There was a feeling that you should make as much money as you could prior to the handover since everything after that would be a big question mark."[119] In this sense, the two films' localism reflects a compulsory socioeconomic condition as much as an aesthetic choice. With the exception of the eighties nightclubs, Kum's assorted shadow worlds—the fishball shops, the massage parlors, her one-woman brothel—all function as contact zones between the men and women of this trapped underclass. She sees them in their moments of tawdry and illicit pleasures, and she sees them on the precipices of self-destruction. In these contexts, de/extinction tropes proliferate, in relation not just to Kum but to the underclass assemblages of her rotating clientele.

The first *Golden Chicken*, for example, opens on December 14, 2002, a few minutes before midnight. Kum is at the bank ATM when she gets held up at knifepoint. When the mugger demands $50,000 from her, she loses her patience and points at her $98.20 balance. "What times are these? $50,000?

Are you nuts?" she snorts. "Do you have \$2? If you do, you can deposit it in my account and withdraw \$100. You need at least that sum for a withdrawal." But before she can sneak out of the ATM vestibule, the power goes out, locking both of them inside. To calm the mugger, Kum suggests they chat and "become friends," and she promises to "entertain" him with the "hilarious" story of her life. This narrative frame, set in the movie's present, sets up the subsequent flashbacks and provides the pretext for Kum's exegetical voiceovers. It also puts in place a cross-gender class bond between Kum and a male counterpart, as both are destitute and barely scraping by. The mugger, it turns out, owes money to loan sharks and has been dumped by his wife. In fact, on the day Kum ran into Professor Chan outside the labor department office, the mugger had been in the long queue of the unemployed, in a modernist instance of missed urban rendezvous. In the movie's closing scene, when the power returns and the two, now friends, part ways outside the bank, the mugger introduces himself, deadpan, as James Bong, or Wan Jan Bong. At this, Kum giggles and giggles, as his English name sounds like "James Bond" while his Cantonese name puns exactly, though with less exotic romance, on the colloquial phrase *wan jan bong*, "looking for someone to help out." When Bong hints that he is suicidal, Kum quickly urges him to *chaang zyu aa* (hang in there), *bei sam gei* and *wan cin* (work hard and make money) so he can *bong can* (patronize) her in the future. The ensuing happy ending is engineered, fairytale-style, when Kum tries the ATM again and discovers, to her shock, that a former client has just repaid his debt to her, seven years overdue but with interest compounded. Suddenly a near millionaire, Kum runs out of the bank looking for Bong. As daylight breaks on the horizon, she finds him sitting forlornly in a tree. She gleefully tells him he has at last *wan dou jan bong*, "found someone to help him out." So, while Bong, like Kum, might hitherto have been a nodal point for multiple extinction tropes—unemployment and crushing debt, wife abandonment and prospective suicide—he, too, is ultimately granted a miraculous reversal of fortune, past the stroke of midnight. His fairy godmother is none other than Kum, her final transformation made possible by the circulations within the city's fringe economies and underclass loyalties.

Not fortuitously, the actor who plays Bong is Eric Tsang, who is also the executive producer of both *Golden Chicken*s. Indeed, the actors who portray Kum's clients are all local celebrities, leading Tony Leung Ka-fai (aka Professor Chang) to comment wryly in the featurette, "Of course this is a good movie: all of Hong Kong's sex patrons happen to be heaven-grade megastars!"[120] In trademark industry fashion, both films capitalize on real-life relationships and celebrity gossip to fuel their reality effects. Aside from Peter Chan and Sandra Ng, Chapman To and Kristal Tin are also well-known to locals as longtime partners, and their characters wind up as a clandestine couple by the first movie's end. Ng is also well-known for her long-standing and unabashed crush on Andy Lau, and both films play on this piece of tabloid lore. The first film stages an all but gratuitous scene of Kum's fangirl encounter with Lau at the massage parlor, and, in a later dream sequence, when Kum was demoralized by the lack of business at her one-woman brothel, what galvanized her was a hallucination in which Lau crawled out from her home television set to personally mentor her on the ethics of becoming a "golden chicken," complete with a lesson on feigning passionate orgasms. With the onset of SARS, the ensemble casting of *Golden Chicken 2* takes on added valence, resignifying the classic genre of ensemble comedy as local popular culture's enduring ability to engineer social assemblages, even in pandemic times. Following its predecessor, the sequel uses the premise of Kum's profession to coordinate a star-studded cast and a spectrum of societal tales, but, this time, fuller focus is given to the present of 2003. Kum's brothel apartment and newly acquired diner now serve as narrative hubs, not just for the lonely and despairing men of the lower social strata but also for those affected by SARS. Kum's habitats, as contemporary reincarnations of the tenement slum, become spaces of temporary refuge for the supposed lowlife and bankrupt elements of the city.

In the first of a series of story lines, Boss Chow (played by Anthony Wong Chau-sang), the owner of a neighborhood *cha chaan teng* or Hong Kong–style café and a frequent customer of Kum's brothel, attempts to choreograph his own suicide in her apartment. Dropping by unannounced on the night of the Lantern Festival, he offers to cook them a late-night meal, in the course of which he becomes maudlin and starts spewing gloomy classical poetry in accented Cantonese, highlighting his immigrant roots. His plan is to burn charcoal in her bathroom and die by carbon monoxide poisoning during sex, but he thoughtfully protects Kum by first giving her an XM-grade gas mask, under the pretext of sex play. When she discovers his ploy and confronts him, he confesses that he is deep in debt and on the verge of losing his café. With no family, no money, and no livelihood, he wants to indulge himself one last time and die a *fung lau gwai*, a dissolute ghost. Filled with pity, Kum offers to lend him some of her savings, and he delightedly reciprocates by proposing to make her a business partner. In a burst of hopeful energy, the two resume intercourse. But Chow, having already been exposed to the charcoal fumes, dies in his moment of climax, becoming a *fung lau gwai* after all. Despite the kinky gallows humor of this story line, it sets up a dark reversal of the deextinction pattern from the first *Golden Chicken*. Here, unlike with Bong, Kum's very first customer fails to come back from the brink, despite the promise of recovery and rebirth, dying a hasty and ironic death in the very moment of renewed desire and hope. And while Chow thereby bequeaths his café to Kum and enables her rise to middle-class respectability as a small-time boss lady, this career upgrade coincides exactly with the arrival of SARS, so that she is compelled to continue her sex work. It is worth noting that this plotline, akin to Boss Hung's in *City of SARS*, avoids an exceptional link between financial suicide and the epidemic, shedding light instead on the daily realities of those ground down and forsaken by local capital. Indeed, Chow's exaggerated possession of a combat gas mask—easily misconstrued here as a satire on face mask use during SARS, a reference to global crisis rather than long-standing local issues—seems to be the film's subtle way of reminding audiences about the metaphorical toxins that preexisted and will outlast the virus, that had already habitually driven locals to self-annihilation and would likely continue to do so.

The next story line is the one most directly tied to SARS, and the one involving the sole character to be infected by the coronavirus in the whole movie. One rainy night, a tall man wearing a surgical mask (played by Leon Lai Ming) comes into Kum's café to order takeout. As he waits, he is recognized by another customer as a physician at one of the SARS hospitals and is immediately shunned by the other diners as well as the cowering staff. He then politely excuses himself to wait outside, shoulders hunched in exhaustion and sorrow. In cartoonish fashion, the elderly janitor jumps out of his path and mops vigorously after him, muttering curses under her breath, while several waiters scramble to carry a table out onto the sidewalk for him alone. By this point in time, the city is on high epidemic alert, and this segment highlights the intense social paranoia at the height of the local outbreak, caricaturing in particular the knee-jerk panic toward frontline medical workers, the demographic hit hardest by SARS in Hong Kong. All told, 22 percent of the city's eventual 1,755 SARS patients were healthcare professionals.[121] Though eulogized in the media, they also faced stigma and discrimination in everyday life.[122] As one local nurse later recalls, "People avoided us as if we were lepers."[123]

162 CHAPTER 3

In the film, Kum is again presented as an ethical paragon. There is a hint that her profession renders her susceptible to infectious diseases too and hence exceptionally empathetic toward those stigmatized by them. She runs outside to invite the doctor back in, and, when he declines and apologizes, she draws him into friendly conversation. She comments that he looks unfamiliar, so he explains he has only recently moved into the neighborhood, renting an apartment nearby so as to avoid going home. "Oh, I saw on TV how pitiful the SARS doctors are, some of them coming home to nothing but a makeshift bed these days in order to protect their families from infection," Kum commiserates. "But I believe [Margaret] Chan Fung Fu-chan: you can only catch the virus through respiratory droplets, right? So, what soup would you like tomorrow night? I'll prepare it for you." With her warm chatter, she wins over Dr. Facemask, as she calls him, and he begins to come regularly for takeout. "Your meals are on the house," she tells him cheerfully the next time. "Give me a chance to support our frontline medical professionals!" In his final visit late one night, just as Kum is about to close up shop, he asks for "stress relief," taking up Kum's earlier offer of a massage. He had gently turned her down before by stating that his wife would give him the occasional massage, so this request is fraught with unsaid implications. As Kum kneads the doctor's tense shoulders and suggests that he try to see his family, even if only to wave at them from a hospital window, he breaks down in tormented sobs. In the next scene, presumably some time later, archival footage of Hong Kong finally containing SARS and being taken off the WHO's list of infected regions flashes across the screen. Business flourishes again around the city, including at Kum's café. But at precisely this moment of citywide recuperation and revival, Kum sees on the news a tragic epidemic epilogue: the death of a frontline physician. As news reports focus on the public reverence paid to this doctor at his funeral by over a thousand colleagues, friends, and family, Kum tearfully recognizes the photograph as belonging to Dr. Facemask. Through this sentimental plotline, the film provides a critical but also heartwrenching reflection on Hong Kongers' fear and small-mindedness during the outbreak itself and their quick about-face afterward, as hitherto pariahs are turned into martyrs. Similar to Boss Chow, in another belated re-reversal, the jubilation of collective survival is tainted by the reminder of a last death.

In the film's longer tragicomic plotline, a man by the name of Chan Saasi (played by Ronald Cheng Chung-kei)—a homonym for "SARS" in Cantonese—moves temporarily into Kum's apartment after his mother's

Amoy Gardens flat gets sealed off. At first, Chan seems to be just another client with perverse sexual habits. Whether in the shower or in bed, he constantly combs Kum's body and living quarters for body hair, examining her armpits with a magnifying glass and tweezers ready at hand, crawling on her bathroom floor and rifling through her trash bin, even licking her shower curtain for stray strands. But he mostly hunts in vain, since Kum had earlier shaved her entire body after hearing a rumor that SARS spreads through body hair. She is initially wary of Chan's strange behavior, but she eventually figures out he is not there for sex but is in fact suffering from a head trauma. Like many other male characters in the two films, Chan has lost his job and is deep in debt, forcing his wife to resume prostitution work. In his final memory of her, he had been on his knees, arms wrapped tightly around her waist, as he begged her not to sell her body. As she pushed away, he was knocked backward and hit his head against the wall. When he regained consciousness, he could not remember her face. But he found one strand of her hair on him, and, ever after, he has scoured Hong Kong's brothels for a prostitute with the same body hair.

Ever the compassionate bodhisattva, Kum takes pity on Chan and decides to help by organizing a citywide "one hair one soup" campaign: all of Hong Kong's female sex workers are invited to her diner for a free bowl of soup in exchange for one strand of their body hair. A long queue soon forms outside Kum's restaurant, snaking down the block into adjacent alleyways, in a visual echo of the first *Golden Chicken*'s scene of jobseekers outside the labor department. But this time around, almost everyone in line is a woman, in one of the most female community spotlighting moments of the sequel. As Kum says sighingly in voiceover, "Who knew so many of my phoenix sisters would show up without embarrassment in public like this, all for a bowl of fresh soup? Times are hard indeed!" The suggestion is that, for local sex workers as for other working-class people in the city, hunger and destitution pose a greater ongoing threat than SARS, as the women brave infection as much as public scorn for a free bowl of soup. Over the next three days, Chan scrutinizes with his magnifying glass all the women who come, but to no avail. At the end of the third day, after the crowds have dispersed, his wife (played by Angelica Lee Sinje) finally materializes. In an inversion of the wife-abandonment trope, she tells Kum the next chapter to their marital story: it is not she who has gone missing but Chan himself. After the blow to his head, Chan was institutionalized at a psychiatric hospital, where he remains a patient. He periodically escapes to go search for his wife, yet he never recognizes her when she finds him, time and time again. This time is no different, and, as she tenderly strokes his hair, he curls up on her lap and affectionately calls her "older sister." Kum sadly accompanies the couple back to the psychiatric hospital, where the staff takes Chan familiarly in hand.

It is telling that, for a movie devoted to narrating the year of SARS, the image of the hospital, the supposedly paramount space of pandemic crisis and disease death, surfaces in relation not to Dr. Facemask but to Chan Saasi. This displacement of the expected scene of epidemic misfortune from the frontline hero and victim to the much more quotidian figure of a homeless amnesiac is consistent with the deflationary treatment of SARS in both Stephen Chow's *Project 1:99* short and Eric Tsang's segment of *City of SARS*. But more distinctively here, Chan Saasi's poignant story couples the extinctionist themes of socioeconomic ruin and marital disintegration with tropes of mental illness and memory loss, intimating that the inability to recollect and recognize one's most beloved constitutes the more heartrending disease. SARS does not decimate lives or relationships here, much less a whole city's population à la some nightmarish apocalypse. Instead, the everyday cycle of underclass struggle and self-debasement, of breakups and breakdowns, at once precede and persist beyond SARS, even for its namesake character.

Memory Lost and Memory Cued

Amnesia may lie hauntingly beneath Chan Saasi's plotline, but the film's speculative frame advances a far more optimistic telos about memory. As in the first film, Kum is narrating her 2003 chronicle in retrospect in the sequel. The year is now 2046, and her putative audience is a young man who, we infer, unbeknownst to himself, is her grandson (played by Chapman To, whose character in the first film had died of cancer at the millennium's turn). The dystopic tinge of this utopian future is more Huxleian than Orwellian, in the film's tongue-in-cheek vision of a capitalist paradise. In the opening shot, far from the disease-ruined planet of climate fictions, Kum's 2046 Hong Kong has developed into a premier world city. It retains the same metropolitan skyline as in 2003 but is now bustling with high-tech aircraft traffic. On Victoria Peak, everyone is dressed neatly in pristine white, from patrolmen to joggers, children, and their Filipino nannies. Even Kum, with her flamboyant outfits and bright orange perm in 2003, appears prim and proper in a white trench coat and headscarf. This uniform whiteness mirrors the later scene at Chan Saasi's psychiatric hospital with its white-straitjacketed inmates, insinuating that local economic prosperity and social harmony have come at the price of a communal cognitive deficit. Hong Kong itself has been turned into a mental health clinic, a consumer hub for purchasable but superficial happiness. Now in her eighties, Kum has paid several million dollars in cosmetic surgery for the face of a thirtysomething. Her grandson, in turn, has bought a supply of memory-erasing pills as postbreakup therapy, and he is about to swallow a handful of these pills, "deleting" years of his life so as to forget a two-month-long romantic relationship, when Kum intervenes just in time. This opening frame serves as the premise for Kum's retrospective narration, as she tries to convince the young man of memory's advantages. As we come to deduce, Kum's intention is to have her grandson, the son of the infant she gave up for adoption and so never knew, hear the story not just of her life but of her romance with the father of his father, a plotline that forms the film's second half and that loops back to the opening sequence of Kum's 2003 "very best fortune" divination.

In contrast to the bleak denouements of Boss Chow, Dr. Facemask, and Chan Saasi, this frame narrative projects, albeit in ironic hyperbole, the ultimate survival and global triumph of Hong Kong. When Kum recalls that SARS killed many Hong Kongers in 2003, her grandson, who has no knowledge of the outbreak, exclaims in disbelief, "People dying of SARS? That's impossible! I myself caught SARS several times just this year. All you have to do is pop a pill." Though the grandson is a comical exaggeration of the amnesia-prone self-medicating millennial, his casual faith in biomedicine's capacity to overcome all emerging viruses gives important voice to the film's imagining of an ever-resilient Hong Kong as a city tougher than any pandemic. And Kum, as the emblem of this resilience, attains her heart's wish by the film's end: she successfully persuades her grandson to treasure his memories and even tricks him into calling her Maa Maa (Grandma). "If you haven't tasted bitterness, how would you appreciate sweetness?" she lectures him, with a moral obviously aimed at the post-SARS local audience. "Hong Kong is also bitter first and sweet after." Thus enlightened, the grandson avers, "I've decided to go look for my girlfriend, Lucy. No matter how mean she is to me in the future, it's still a memory, right? Actually, we had a date tonight to go watch the debut of 2046. The movie is finally screening!" This snarky dig at Wong Kar-wai's art-house epic, which took four years to produce and was released the following year in 2004, can be taken as a metacommentary on *Golden Chicken 2*'s own commitment to locality. Wong may be the stylish auteur adored by international film critics and festivals, this jibe implies, but, by the time his masterpiece gets released, the contemporary history of Hong Kong and the memories of recent experiences, including those of SARS, will have been completely "deleted" by local viewers, who will likely be a new generation existing in a new eon. (In fact, it was precisely due to his prioritizing *2046*'s production that Wong failed to complete his short in time for *Project 1:99*'s release.)[124] So, while both *2046* and *Golden Chicken 2* tackle themes of memory and amnesia, the latter represents an alternative aesthetic and filmic ethic: quicker and messier, commercial and crowd-pleasing, yet still artistically scrupulous and thematically rich, and, above all, staunchly devoted to the thickness and presentness of local life, to the stories of the here and now.

In the film's closing fantasy sequence that parallels the first *Golden Chicken*'s, in a self-reflexive recollecting of its own predecessor, Kum has another quasi hallucination of Andy Lau—still playing himself, but now promoted to the role of Hong Kong's chief executive. In a state-of-the-union hologram broadcast to the public, Lau announces that, at the entreaty of the American president, he has agreed to reinstate currency exchange between Hong Kong and the United States, setting the new exchange rate at HK\$1 to US\$7.8 (a cheeky inversion of the real-world ratio). "Moreover," Lau continues, "our local oil production levels have reached the third highest in the world, and, for a fifth consecutive year, local unemployment rate is at 0 percent. Given our city's boundless reserve, I have decided to eliminate taxes for the next twenty years!" He pauses for imagined applause. "In addition, everyone is entitled to unlimited free education, housing, healthcare, and senior services. As long as you carry the three-star Hong Kong ID card, you will be guaranteed a lifetime of benefits." This 2046 Hong Kong, it turns out, is a true paradise after all. Under the leadership of a former Cantopop movie star, it has prospered for fifty years and achieved a merger between capitalist means and socialist ends. This, at least, is Kum's fangirl view, as she cheers on her favorite idol. "I can still sing all your songs," she gushes to Lau's hologram, breaking into one of his melodies. Lau looks down briefly in Kum's direction, with an expression of mild amusement and forbearance. "Do you think you'll release a new album?" she continues excitedly. "Geez, other people are singing stars, too, but you sing-star your way to becoming chief executive. No wonder I love you so much!" While other directors have envisioned 2046, this resonant year leading up to the official termination of Hong Kong's autonomous status, as an ambiguous nightmare, *Golden Chicken 2*, in this self-indulgent final moment, catapults one of its own industry superstars into the center of an imagined new world order, with Hong Kong and Cantophone culture at the summit of not just regional but global power. Per Lau's instructions, Kum closes her eyes for a minute and holds in her mind's eye the image of her "most beautiful Hong Kong." When she opens her eyes again, she beholds, magically, the nocturnal skyline of the city in 2003, revivified in the film's last reverie of its own world's deextinction.

Psychologists make a distinction between retrospective memory and prospective memory: the former involves recalling past events, the latter planned intentions. The futuristic frame narrative of *Golden Chicken* 2 may be construed as expressing a longing for Hong Kongers' prospective memory of self-retrospective memory—a longing to remember to remember themselves. In this most memorable of years, as the film's crew called 2003, future memory cues have already been proliferated by SARS itself. Yet the desire for remembrance here, as in the first *Golden Chicken*, stretches beyond a single outbreak to encompass the span of Hong Kong's modern past, from the prelude to its golden age to this age's coda. The fear is not of momentary forgetting, of a short-term memory lapse, but of an irrevocable long-term memory loss and a second-order loss of the very impulse to remember. What if the city's collective memories, however vivid once, however deeply encoded once, become inaccessible in the far future? What if the 2046 Hong Konger, with Kum's grandson as proxy, does not even know *that*, much less *what*, he is supposed to recollect?

It is within this framework of local memories' fast loss but hoped-for long retrieval that we can understand the assertive use of Cantopop in the two *Golden Chicken*s. Their soundtracks are chock-full of enclave references, some overt, others oblique and detectable only by Cantopop followers. But more than just inside nods, and more than just vehicles of nostalgia, these songs function as aural memory cues for audiences, what Linda Lai calls "mnemonic schemes."[125] The songs are meant to shore up an embodied sense of cultural community and local history, one that is not merely intellectual, textual, or visual but multisensorial, emotional, visceral. According to the psychological theory of retrieval failure, information in long-term memory "is said to be available (i.e., it is still stored) but not accessible (i.e., it cannot be retrieved) . . . [when] retrieval cues are not present."[126] Music, as we know, can be a powerful mnemonic and retrieval cue. The films' repetition of Cantopop thus serves to trigger memories of a vanished past for local audiences and deextinct, if only for the duration of a tune and in the echo chamber of a listener's head, a bygone Cantophone epoch. Not fortuitously, many of the songs included in the two films are the themes to popular television serials from earlier decades and onetime household tunes. Their sounds reverberate with sentimental evocations of the serials themselves, and hence of a multimedial milieu when local television programming still dominated the cultural psyches of Hong Kongers.

In *Golden Chicken 2*, one scene exemplifies this self-conscious deployment of Cantopop as Cantophone retrieval cue: that of Kum's first kiss. With SARS successfully contained by the summer, the second half of the movie shifts focus to Kum's decades-long, on-again-off-again relationship with her money-obsessed maternal cousin from Guangdong, Kwan (played by Jacky Cheung Hok-yau). After a ten-year absence, Kwan shows up unexpectedly on Kum's doorstep one day in mid-2003. This extended plotline then retraces the narrative steps and time periods of the first *Golden Chicken*, inserting itself into the original script's gaps while spinning out another layer of memory, nested matryoshka-like inside the first movie. In effect, this plotline repeats the original movie's repetition of local history, with scenes from it now integrated as archival footage into a hitherto repressed romance. Audiences are taken back to Kum as a pigtailed fishball girl in the late seventies, when Kwan first emigrated from the mainland to pursue his dreams of wealth in Hong Kong. He moved into her family's apartment, sharing a bunk bed with Kum in the tiny space of her curtained-off makeshift bedroom. As the two grew older, they became each other's closest friend and erstwhile love interest. We learn that Kum's motivational dance and mantra "Ah Kum *wan dou sik*," her signature refrain from the first film, was in fact derived from Kwan's personal motto. Despite their mutual attraction, Kwan's manic pursuit of riches left Kum disappointed time and again. It is revealed that the child Kum had given up for adoption was fathered by Kwan, a fact she withholds from him until nearly the end of this sequel, in the very moment when the two cousins are physically torn apart at the airport as he is dragged away on embezzlement charges by mainland police. As he shouts out his love for her, the soundtrack erupts into one of Jacky Cheung's own signature operatic ballads, "Love Is Eternal" ("Ngoi si wing hang"/"Ai shi yongheng"). Familiar to most Cantopop listeners, this is one of the themes to Cheung's 1997 musical *Snow.Wolf.Lake*, first heard when the male protagonist (played by Cheung himself) declares his love for the female protagonist. The intertextual web amplifies the emotions of this scene as Kum and Kwan at long last let down their guard with each other and throw propriety to the wind.

The scene of Kum's first kiss with Kwan is much more delicately crafted, with layers of Cantophone memory cues. One day, Kwan was trying to repair the family's broken television set. When the static cleared, a scene from the popular 1981 TVB drama *The Fate* (*Fo fung wong/Huo fenghuang*, literally "fire phoenix," with a silent wink to Kum's later profession) appeared on the screen. It was the climactic scene in which the male and female protagonists, played by Chow Yun-fat and Carol "Dodo" Cheng Yu-ling, the archetypal couple of late seventies and eighties television dramas, embraced in a passionate kiss. Viewers are further cued in to this local media memory by the soundtrack, as the rousing melody of the serial's theme song "Fate" ("Ming wan"/"Mingyun") blasted forth for a few seconds. Then, abruptly, the television set exploded in fire and smoke, in a hyperbolic and parodic image of Cantophone culture's blazing demise. Lest audiences are left still clueless, Kum came bouncing home in her school uniform in that instant. "Did you see *The Fate*?" she asked Kwan excitedly, naming the show for forgetful viewers. He answered by naming the two lead actors' full names, half showing off his familiarity with Hong Kong popular culture and half showcasing his migrant status by not referring to them by their local nicknames. Wistful audiences are thereby quietly reminded of a time when local shows carried that kind of cultural cachet in the sinophone world. Kum then continued, "They kissed for an entire minute! It was so satisfying. You could see their drool splattering everywhere. Why don't we try it too?" The two cousins then bawled out the opening melody together before embracing in mock reenactment of the on-screen kiss. After several seconds, their passion turned genuine.

In this moment, as the mood shifts from high-spirited roleplay to authentic tenderness, the soundtrack provocatively switches to another song, one that has been cited by local music critics as a representative work of Hong Kong Cantopop, "Ask Me" ("Man ngo"/"Wen wo"):

> You ask me how many sounds of joy there are, [*man ngo fun fu sing jau gei do*]
> you ask me how many sounds of sorrow there are. [*man ngo bei huk sing jau gei do*]
> How can I [*ngo jyu ho nang gau*]
> count them one by one? [*jat jat heoi sou cing co*]
>
> You ask me why I'm happy, [*man ngo dim gaai wui gou hing*]
> why exactly I suffer. [*gau ging dim gaai jiu fu co*]
> I smile and answer [*ngo siu zyu wui daap*]
> in brief, "I am me." [*gong jat seng ngo hai ngo*][127]

The tune and lyrics of this song evoke a very specific phase in the development of Hong Kong popular music. First introduced as part of the soundtrack of the 1976 film *Jumping Ash*, the song was composed by Michael Lai Siu-tin with lyrics by Wong Jim.[128] Lai was an industry giant who composed over seven hundred songs for local television and cinema, while Wong was a legendary all-around talent who wrote lyrics for over two thousand Cantonese songs in his lifetime. Originally sung by Grace Chan Lai-sze, "Ask Me" has been covered by countless local artists, with renditions by everyone from Wong and Lai themselves to Leslie Cheung. In May 2003, amid SARS and nineteen months before his own death from cancer, Wong completed a doctoral dissertation on Cantopop, his final contribution to what he saw as a fast-fading musical world. There, Wong divides the historical evolution of Hong Kong popular music into four phases, with "Ask Me" as his chosen representative work for the third phase, from 1974 to 1983: "This was the period when Hong Kong local consciousness became established, so I use the last line of 'Ask Me'—'I am me'—to designate this era when Hong Kong pop music found its own voice."[129] Cantopop came into its own in this period because local lyricists, prime among them Wong himself, consciously cultivated a Hong Kong vernacular style. As Wong explains, "Old-fashioned terms of address such as *hing* (dear), *go* (older brother), *mui* (younger sister), *long* (husband), *gwan* (sir) were no longer used, replaced instead by the more direct *nei* (you) and *ngo* (me). This gave off a more contemporary feel . . . a more modern sense of 'self.'"[130] "Ask Me," like many classics in the Cantopop canon, "used contemporary people's speech to express contemporary people's thoughts and feelings, frank and forthright, with no false fronts and no polite concessions. . . . That's why Cantopop," Wong sums up, "can travel to every corner of the earth and still meet with recognition and sympathy by music fans everywhere."[131] This last comment underscores again the subimperial dual consciousness of Cantophone elites: at once top dog and underdog, claiming universality for local cultural goods even while bemoaning with one's last breath, "It's a pity that the [golden] era is gone, that Cantopop sounds will pass into oblivion any time now, and, other than people's memories and a few dusty vinyl records, this music may not resonate again for the next generation."[132]

Golden Chicken 2, though, is at once less melancholically resigned and less anchored in a position of onetime privilege. By tying the rise and fall of the Hong Kong Cantophone to the romance of two underclass marginals, the film also allows the former to live a displaced afterlife through the latter, through the fringe narratives Cantophone culture has helped spawn. So it is against the multiply recycled backdrop of TVB images and Cantopop sounds that Kum and Kwan's love took its first step, in a lifelong relationship that would culminate in their grandson of 2046. Theirs is not simply an imitation of hollow simulacra. Rather, local songs and local shows make up the multimedial environment within which local feelings sprout, grow, and are given license to be acted on, even if without design, even if faced with a precarious future. In that future, whether the 2003 of the film's historical present or the 2046 of its diegetic present, those old songs may seem sappy and formulaic, those old shows outdated and clichéd, but they will continue to perform their task as local retrieval cues, unlocking the memory vaults of the heart's homegrown affections. The trick is to remember and replay those oldies with heart, without shame, along the model of both *Golden Chicken*s. Even as the two films reconstitute a Cantophone heritage in their multimedial scenes, they stitch themselves into and prolong the memory fabric of that inheritance, giving extended life to the music scores of a sonic memoryscape and the visual collage of a graphic archive. In this way, the films make themselves into a bricolage reservoir of emocognitive triggers for the post-Cantophone Hong Kong future. To love a vanishing local is to want to recapitulate it, to reenact its most memorable scenes and hum its most lingering songs, in gratitude and homage, and with full embrace of its cheesiness and hubris. What gets mistaken for mere nostalgia is actually one way of warding off amnesia, of expressing one's wish to remember and hold on to bygone love.

Even when death has taken its toll on this realm, Cantopop can be beckoned as tacit elegy, even enlisting the filmscript itself as a metatextual temple. Most prominent in this regard is the two *Golden Chicken*s' inclusion of several songs by Danny Chan Pak-keung. Chan was a Cantopop idol who rose to popularity during the late seventies and eighties, a young talent who sang and composed some of the most memorable songs of that period, including several hit themes to TVB dramas. He died in 1993 at the age of thirty-five, from a depression-induced drug overdose. At the time, Chan's death had dealt a blow to local entertainment circles, prefiguring Leslie Cheung's suicide a decade later. By 2002, however, the memory of this tragedy had been somewhat ameliorated, so Chan's songs could be recuperated with some emotional distance, as a metaphor for premature loss as well as a vehicle for conveying the broader sense of Cantophone extinction. So, in the first *Golden Chicken*, Chan's "Just Loving You" ("Pin pin hei fun nei"/"Pianpian xihuan ni"), perhaps his most iconic ballad, plays in the background throughout the scenes immediately after Kum gave up her infant for adoption. Mourning at home, Kum bawled and shrieked, banging her head repeatedly against the wall, in a bittersweet literalizing of the Cantonese expression *ham tau maai coeng*. When she tried to rush to the airport to see her son off to America one last time, even the heavens thwarted her passage, as a tropical cyclone swept in and turned into hail. "It's a miraculous sight, miss!" exclaimed the taxi driver, turning the car around to take Kum home. As if on cue, as soon as she stepped out of the taxi, the sky cleared and the rain abated. "This was the worst decision of my life," she says in voiceover. The film, though, hints that her lifelong separation from her son is karmic, a matter more of providential logic than personal choice. For, rather than an isolated miracle, this sudden storm followed a series of earlier celestial interventions, when a typhoon would break out every time Kum headed out the door for her scheduled abortion. When Kum reported the eerie phenomenon to her aunt, an ex-prostitute and a motherly mentor to her, calling it *ce* or demonic, the aunt interpreted it instead as a manifestation of *gun jam sung zi*, "Kwan Yin gifting a son." Now the aunt reuttered the adage and the word "gift," explaining to Kum that something divinely given is also something to be divinely taken away, two sides of the same coin and an arrangement that lies beyond human control. Fittingly, Danny Chan's voice echoes in the background throughout this tale of destined loss of one's young—as if enigmatically whispering to Hong Kong listeners, from beyond the veil, that they, too, must accept the coming and passing of local talents. The Cantopop soundtrack therefore performs more than "narrative functions" to supplement the meanings of its fictional script.[133] Here, the filmscript itself conversely supplements the soundtrack, with Chan as a ghostly proxy for the Cantophone and its uncontrollable fortune.

Reinforcing these suggestions is both films' closing invocation of Chan's other famous song "What Does One Ask for in Life" ("Yat sang ho kau"/"Yisheng he qiu"). This was the opening theme to the 1989 TVB drama *Looking Back in Anger*, one of the most watched serials of the decade starring Felix Wong, the same actor who now plays Richard, the adoptive father of Kum's child. In the opening episodes of that drama, a poor pregnant woman is scapegoated for murder and sentenced to death by hanging after giving birth in prison, leading her husband to commit suicide and leaving their two young sons orphaned. That haunting story line lurks unspoken behind Kum's maternal trials, and, for viewers who remember, their memory is cued and the aura of real-life tragedy enhanced by Chan's song. In *Golden Chicken*'s final scene, when Kum runs out of the bank and down the dawn-bathed streets searching for Bong, the film splices together a montage of its ensemble cast, in a highlight reel set to Chan's ballad. The lyrics amplify the notes of wistful retrospection and life review, underdog struggle and bewilderment, unexpected gains and irrevocable loss:

> How can life's changing fortunes rest?
> When I look back, how many autumns have passed?
> I have lost what I searched everywhere for
> yet hold in my hand what I never expected.
> I have gained nothing,
> cannot explain my successes, failures, or mistakes.
> As soon as I hear or see it, things have already changed,
> and I don't know where to look.
>
> What does one ask for in life?
> There are constant decisions about what to give up and what to keep.
> I have exhausted my whole life,
> but before I can grasp it, it's already fled.
> What does one ask for in life?
> I can never see clearly through this confusion.
> But who knew that what I have lost
> is actually everything I have.

The penultimate moment in *Golden Chicken 2* also returns to this song for its ending montage, accruing yet another layer of filmic self-reference and self-repetition. After summing up her recounting of 2003, Kum and her grandson behold a spectacular fireworks display in the night sky. The date happens to be the fiftieth anniversary of the handover. Against this backdrop, "What Does One Ask for in Life" is queued again, this time assuming wider significance as an anthem to the city's life review and historical reckoning but also its potentially renewable future. The lyrics now speak not just to Kum's travails or the Cantophone's dissolution but to Hong Kong's collective experience of searching and disorientation, attainment and loss. Channeled through the voice of the prematurely dead, this song from Cantopop's golden era, when replayed in the sequel, poignantly captures the paradox of a passing and a return—and hence a hope, too, that memory cues may beget new life.

For those most in tune with Cantophone sounds, one other elegy may be heard between the lines. Some critics have opined that, for a work so steeped in the contemporary past and local popular culture, it is odd that *Golden Chicken 2* fails to mention Leslie Cheung's death.[134] But perhaps, for a crew with so many connections to the core of local show business, the sounds of homage are not missing at all, just submerged, made private. In the Chan Saasi plotline, when Kum hits on the idea of a "one hair one soup" campaign, what plays triumphantly in the background is "Gone with the Wind" ("Fau saang luk gip"/"Fo sheng liu jie"), the theme song to the 1980 ATV serial of the same name. Like *Golden Chicken*, that drama focused on recent local history, charting the fates of refugee migrants and their families' changing fortunes from 1950s to 1970s Hong Kong. Those who are familiar with Cheung's career will recall that he entered the entertainment industry not through TVB but its rival station ATV. Cheung's role in that serial, as the youngest son of a Shanghainese tycoon, was one of his early standout performances, years before his music and film career took off locally and internationally. *Golden Chicken 2* teasingly plays this song in the background as Chan Saasi hunts for his missing wife by scrutinizing the line of prostitutes and their body hairs with a magnifying glass. It is as if the film is gently telling those viewers hunting for minute traces of Cheung that he, though ostensibly missing from the script, may be found, too, if remembered by other means.

Coda: From *Golden Chicken SSS* to Sam Hui's COVID-19 Concert

Despite the two *Golden Chickens*' deextinction efforts, 2003 could be considered the beginning of the end for the Cantophone subempire's restoration dramas. By all numerical measures, Hong Kong cinema post-SARS has shrunk to a fraction of its former self. In 1993 the industry released an all-time high of 234 local films.[135] Ten years later, that number had dwindled to 76 by one count and 54 by another.[136] Nor was SARS an anomalous year, for the lower 2003 estimate has now become the industry norm. Since 2003, the number of annual domestic productions has averaged in the low fifties.[137] In both 2017 and 2018, only 53 Hong Kong films were produced each year—contrasted with 278 and 300 foreign films released in the local market in those same years, respectively. In effect, every year is a SARS year for the native cinema now. COVID may have further accelerated this decline, as 2022 saw only 27 local films released, compared to 190 foreign ones.[138] In this light, it is no exaggeration when Michael Curtain laments, in the language of species extinction, that Hong Kong, "once the capital of Chinese cinema . . . is littered with the corpses of film companies that have been unable or unwilling to adapt."[139]

For some, Hong Kong cinema's adaptation to this newer brave world has meant a strategic transformation of its earlier aesthetic of subimperial melancholy and underdog spirit. The 2014 sequel to the two *Golden Chicken*s, *Golden Chicken sss* (*Gam gai sss/Jin ji sss*), is one example. The three *s*'s in the title signal not just the film's status as the third installment in the franchise but also its upgraded and glossier packaging, with the "sss" resembling silver-studded dollar signs ($$$) on promotional material. Sandra Ng was the prime mover behind this second sequel, and, this time, she took over the role of producer, in her first solo production credit. Ng jokingly recounted the behind-the-scenes story to local tabloids as follows: since 2003 both *Golden Chicken*s had become rerun classics on local television and Kum's character had grown into a beloved icon, and, every time she rewatched those movies, she felt nostalgic about the part and wanted to reprise it one more time, especially since Kum gave Hong Kong audiences so much joy at the time. But Peter Chan was the one with funding power in their partnership, and he rejected her proposal at first. "Because the subject [of *Golden Chicken*] can only work in Hong Kong," Ng said, "Peter Chan felt it would lose money for sure, so initially he wouldn't lend me the money to make the movie."[140] Chan has long since moved on from a Hong Kong–centered production model, and, since the late 2000s, he has also largely abandoned his pan-Asian Applause Pictures in favor of coproductions with mainland companies, founding in 2009 the more broadly China-oriented We Pictures. But at Ng's persistence, he relented and agreed to underwrite *Golden Chicken sss*. To staff the star-studded cast, Ng relied on personal friendships within the industry, relationships she had cultivated and deepened through the decades. "They are all megastars," she reported in an interview. "How could I [pay them]? The box office cannot support their salaries." So she bought each actor a thank-you card and enclosed a red packet with several hundred dollars in lucky money as surrogate wages. It is a testament to the industry's enclave intimacy, and perhaps the performers' loyalty to the symbolic localism of the *Golden Chicken* concept, that they accepted Ng's invitation. "Everybody came to this movie and their cameos for fun, for a party," Ng proclaimed. "This is really Hong Kong spirit."[141]

If this ensemble casting and Ng's explicit homage to "Hong Kong spirit" harken back to the two earlier *Golden Chicken*s and their zeitgeist, *Golden Chicken sss*'s themes and tone show clear signs of that spirit's aging. Most conspicuously, Kum is no longer the ugly duckling or Plain Jane of old, much less the struggling underdog representing the city's underclass masses. Now in her fifties, she has retired from the one-phoenix brothel business and graduated to top mamasan status, with a multiracial fleet of sophisticated young women as her call girls and a rotation of well-to-do men as her clientele. Her habitats are no longer the tawdry underbelly of the post/colony but its shiny facades: chic fitness clubs and designer salons, five-star hotels and private wine cellars, exclusive beach spots and seaside mansions. Hers is now a full-service enterprise catering to the high-end needs of high-end patrons, and the film defines Kum's success in the post-1997 economy in terms that reinforce rather than critique neoliberal ideals. What she calls the "new challenges" of Hong Kong's sex trade now serve to entrench regional power elites, including mainland business bosses, while naturalizing their class privilege as mere erotic quirks.

Equally troubling is Ng's perceived need to convert Kum's, and by extension her own, body into a cinematic object of male lust. At the time of its release, *Golden Chicken sss* was heavily promoted as Ng's breakout role as a voluptuous beauty, as the new Kum has been upgraded in not just income and style but breast size. Ng expressly hired a top makeup artist to enhance her breasts to 38G, spending hours on the set each day having "augmentation engineering."[142] Whether this publicity stunt contributed to the movie's runaway box office success, Ng's makeover efforts clearly reflected the industry's ongoing ethos of cultural survival—the lengths Hong Kong cinema would go to in order to remain fashionable and amusing, servicing the tastes and heightening the pleasures of newer elites, in a regional world where Cantophone works are becoming ever more outdated. Indeed, this ethos is not so different from many Stephen Chow comedies, where a spectacle of artificial manic cheer hides profound self-abjection. But if the earlier *Golden Chickens* unapologetically and uncompromisingly gave the spotlight to Kum and Ng sans glitter, by 2014 *Golden Chicken sss* seems to have lost confidence in that down-home aesthetic and its ability to captivate even local audiences.

Fortuitously, as I was wrapping up this chapter in April 2020, COVID-19 was unfolding in a timeline nearly parallel to that of SARS. The figure who emerged again as the face and voice of Hong Kong's pandemic resilience was Sam Hui. Having officially retired in 1992, Hui decided to resume performing in 2004 to help boost Hong Kongers' morale after SARS. His concert series "Keep Smiling with the God of Songs," held in the Hung Hom Coliseum that year and extending over four months into thirty-eight sold-out shows, was

PANDEMIC RESILIENCE   177

attended by a record-breaking 500,000 fans and triggered a wave of Cantopop nostalgia across the city. He conveyed with his very presence the hopeful message that Hong Kong, too, would make a comeback. Moreover, to show that Hong Kong had a younger generation with talent and heart, he composed two new ballads, his first in fourteen years: "Keep Smiling" ("Gai zuk mei siu"/"Jixu weixiao) and "04 Bless You" ("04 zuk fuk nei"/"04 zhufu ni"), which he sang with a group of ten female apprentices he called his "Angels."

In 2020 Hui was originally slated to hold another concert series at Hung Hom in July, but COVID suspended those plans. At his production director's suggestion, he moved the show forward and online, to be livestreamed free of charge. On Easter Sunday, Hui gave a one-hour miniconcert evocatively entitled "Riding in the Same Boat" ("Tung zau gung zai"/"Tongzhougongji"). This is the name of a song he wrote in 1990, in response to the mass exodus ahead of the 1997 handover, meant to "encourage Hong Kong people to face the political change positively, to have faith in Hong Kong and to stay and build [their] home here."[143] The music video had showcased Hui playing his iconic guitar, first on the open deck of a boat in Victoria Harbor, then on an open-top bus. Now as then, rather than broadcasting from a home studio, Hui performed in the open air, at the Tsim Sha Tsui waterfront with Victoria Harbor behind him, accompanied by a simple orchestra, his guitars and harmonica, and, at one point, his son Ryan on electric guitar. To discourage fans from mobbing the area and breaking social distancing rules, event organizers advertised the concert locale as "all major global new media and Hong Kong media outlets." Since Hui himself does not use social media, his sons helped him post a message on his Instagram and Facebook accounts: "To all my dear fans, I know you really want to see me in person and live in concert, but because of the seriousness of the outbreak, I want to use my music to bring positivity and strength to you and all Hong Kongers, but I hope you will all behave and stay home to watch me, so we can fight the epidemic from home together!"[144] His fans complied, and a purported 2.5 million viewers tuned in for the concert.

This feat of lifting Hong Kongers' spirit, what Hui and the local press called *daa hei*, is all the more remarkable in that Hui is now in his seventies, part of the older vulnerable population advised to shelter in place. Not only was he not profiting from the disaster, but, ever mindful of the pandemic's economic impact on local workers, he had also pledged to donate HK$250,000 to his sound production company's staff.[145] In this one hour,

178   CHAPTER 3

a fleeting note of extinctionist melancholy crept in when Hui prefaced the song "Silence Is Golden" ("Cam mak si gam"/"Chenmoshijin") by recalling that he had sung it as a duet with Leslie Cheung, and many listeners would recall that this song was composed by Cheung with lyrics by Hui, an enduring emblem of their legendary friendship. Aptly, though, Hui looped back in his closing anthem to his concert's eponymous ballad, with its original 1997 reference palimpsested now by COVID—but still filled with Cantophone vernacular wit, little-guy sassiness and fighting spirit, and an undying faith in the strength of local peopleness:

> Hong Kong is my heart, [*hoeng gong si ngo sam*]
> an unchanging heart. [*jat fo bat bin sam*]
> I'd really hate to [*sat zoi gik bat jyun*]
> immigrate and become a second-class citizen. [*ji man ngoi gwok zou
> ji dang gung man*]
> Gotta have confidence [*bit seoi pou zyu seon sam*]
> and set a strong foundation. [*baa gei co daa wan*]
> Then if I do my best to do my part, [*zeon lik dei zou ngo bun fan*]
> I'll surely overcome the darkness. [*ding nang dat po zin sing hak am*]
>
> Hong Kong is my home. [*hoeng gong si ngo gaa*]
> How can I bear to lose it? [*zam se dak sat heoi taa*]
> I'd really hate to [*sat zoi gik bat jyun*]
> immigrate and just serve dishes and pour tea. [*ji man ngoi zou dai
> coi za caa*]
> I hug my guitar tight [*gan gan pou zoek gat taa*]
> and pour out my soul, [*king ceot ze sam leoi waa*]
> hoping that through these words [*daan jyun zik zoek ze faan waa*]
> I can vent a little with you together. [*cai cai gung nei faat sit jat haa*]
> In the days ahead under the Lion Rock, [*daan jyun jat hau si zi saan
> haa*]
> may everyone rally [*jan jan tyun git*]
> and never break apart. [*wing bat fan faa*]

Pandemic First Patients
Deperilizing the Anglophone SARS Archive

Pandemic Origin Stories

Throughout the COVID-19 pandemic, SARS-CoV-2's origin has remained a hotly contested issue, on both scientific and geopolitical grounds. Although the prevailing hypothesis from the outset has been that a naturally evolving virus jumped from some animal host to humans, conspiracy-shaded theories about the coronavirus's man-made origins have circulated in global news since as early as January 2020, particularly concerning a possible bioweapons laboratory leak at the Wuhan Institute of Virology.[1] Countering these allegations, some of which came from the US government, Chinese state media has in turn promoted the alternative theory that the coronavirus originated from a bioweapons leak within the US military, at the US Army Medical Research Institute of Infectious Diseases at Maryland's Fort Detrick.[2] In this battle over narrative control of pandemic origins, even the zoonotic thesis about natural viral mutations, presumably the most science-based and least politically invested of the available hypotheses, is rarely free of bio-orientalist tendencies—especially when the trope of "wet markets" is invoked.

Two studies published in *Science* in July 2022, for example, conclude that, contra the lab leak theories, SARS-CoV-2 did in fact emerge "via the live wildlife trade in China" and that it likely involved two "zoonotic jumps from as-yet undetermined, intermediate host animals at the [Wuhan] Huanan market."[3] This news quickly prompted another flurry of international headlines on Wuhan's "wet markets," which had been in the global spotlight during COVID's early days. Strikingly, this time around, the scare quotes around "wet markets" have largely been dropped, in both scientific and popular journalistic outlets, as if the English term is now standard global nomenclature. One of the *Science* studies, for instance, uses the term without quotation marks while offering multiple descriptions of these markets' "live, wild-captured or farmed, mammal species" with barely veiled disgust.[4] As part of its evidence, the article summons an anecdotal and nearly decade-old eyewitness account and photograph by one of its authors, from a 2014 Wuhan visit, of "live raccoon dogs housed in a metal cage stacked on top of a cage with live birds."[5] Amid the georacial politics of pandemic origin stories, the impulse to testify to a Chinese primal scene, replete with ecogothic images of captive and contaminated exotic creatures, runs deep in the Western world. Yet it is not new.

As Mei Zhan has analyzed, global media coverage on SARS throughout 2003 also fixated on "wet markets" and their "wild animals," especially the civet cat, as outlandish fare for the southern Chinese. These sensationalized reports recycled "racialized Orientalist tropes that produce various exotic Others through their excessive pleasures and enjoyments . . . visceraliz[ing] the traditional and the uncanny as the origin of a culturally specific disease that—if not contained—threatens to destroy the global." International debates about SARS's zoonotic origin thus "did not blame nature itself for the SARS outbreak; what went wrong was the Chinese people's uncanny affinity with the nonhuman and the wild," their "strange entanglements of human and animal bodies, and the deadly filthiness of such entanglements" that "breed disease and viruses."[6] As Zhan notes, the term *wet markets*, which "emphasizes the wet and slippery floors—and filthiness, by association—of these markets," soared in English usage during SARS.[7] While this term is also commonly used in anglophone Asian countries, where such traditional open-air food markets are sometimes upheld as a cultural heritage—Singapore's National Heritage Board, for instance, calls them "a microcosm of Singapore's multicultural society" and a treasured "community experience"—the term takes on uniquely bio-orientalist overtones when applied to China.[8] As Christos Lynteris observes in his study of SARS-era epidemic photography, "Wet markets have been singled out as exotic, oriental sites in Euro-American guidebooks and media coverage of China ... synonymous with disorderly human to non-human animal relations and zoonotic emergence." The representation of China as "home to bizarre animals that fail to fall under usual taxonomic categories" has roots in "the colonial construction of the Qing Empire as a kingdom out of joint with the rest of the world," and it "made a comeback during the SARS outbreak, in the shape of widespread media fascination with the masked civet cat."[9] With COVID, this discourse resurges again. As Lynteris and Lyle Fearnley reiterate early on during this pandemic, "In western media, 'wet markets' are portrayed as emblems of Chinese otherness: chaotic versions of oriental bazaars, lawless areas where animals that should not be eaten are sold as food, and where what should not be mingled comes together.... This fuels Sinophobia" by "communicat[ing] a sense of disgust toward the eating habits of the Chinese" even as it "misrepresents the material and economic reality of these markets"—most of which do not sell wild poached animals at all.[10] Indeed, as Yunpeng Zhang and Fang Xu point out, the term *wet market* does not even have an equivalent word in Mandarin Chinese.[11] Hence there exists a fundamental gap between dominant anglophone terminology and domestic language at the pandemic's original epicenter, one that continues to produce and reproduce georacial fractures and discursive power inequities.

This intense focus on zoonotic origins, however, does nothing to shed light on the human dimensions of pandemic experience at the first outbreak sites. What happened to the human origin stories, and why is there so little global attention to them? So eager is the world to hunt down cardinal culprits that the humanity of Chinese first patients has been eclipsed, supplanted by ecogothic stock figures of barbarous animal dealers, bloody-handed butchers, and rabid eaters. In this respect, COVID bio-orientalism is a repetition of SARS bio-orientalism, in its disfigurements as much as ellipses and oversights. This chapter thus takes up the questions: Who were the first SARS patients, what were their experiences, and how did they make sense of their illness? Did they survive, and, if so, what were their post-illness practices, and if not, who kept them company and survived them? In the following pages, I focus on three index cases: in Foshan, Hong Kong, and Singapore. If the previous chapter showcases how deextinctionist resilience is fought hard for and hard-won for Hong Kongers, global pandemic crisis discourse by contrast made easy deaths of SARS's first Chinese patients—even when they did not die. Vis-à-vis SARS's first known index case in particular, anglophone accounts are chock-full of inaccuracies, distortions, and prejudices, premised precisely on zoonotic origin stories that link him to dubious animal farms and "wet markets."

Foshan: Pang Zuoyao

Anglophone Misinformation

If one were to do an internet search on SARS in English today (and I am updating this narrative in December 2022), one of the top hits would likely be the Wikipedia entry on it. There, under the subheading "Outbreak in South China," pandemic origins are narrated as follows: "The SARS epidemic began in the Guangdong province of China in November 2002. The earliest case developed symptoms on 16 November 2002. The index patient, a farmer from Shunde, Foshan, Guangdong, was treated in the First People's Hospital of Foshan. The patient died soon after, and no definite diagnosis was made on his cause of death."[12] A separate Wikipedia entry on "2002–2004 SARS outbreak" provides this companion timeline: "On 16 November 2002, an outbreak of severe acute respiratory syndrome (SARS) began in China's Guangdong province, bordering Hong Kong. The first case of infection was traced to Foshan. This first outbreak affected people in the food industry, such as farmers, market vendors, and chefs. The outbreak spread to healthcare workers after people sought medical treatment for the disease."[13] As I have surveyed elsewhere, numerous other websites on the anglophone internet, not surprisingly, have replicated this narrative, sometimes verbatim.[14] During COVID, anglophone news outlets spanning the United States, the United Kingdom, Europe, and Asia have retrospected on SARS by repeating this very story of its first index case as an anonymous dead farmer from Foshan, Guangdong. Given the widely accepted thesis on SARS's zoonotic origins, contemporary readers are left to connect the dots between the virus's animal hosts and the Chinese farmer who first contaminated himself by living in close proximity to them. In line with Zhan's argument, the dead farmer story subtly implies a "deadly filthiness" to the Chinese's "strange entanglements of human and animal bodies."

Nor is this narrative restricted to online sources. Print references to SARS's primal farmer have long appeared in English-language scientific and academic venues, from a 2005 *Pediatric Annals* article on animal viruses to a 2006 *Urban Studies* article on global cities and infectious disease to a 2007 *Lancet* book review. By now, the notion that the world's first SARS patient was a Foshan/Guangdong farmer has entered into anglophone pandemic lore, dispersed across, among other things, a virology textbook, a guide on sustainability and corporate responsibility, a crisis management reference work, a mathematical engineering study, as well as myriad mass-market books on climate change, emerging viruses, and pandemic outbreaks.[15] Even Ali Khan, the former director of the US CDC Office of Public Health Preparedness and Response, affirms this version of events in his 2016 book *The Next Pandemic*: "The official narrative" for SARS, he writes, "traces the first reported case to Guangdong Province, China. This was mid-November 2002, and the patient, a farmer, was treated in the First People's Hospital of Foshan, and then promptly died."[16] What further unites all these anglophone accounts is the allegation, sometimes explicit, other times strongly insinuated, that the farmer not only infected himself and those around him but initiated a nuclear chain infection that ultimately culminated in a catastrophic global pandemic.

The problem with this "official narrative," however, is that it is replete with egregious errors and orientalist biases. In reality, SARS's first known patient was *not* a peasant farmer, he was *not* at the center of an explosive outbreak cluster, he did *not* kill anyone, and, above all, he did *not* die from the virus. In reality, he was an elected local official with an administrative office job; he directly infected only two family members but no healthcare workers; this was a contained cluster with five infections total and no fatalities; and he lived on to tell his tale ten years later.

Reconstructing Pang's Life

His name is Pang Zuoyao. In November 2002, he was the deputy chief of Bitang Village. Though categorized as a village, Bitang is a thriving industrial town in the heart of Foshan, a city of over three million by the early 2000s. "The people in this village are quite wealthy," according to migrant workers who come here looking for factory jobs, "and you can earn a lot just with annual bonuses."[17] Pang's was an elected position, one that he would continue to hold for at least another decade. At the time, he was also vice chair of the local shareholding economic cooperative.[18] By the early 2000s, most local enterprises had been privatized, so Pang's work consisted mainly of managing real estate and sometimes overseeing family planning issues.[19] He was relatively well-to-do, living with his wife and four children in a four-story house.[20] His oldest son was applying for college that year, his daughter was about to enter high school, and his youngest child was a rising fifth-grader.[21] By all indications, he was a low-level cadre leading a comfortable middle-class life in China's liberalizing economy.

It was also this set of personal circumstances that afforded Pang and his family access to advanced healthcare and that led to their surviving SARS. On November 16, Pang developed a high fever, headache, dry cough, and weakness and was rushed to the hospital closest to his house, the second-tier Shiwan People's Hospital. After nine days, his fever persisted, so he was transferred to the top-tier Foshan No. 1 People's Hospital. There, he was admitted to the isolation ward and then transferred to the intensive care unit, where he was put on a ventilator—all treatments available only to those with financial means.[22] Throughout that period, Pang's family visited him at the hospital every day, and, since no one knew to take precautions, he infected both his wife and his maternal aunt, and the latter in turn infected her husband and daughter. All five family members were hospitalized, but, in the end, all recovered, and Pang himself was discharged on January 8, 2003.[23] None of his children at home caught the virus, nor did any of his Bitang neighbors or hospital workers who cared for the family. According to several early epidemiological studies on SARS, this Foshan outbreak, the first one known to us, was an intrafamilial cluster with only five patients, and the transmission chain ended there.[24] So, despite being SARS's first known cluster, it was not the spark that ignited a global infection chain. As one of Pang's physicians commented afterward, this case could be considered a "miracle."[25]

Later on, Pang would be identified as the world's first known SARS patient, the pandemic's first index case. At the time, though, no one knew this was a new virus, least of all Pang himself. Even the ICU director at the Foshan hospital who oversaw Pang's case remembered calling it simply a "respiratory infectious disease of unclear cause."[26] Pang was never formally diagnosed with SARS, and, in fact, according to his wife, the hospital's initial diagnosis was food poisoning.[27] Technically, Pang was SARS's first index case but not its primary case: the former term refers to "the patient in an outbreak who is first noticed by the health authorities, and who makes them aware that an outbreak might be emerging," whereas the latter refers to "the person who first brings a disease into a group of people."[28] With SARS as with many other infectious disease outbreaks, the primary case may never come to light, insofar as we do not know who was the new coronavirus's first human host who transmitted it to others. But in the world's eagerness to hunt down a primal human causal agent for the pandemic, narratives of Pang such as the dead farmer one tend to frame him as primary rather than index case, effectively suppressing the possibility that he, too, might have been the unsuspecting victim of human infection.

For his part, Pang's processing of his own disease experience was protracted and traumatic. A few months after his discharge, after the coronavirus had been identified and as the pandemic raged worldwide, Pang and his family still found it hard to believe that what they had suffered was SARS. "I don't even know if I am related to what happened elsewhere," he told a *Los Angeles Times* staff writer over the phone in April. "The day I left the hospital, they said they didn't know what I had."[29] Likewise, Mrs. Pang told the *South China Morning Post* journalist Leu Siew Ying in person that month, "I find it baffling [that people say we had SARS] because no one in my family has the illness. My husband's parents and his seven siblings and my parents and my own four siblings spent time with him during the day or visited him regularly. None of them fell sick." Pointing to the town traffic, she speculated, "I think it is the air pollution that is making us ill."[30] To reporters from Guangzhou's *21st Century Business Herald* (*21 shiji jingji baodao*), Mrs. Pang pleaded, "[My husband] is very busy with work, and he has a stress prone personality . . . so please don't bother us anymore."[31] Another few months later, Pang himself remained terse with reporters both domestic and foreign. "I have completely recovered," he declared to Leu on her follow-up visit, with an emphasis on recovery that had become a refrain for him. "If you are concerned about sick people go to the hospitals. You are wasting your time with me."[32] "Let the past be the past," he implored several other journalists from Guangzhou's *Southern Weekend* (*Nanfang zhoumo*) who tracked him down in 2006. More resigned now to the SARS diagnosis, he told them, "I don't want to think about it anymore. I myself have no idea why I caught SARS. When I got sick, there wasn't yet the term 'atypical pneumonia.' Properly speaking, I was only retroactively labeled a SARS patient."[33] One oft-cited comment by the respiratory specialist and "SARS hero" Zhong Nanshan— whose investigative team first coined the term *feidian*—is that 96 percent of China's SARS patients had no clear contact history, so for them, the whole episode was like "bafflingly having a nightmare."[34] For Pang especially, the virus must have struck like something utterly out of the blue, supernatural and uncanny. If the disease itself left, the stain of it lingered, branding him the global index case, a designation he had no power to reject. He had little time to narrate the experience for himself and to give it personal meaning before the external world descended to take over his story.

For much of the decade after SARS, Pang kept a low profile, dodging all media attention.[35] For a period that summer, his family even vacated their Bitang house and went into hiding.[36] What little we know of his actual post-SARS life comes from a handful of articles based on the few interviews he and his family granted over the years, primarily to journalists from southern China. One significant impact the disease episode had on him and his family, as he related to provincial reporters, was economic. The medical bills for his family had come to 400,000 RMB, a not insubstantial sum for a village-level official, even a well-off one like Pang. "At the time I thought, out of nowhere came this strange disease, and, just like that, 400,000 yuan gone. What a waste," he said. "But then I thought, if you lose your life, what's the point of mourning the loss of money?"[37]

Indeed, SARS had a deep and lasting impact on Pang's lifestyle and value system. In the half-year following his hospitalization, he remained physically weak and would gasp for breath after climbing a few flights of stairs.[38] He became much more health conscious as a result, quitting smoking and giving up alcohol, taking up regular tai chi and long-distance jogging. He also stopped dining out, and, every day at noon, he unfailingly drove home from work to eat a lunch prepared by his wife, meticulously washing his hands before every meal.[39] Ten years on, he kept up these habits. By then in his mid-fifties, he continued to serve as Bitang's deputy chief. As he remarked to a reporter from *Blog World* (*Boke tianxia*) in 2012, "I take my work seriously every single day, and I intend to work hard until my retirement. If there's a change in me, it's that I give greater importance to health and family now."[40] SARS also made him more fastidious about hygiene. Guangzhou reporters from *Information Times* (*Xinxi shibao*) noted in 2013 that, after receiving guests in his office, Pang would wash all the cups by hand and then sterilize them in a disinfecting cupboard next to the sofa.[41] All these routines grew out of Pang's brush with SARS, the small residual effects of his disease experience and the enduring transformations of his everyday life thereafter.

At the same time, these self-care practices may have embodied Pang's coping mechanisms for the physical trauma of the ordeal and its various mental health side effects. One Hong Kong study found that 45 percent of recovered SARS patients developed one or more mental illnesses within three weeks of discharge: 13 percent suffered from organic mood syndrome, 11 percent from major depression, 11 percent from adjustment disorders, 7 percent from posttraumatic stress, 5 percent from generalized anxiety, and 2 percent from transient delirium or psychosis. Those who had been in an ICU had a higher likelihood of developing one of these conditions, and many survivors additionally "complained of profound lethargy and disturbing forgetfulness."[42] There is no public record of Pang ever seeking professional therapy, but the person who emerges from these published accounts fits the profile of someone struggling with posttraumatic stress and anxiety as well as someone who eschewed institutionalized treatment in favor of alternative self-healing.

In his case, disease survival was compounded by the stigma of being the world's first known SARS patient. When the WHO investigative team to China visited Pang's house in April 2003, word got out and "it was clear to everyone in his neighborhood that it was him," according to Robert Breiman, the team's leader. "He told me that this created many problems."[43] As some of Pang's neighbors admitted to reporters later that summer, "At first, we didn't know who [the SARS patient among us] was. After we knew that he got SARS, we didn't want to have any connection with him."[44] Years later, the family still remembered how their neighbors gossiped about and blamed Pang for unleashing a global plague. In one workplace dispute, Pang's SARS diagnosis was brought up against him, an incident that put him on guard thereafter for political rivals weaponizing his medical history against him.[45] In the post-SARS decade then, Pang rarely spoke of his SARS history and hid it from most coworkers, even deliberately distancing himself from the doctors and nurses who had treated him and his family. His attending physician at the time sympathized with this evasion: "Foshan people are very practical and low-key. Besides, this isn't something anyone would want to grab the limelight for," the doctor commiserated.[46] Over time, to Pang's longtime colleagues and relatives, it seemed as if SARS had never happened, as if it had been wiped clean from his memory, whether by design or repression.[47] These, then, were also things that lived through SARS and trailed Pang for years: ostracism and stigma, uncertainty and suspicion, forgetting and self-silencing.

Perhaps what gnawed at Pang the most was the accusation, and the possibility, that his own dietary habits did in fact cause a new deadly human virus. Like many of his neighbors, Pang used to enjoy eating wild animals, or *yewei*. About a month or so prior to falling sick, he had traveled with a friend to Guangxi Province and brought home some game meat.[48] And about a week before his hospitalization, he had dined on "wild cat meat" with a friend twice and again brought some home for his family.[49] During that period, he also prepared various meat dishes at home, including "chicken, domestic cat, and snake."[50] But, significantly, none of those who shared these meals became infected.[51] "My husband ate mutton and cat meat before he fell ill," recalled Mrs. Pang. "He said cat meat was good for his backache, so sometimes he has cat meat outside and sometimes I cook it at home. Most people here eat cat meat, but nobody has SARS."[52]

As Judith Farquhar suggests in her "anthropology of the mundane," everyday consumption practices in the reform era may carry a posttraumatic as well as postmemorial residue tied to the deprivations and starvations of the Maoist past, whereby eating itself becomes a set of personal reckonings with historical "excess and deficiency." She captures the mental calculus around eating thus: "How much enjoyment or bulk is justifiable for the fortunate in a world where starvation is all too real for some of their neighbors? Is there value in 'high' civilization (gourmet food, for example) if many of the socially 'low' have no access to its sophisticated pleasures? Can past famine justify indulgence in present and future gluttony?"[53] The Pangs, born right before and during the 1958–61 Great Famine years, would have lived through this history, with SARS as the latest event in an ongoing national dialectical grappling with lack and surplus. Maybe, to some degree, the pandemic interrupted their reliance on that calculus and helped redefine well-being from endless consumption to equilibrium upkeep. In any event, the Pangs abandoned their wildlife diet after their infection, opting instead for healthy dishes such as plain steamed fish.

According to their daughter, though, Pang never accepted the zoonotic thesis about SARS, despite mounting scientific consensus. In the ten years after, he never ceased searching for an alternative cause for the coronavirus. Like his wife, he pointed to environmental factors such as industrial pollution as the root of his illness. He often suspected that the exhaust gas from a funeral parlor near his workplace was the true culprit, and he repeatedly campaigned to have the funeral parlor relocated, even enlisting for help the media he so assiduously avoided otherwise.[54] This, too, merits consideration

PANDEMIC FIRST PATIENTS   189

as a small act of local eco-activism, as epidemic experience bred skepticism toward the state's economic development goals and an awareness of the human reverberations of environmental contamination.

First Patient Microagency

I patch together this reconstruction of Pang's story in order to highlight that, even for its first patient, SARS infection and survival can be narrated in the terms not of perpetual emergency and pandemic crisis but of ordinary resilience. Medical authorities and experts might reach for the magical or the occult to explain the scientifically inexplicable aspects of SARS and Pang's case—a "miracle," a "nightmare"—but Pang himself seemed to want nothing more than a restoration of the normal and the prosaic. Not so unlike Ru Yan in Hu Fayun's *Such Is This World*, Pang lived beyond SARS by turning to aspects of his domestic life that allowed for small and everyday agency, such as quitting risk-raising old habits and initiating new self-nourishing routines. Indeed, his reformed lifestyle resonates with Western biomedical paradigms that emphasize personal health regimens such as diet, nutrition, and exercise to prevent endemic disease. In the process, he reoriented himself away from the raw accumulation of economic, political, and social capital toward bodily self-care and familial care. These mundane changes in his daily life did not carry any noticeable impact on the national or global stage, nor did they amount to any grand gesture of revolution or resistance. As a whole, Pang's story does not lend itself so easily to either prefabricated cautionary tales of disastrous contagion or geopolitical critiques of communist totalitarian biopower. In a much quieter but not quietist way, his story bespeaks a rebuilding of personal world, a form of autopoietic resilience, where survival is not a passive condition but a process of corporeal maintenance, to be continually enacted through everyday embodied practices. These in turn facilitate a transfer of sentimental attachment, an affective shift away from the rationales of both the party-state system and the postsocialist neoliberal market, toward a self-valuing ethics and deeper kinship intimacies.

Rather than interpret these living practices cynically, as a naive buying into the false promises of the good life in an individualist capitalist society, what Lauren Berlant would call the slow death of cruel optimism, we might see in Pang a conscious embrace of a nonelitist biopolitics of care, salvaged from the postcrisis scene of epidemic illness. If Anna Tsing glosses "conditions of precarity" as "life without the promise of stability," then a nonexceptionalist ethics and self-organizing biopolitics such as Pang's testify to a desire for postprecarity, a faith in the possibility of everyday life's meaningful continuance, after disease catastrophe, through small acts of recreated stability.[55] Similar to Ru Yan's decision to not resume her internet writerly persona at the end of Hu's novel, Pang's post-SARS life was marked by his decision to eschew media attention, which was also an act of not relinquishing his right to live beyond his illness on his own terms, of not ceding his epidemic story over to those already endowed with an inordinate share of power in constructing macro pandemic narratives.

While many scholars have analyzed the racist and orientalist dimensions of the SARS outbreak, few have heeded the Chinese index patients themselves, particularly how surviving first patients such as Pang went on to embody new practices and reshape their own living relations to animals and consumption, thus modeling the transition to postepidemic renewal at disease epicenters. These modifications in bodily conduct toward self and others, both human and nonhuman, deserve attention as *re*emergent forms of life. Rather than flashy bioforms at the frontiers of cybernetics and biotechnology, here we observe precisely a retreat from translocal hybrid networks both human-social and human-animal. We observe a forgoing of participation in anthropocentric cultures of species extraction, displacement, and incorporation, and a deliberate return to smaller scales and more proximate relations of living. Even micro decisions and inner commitments—such as a determined letting go of one's appetite for certain foods, or of one's involvement in certain toxic networks of mediatized social community—can encapsulate profound ethical responses to pandemic assemblages and crises. Withdrawing from one's neighboring regimes of ingestion and refocusing on the locality of one's household, leaving be and dwelling alongside the creatures deemed ingestible, releasing attachment to limitless wealth concentration and historically compensatory pleasure, and carving out the parameters of what one considers actually livable togetherness—these, too, constitute performances of Tsing's "collaborative survival," the ordinary and minute navigations of personal "living-space entanglements."[56] In the wake of pandemic ruin, these, too, instantiate means of recovering life, of rethinking living.

Perhaps most of all, I insist on reconstructing Pang's life because it is startlingly absent in English. As far as I know, this narrative arc of Pang's encounter with and survival of SARS—though fragmentary and mediated, and slim by any serious biographer's yardstick—is missing from the anglophone archive altogether. Of course, anglophone discourse is not homogeneous, and I am not suggesting that no writer in English has given an accurate and good-faith rendition of Pang's story. Among anglophone journalism on SARS, aside from Leu Siew Ying's conscientious investigative work for *South China Morning Post*, Hong Kong–based Thomas Abraham's *Twenty-First Century Plague* also stands out for its impartial style that refrains from sensationalist pandemic tropes and bio-orientalist conventions. In this book, Pang, though unnamed, is correctly identified as "a 46-year-old local government official," and the Foshan outbreak is correctly described as involving five family members and no hospital staff and not spreading beyond the city.[57] Abraham's work, though, is more the exception than the rule in anglophone journalism on SARS. One might expect that, as the world's first known patient of this century's first global pandemic, Pang Zuoyao would be a familiar name in the annals of SARS, or, at the very least, that the outlines of his lived experience would have been documented by someone, whether through direct investigation or translation, for an anglophone readership. Yet the exact opposite is true. On a most basic level, his name has largely vanished from the anglophone public record. This erasure may have partly come about from a well-intentioned assumption that anonymity protects the patient and his family, though in practice it has mostly enabled the replication and recirculation of false narratives about him.

More insidiously, this erasure feeds contemporary bio-orientalist perceptions of China as a totalizing terror state. One best-selling and critically acclaimed mass-market book on human pandemics, David Quammen's *Spillover*, for example, strongly intimates that the first patient's "name goes unmentioned" in all of the author's research because the Chinese government has censored Pang's story.[58] This claim echoes tabloid news that entrenched the idea for anglophone readers that the "identity of the first recorded victim remains a closely guarded secret"—when the sinophone sources I draw on here are readily available on the Chinese internet.[59] The politics of SARS representation in the anglophone realm thus remains profoundly caught up in a post–Cold War ideology of China as the West's totalitarian other, and index case narratives often reiterate Xiaobing Tang's dissidence hypothesis. This dynamic was exacerbated at the time by the anticommunist activism of certain high-profile diasporic elites such as the Chinese Canadian journalist Jan Wong. Writing for the Toronto *Globe and Mail* that spring, Wong declared that "these first deaths [from SARS] went unremarked" by the Chinese government because "life is cheap, apparently, when there are 1.4 billion lives," especially when these lives belonged to peasants in "a third-world city" like Foshan.[60] When writers such as Wong refer to "a cover-up," they generalize beyond actual acts of censorship and end up replicating global misinformation or suppressing even well-known accounts circulating publicly within sinophone platforms. Indeed, had anglophone researchers delved into the epidemiological literature on Guangdong's early outbreak clusters, some of which were already published in English-language science journals by late 2003 and 2004, they would have learned that none of the index cases were "farmers handling livestock or poultry" or "commercial farmers," and that "living near a farm" was not "associated with increased risk."[61] The recognition of this one scientific finding would have dispelled the dead farmer myth for good.

Yet, not only was the farmer template left to stand intact, but, within a decade, another set of wildly fallacious and deeply orientalist stories surfaced about Pang—including accounts of him as a businessman or salesman, a wild animal trader or dealer, and an exotic game restaurant chef.[62] This specific discourse proliferated a lexicon whereby terms such as *wet markets, exotic animals, wild animals, animal dealers, animal traders,* and *food handlers* all became interchangeable, functioning as synecdoches for a larger script about SARS's cultural origins in China's perverse consumptive habits. In anglophone journalistic accounts at the time, even as horrified Westerners voyeuristically obsessed over the ghastly filth and gore of China's "wet markets" as the explosive hubs of emerging viral outbreaks, the accusatory focus was more often than not on the Chinese who captured, caged, maimed, slaughtered, cooked, and ate those poor wild creatures rather than the creatures themselves as disease carriers.[63] The unstated judgment against Chinese brutality in the gourmet wildlife trade was staged on anglophone writers' and readers' shared sympathy for the doomed animals, not SARS's human victims. The underlying message often seemed to be that the animals themselves were morally faultless and would have remained biologically harmless, too, had they been left alone in their natural habitats, and that the agency to be feared and scorned rested squarely with the aberrant Chinese who dislocated, trafficked, and consumed these animals out of profit-seeking and self-indulgent gustatory pleasure; indeed, if SARS's first cases were animal dealers and wild game chefs, then they karmically received what they had meted out. This bio-orientalist script brought SARS first patients ever closer to an imagined zone of heightened contagion and blurred boundaries between human and beast, civilization and wilderness, proper and transgressive interaction with the nonhuman world. Pang, for one, was transfigured from someone who occasionally dined out on *yewei* with friends and prepared it at home for family into a professional agent complicit in the fetid system of wildlife exploitation. These stories were told and retold, taking hold of the popular anglophone imagination until they bore almost no resemblance to the real Pang, who lived on as if in a parallel universe.

Heyuan: Huang Xingchu

Before moving on, let me briefly draw out the parallels between Pang's story and that of Huang Xingchu—SARS's second known index patient, the first case in the Heyuan outbreak cluster and the one around whom the animal chef or trader myth devastatingly coalesced. In 2002 Huang was in his mid-thirties and in good health. He was a resident of Heyuan, a Guangdong city of about three million, and a chef who worked in a Hakka restaurant in nearby Shenzhen.[64] Like Pang, unbeknownst to himself, Huang somehow contracted SARS and fell ill around the first week of December and was later admitted to a local hospital; two days later, he was transferred to the top-tier Guangzhou Military General Hospital.[65] Like Pang, he survived and was discharged on January 10, just two days after Pang's discharge in neighboring Foshan.[66] And like Pang, he unwittingly infected several people around him, in his case seven healthcare workers. But here, too, everyone recovered, and the outbreak remained a contained cluster with no fatalities.[67] As the local hospital director remarked years later, "One thing that makes me proud is that, even though Heyuan had the first [*sic*] global case of SARS with nineteen infections afterward, not one person died."[68]

Crucially, Huang's work did not involve the handling and killing of wildlife. At his restaurant, he might have come into "regular contact with several types of live caged animals used as exotic game food," according to one early epidemiological study, but a later study lists his animal contact history as "unknown" and further notes that his work was "mainly stir-frying and did not involve killing animals."[69] This latter task was left, Huang himself explained, to "unskilled laborers."[70] Yet, because of his occupation, he was soon branded "Poison King" (*duwang*) by both the domestic and international press, which jumped to the conclusion that he must have been exceptionally tainted by the virus. From the early months of SARS to the decade after, alongside the dead farmer narrative, anglophone journalism as much as academic and scientific literature entrenched the idea that the new coronavirus "first appeared among chefs and butchers working with exotic meats in the Guangdong province of southern China."[71] As a Guangdong chef who had the misfortune of being the index case of an early cluster, Huang was hit hard by these rumors. As the primary earner for his family and someone dependent on a jobs economy, he, more so than Pang, had to endure the impact of this disease misinformation on his employment and livelihood. After his recuperation, he went back to work at his old Shenzhen restaurant, hoping to resume a "normal life," but his return triggered a dramatic decline in the restaurant's business, as patrons learned that the "Poison King" worked there and stayed away. He lost his job and was wracked with hopelessness and guilt about being a burden on those around him, including his former boss.[72] "I am a normal man and my greatest wish is to have work at once so as to support my family," he told the Chinese state media that summer. "I sincerely hope that society won't despise people who have fully recovered just like me. We are healthy people. This is one of the reasons why I met the media with courage today."[73] In the years after, however, he too, like Pang, started to dodge media attention. A decade later in 2013, he would continue to protest, "I was not the origin of SARS, I was a victim." Echoing Pang's words in letter and spirit, he pleaded, "I have no idea when and where I contracted the illness.... I have avoided approaching most old friends and workmates I knew for years. And I seldom even go back to my hometown, the village where I grew up. I just don't want to bring up the matter of the past. I would like to do everything to let the world just forget me."[74]

For Huang, the myth of an originary wild game chef who sparked a worldwide plague brought damaging consequences close to home. While he did not directly or indirectly cause anyone's death, he nonetheless felt "tormented by a guilty conscience" months and years later.[75] This was one trickle-down effect, perhaps, of macro pandemic narratives that, however much he knew them to be untrue, persisted in impugning him with primal responsibility for global deaths. And in the confused anglophone reporting on SARS, the conflation of Pang with Huang, and of Huang with another chef from Zhongshan as well as a Guangzhou seafood merchant who later also came to be called "Poison King," all led to the impression that this shadowy composite figure from southern China was the precursor "patient zero" who infected Liu Jianlun, Hong Kong's index case. The rest, presumably, was history.

Hong Kong: Liu Jianlun

If Pang Zuoyao's name has largely been lost to the anglophone SARS archive, Liu Jianlun's, by contrast, is a narrative staple. Compared to Pang, anglophone accounts of Liu are not as outrageously erroneous or contradictory, and there exists a relatively stable story with relatively accurate outlines: Liu was an elderly doctor from Guangzhou who contracted the virus while treating hospitalized patients there and then transmitted the disease to a number of others at the Metropole Hotel in Hong Kong, where he stayed overnight on February 21, 2003; from there, those infected by Liu traveled home or farther abroad, precipitating major outbreaks in Hong Kong as well as Hanoi, Singapore, and Toronto. Liu himself died of SARS on March 4. But here, even more blatantly than with Pang, bio-orientalist and sinophobic biases shape the central narrative, through selective omissions and slanted framing of details bent toward the sinister. This narrative tends to portray Liu as a blameworthy foreign agent who globalized the virus and endangered the entire planet. What Alan Kraut calls "medicalized nativism," whereby "pre-existing nativist prejudices" against immigrant groups are justified through a public health paradigm linking the foreign-born to disease and contamination, has itself become globalized in the new millennium.[76] Now, the remote foreigner does not have to enter into a host country to be perceived as a domestic threat, needing only to step into a city hotel elevator or take a cross-border bus on the other side of the world to be deemed a transgressor of global health and a jeopardy to global biosecurity. No surprise, then, that such a racialized ecogothic imagination, when coupled with the fear effect of pandemic crisis epistemologies, leaves room for a few conspiracy theories to thrive and persist about Liu.

Key to this narrative of Liu are two tropes in contemporary infectious disease discourse: *patient zero* and *superspreader*. These terms, unlike the more neutral *index patient* or *index case*, are freighted with connotations not just of superlative deadliness but also of a measure of biological and moral malice. Constructed not just as Hong Kong's index case but as the global pandemic's "patient zero" and original "superspreader," Liu came to symbolize an uncanny biological villain within the hyperconnected terrain of globalization. These constructions exemplify what Megan Glick calls "infrahumanist ontologies," turning Chinese first patients such as Liu into "forms of nonvaluable life."[77] In turn, SARS took on the quality of a new mutated variant of an old civilizational menace, reinvigorating a yellow peril worldview that fanned

196   CHAPTER 4

social discrimination against Chinese and other Asians around the world during the pandemic, especially those perceived as coming from outbreak "hot spots."[78] Stories of Liu enacted and validated such georacial targeting, epitomizing the disease bio-orientalism that we see resurging today amid COVID.

"Patient Zero" and "Superspreader"

In the anglophone news media in 2003 as in 2020, Liu Jianlun remains the person most often identified as SARS's "patient zero." The meaning of this term is not always clear or consistent. A 2013 CNN article on "SARS Fast Facts," for instance, updated in June 2020, names Liu as "patient zero, or the first person to die of the disease," and he is said to have developed symptoms "on a trip from Huang Xingchu in the Guangdong province to visit family in Hong Kong" and then died of the disease there.[79] Aside from confusing Huang Xingchu for a place name, this article is obviously flawed in logic since there were other SARS fatalities before Liu, contradicting even the article's own timeline of events, which states that five people died of SARS in Guangdong from November 2002 to February 2003. The use of the term *patient zero*, then, serves an alternative purpose, operating as a convenient signifier to launch the narrative of global pandemic crisis and endowing it with the aura of an absolute beginning. From the perspective of global health, Liu is the index patient who matters—as opposed to the often unnamed Pang, who can henceforth be relegated to a mysterious prehistory. As one April 2003 *Guardian* article puts it, Liu as SARS's "patient zero" was "the human conduit who unwittingly turned a personal tragedy into a global threat," on what the article's title quips as "the day the world caught a cold." Here, the "patient zero" trope enables a mode of brisk storytelling that draws a straight vector from Liu to "the world" and then "global threat." Despite the seemingly forgiving "unwittingly," the article conjectures that perhaps Liu did not journey to Hong Kong simply to attend a family wedding but had wanted to seek medical treatment there, hence insinuating that Liu *did* know he was "harbouring something local medicine could not cure" and then knowingly carried it across the China–Hong Kong border.[80] It is this double-edged zone of signification, implying simultaneously woundedness and culpability, a liminal state between victim and killer, that the language of "patient zero" puts into play.

    Patient zero also conjures up the cognate term *ground zero*, with its overtones of nuclear explosions and, increasingly since 9/11, terrorist attacks. In this rhetorical echo chamber, it is as if an index patient were not so much human as human bomb, the tool of a biomilitary assault and disaster. One 2020 CNBC report typifies this usage by referring to the Metropole Hotel as "a SARS hotspot and a ground zero for the disease that spread across the globe after Liu's stay." The idiom of destructive magnitude, of the numerical enormity of Liu's global reach and detonation effect, swiftly enters in, as the article emphasizes that "roughly 4000 of the world's total SARS cases (about half) during that outbreak could be traced back to Liu's stay at the Metropole Hotel."[81]

Richard McKay, writing on the revival of the *patient zero* term during COVID, observes that these stories may "seem motivated by science," but "scratch a little deeper . . . and you will often uncover a desire to assign blame."[82] As he explains, the term *patient zero* was first coined via a procedural accident, when AIDS researchers misread the labeling of an "Out-of-California" patient and the letter "O" as the number "0" in a study of a Los Angeles outbreak. Randy Shilts's bestseller *And the Band Played On*, however, decisively sensationalized the term by tying the global spread of HIV/AIDS to a single "Patient Zero," the French Canadian flight attendant Gaétan Dugas, whom Shilts portrayed as a reckless gay man who ignored public health warnings about unprotected sex because he wanted to infect as many people as possible.[83] As Priscilla Wald notes, discursive constructions such as "patient zero" and "superspreader" are part of the formulaic conventions of a modern "outbreak narrative": the "unwitting role in the spread of the new virus turned these unfortunate sufferers into stock characters of a familiar tale . . . from victims to agents—and embodiments—of the spreading infection."[84] Through Shilts's book, Dugas transforms from an early patient into a "human-virus hybrid" and a "foreign agent whose behavior posed a threat to the body politic that required his excision," in an interlocking of homophobia, xenophobia, and racism.[85] In the lineage of global pandemic discourse, Dugas is an ancestor to Liu: even posthumously, both men continue to be constructed as racialized aliens with potentially perverse motives, transgressive border-crossers who kindled global outbreaks with some degree of conscious intent.

Even more so than "patient zero," Liu is often identified in anglophone sources as the supreme "superspreader" who globalized SARS—"among the most famous 'super-spreaders' of modern history," as one virologist puts it.[86] According to the *Oxford English Dictionary*, the word *superspreader* first appeared in the English language in 1973, in a *Journal of Infectious Diseases* article on influenza. But the term was not widely used until SARS, when it was popularized by health officials and science journalists, taking on the quality of a distinctly contemporary phenomenon. When the SARS virus first emerged in China, it was predominantly a sinophone disease, a topic discussed primarily in Chinese, but, by March 2003, it had become internationalized as a global health issue. With WHO's involvement, SARS became definitively anglicized. In early April, after the WHO investigative team was given access into Guangdong, the lead investigator Robert Breiman reported that his team was especially interested in "the phenomenon of 'super spreaders'—people who seem to spread their disease to a lot of other people," a remark that was then extensively repeated by anglophone news outlets worldwide.[87] David Heymann, who directed WHO's global SARS response, soon echoed this emphasis on the need to determine "why some people appear to be superspreaders and others are not," further entrenching the impression that the term had become official within top public health circles.[88] Even though some WHO officers at the time tried to debunk its use and put forth "superspreading event" as a less stigmatizing alternative, by mid-April and May the term had become ubiquitous in anglophone news media.[89]

For the most part, writers did not have a standard definition for the *superspreader* concept and used the word loosely, and, in the absence of precise meaning, they often resorted to fear-provoking metaphors. One *New York Times* article in mid-April 2003, for example, opened with the alarming similes that "some people are hyperinfective, spewing germs out like teakettles while others simmer quietly like stew pots," and its sinister headline "How One Person Can Fuel an Epidemic" itself fueled the impression of exceptional singular causation.[90] This same article was reprinted on subsequent days by other newspapers around the world that carried similarly ominous headlines such as "Doctors Worry That 'Superspreaders' Are Dotting the Map with SARS" and "Tracking Typhoid Marys: One-Person Epidemics."[91] Ironically, in the anglophone world, the lexicon of *superspreader* was much more pervasive than the actual empirical phenomenon it referred to, haunting even countries with single-digit cases and/or no fatalities. Its ubiquity in anglophone news, however, especially in major American media outlets, was instrumental in disseminating the fear effect of pandemic crisis discourse, putting into global circulation and cementing a set of themes about the fragility of the globalized world, the rapid reproduction of microbial threats, and the moral necessity of fear.

Anglophone accounts on Liu not only have been key to this pandemic crisis discourse but have helped to georacially sinicize it. Later that April, the *New York Times* ran a front-page feature on SARS with the headline "From China's Provinces, a Crafty Germ Breaks Out," thereby anthropomorphically marking the virus as Chinese. The article identified several "super-spreaders" and explicitly named Liu as the person who "unleashed [SARS] on the world." This time, the people Liu infected were described as "dispers[ing] on airplanes like bees carrying a deadly pollen, seeding SARS locally and to far corners of the world."[92] The article title already set into motion a rhetoric of evil intelligence and fugitive deceit, but the trope of killer bees further racialized the virus, as these insects are commonly called "Africanized honeybees" and sometimes "murder hornets" in English. Evoking the ecogothic plotlines of biohorror movies about animal vengeance, this trope subtly affiliated African and Chinese life-forms as homicidal alien invaders. Simon Estok has theorized that, beneath the popular discourse of ecophilia or our supposed human love of nature, there often lies an unrecognized "ecophobia"—the "contempt and fear we feel for the agency of the natural environment" as "an opponent that hurts, hinders, threatens, or kills us." This ecophobia, he suggests, is "thoroughly interwoven" with social power structures based on "irrational and groundless hatred" such as "racism, misogyny, homophobia, speciesism."[93] Anglophone SARS reporting on Liu illuminates the bio-orientalist dimension of this ecophobia. Indeed, long before Donald Trump dubbed SARS-CoV-2 a "China virus" and "China plague" in 2020, that sinophobic vocabulary was already flourishing in anglophone coverage on SARS, with multiple news outlets worldwide labeling it the "Chinese virus" and "Chinese plague," in a direct prehistory to our pandemic present.[94]

If we were to exonerate headline news and digital media for resorting to narrative shortcuts, it is the full-length humanistic investigative works that arguably most incriminate and dehumanize Liu. In my analysis of *City of SARS* in the previous chapter, I touched on how the urban elevator represents a zone of heightened disease danger in SARS iconography, a spatial synecdoche for the overpopulated global city and a metaphorical "ground zero" for planetary contamination. One example of this elevator chronotope that ties directly to Liu appears in the 2008 documentary *The Silent Killer: SARS*, produced by the New York–based Films Media Group. In a dramatic reenactment of the Metropole Hotel outbreak, the documentary depicts a hypothetical scenario in which a sickly Liu coughs violently, open-mouthed, inside a filling hotel elevator. An "outbreak expert" then states that "approximately 50% of all the SARS cases in the world were epidemiologically linked

200   CHAPTER 4

back to this Chinese physician from Guangdong province," thereby casting Liu as a hyperinfectious hub and pandemic first cause.[95] Crucial to the tacit impugning of individual responsibility here is the portrayal of Liu as an already symptomatic body: the film visually implies that, as a physician, Liu should have known better than to travel while sick and that it was his lapse in professional judgment as much as his social inconsiderateness that exposed global others to "killer" germs.

An earlier anglophone source for this elevator trope is Karl Taro Greenfeld's oft-cited mass market book *China Syndrome*, an in-depth week-by-week chronicle of SARS. Despite its nonfiction classification, the book's style unabashedly blends fact with fancy, and the chapter on Liu exemplifies this mode of ambiguous storytelling. Liu is at first portrayed intimately and even affectionately as an elderly doctor with a "kindly round face" and somewhat befuddled grooming habits, and his trip to Hong Kong is described as motivated partly by relatable desires for "a little shopping, mahjongg, and karaoke." But then the narrative begins to blur the line between empirical history and creative extrapolation. Burrowing into Liu's interiority, Greenfeld writes that, even before his trip, Liu "had been feverish for a few days, with some mild body aches and a dry cough, causing him to regret not having taken Tamiflu prophylactically." On the bus, he "was again feeling a bit feverish but swallowed two Panadol and tried to nap," though when "his dry, hacking cough recommenced," he was surprised to notice it was "unproductive . . . and he was a little distressed at feeling severely out of breath after each fit of coughing."[96] The initial humanizing touches now take on a more accusatory inflection: the reader gets to glimpse Liu's internal reasoning around his illness, his downplaying of symptoms to himself, and his unwisely continuing with the journey on public transit despite his own troubling medical observations. As in *The Silent Killer*, the spotlight is on Liu as an already symptomatic body. Though Greenfeld does not label Liu a "superspreader," later in the book he elaborates that what made SARS so "sinister" was precisely its ability to inhabit human bodies without triggering severe enough symptoms to prevent travel: "That man next to you on the train, that lady coughing across the aisle—suddenly the means and modes of transit were rife with potential superspreaders . . . the stocky Italian man with the bright eyes and round face would turn out to be just such a carrier."[97] In retrospect, Greenfeld implies, beneath the innocuous surface of the Chinese doctor's avuncular "round face" lurked exactly this mortal viral threat.

Greenfeld then recreates Liu's stay at the Metropole Hotel, again augmenting his account with unmarked embellishments, and it is here that the iconic elevator scene assumes dramatic life:

> Room 911 . . . Liu still felt fatigued and considered taking a nap. Instead, he slipped on his jacket and went to the elevator bank, where several other guests were already waiting. In the elevator, he was seized by a coughing fit so severe that the other passengers would later recall being alarmed. Still, the doctor was determined to head out for a shopping trip. Amazingly, despite again feeling feverish and, now, nauseated, he made his way to Nathan Road and eventually bought a new windbreaker from one of the discount shops there. Upon his return to the hotel, he felt so weak he had to sit down in the lobby and then lean against the wall in the elevator for support. On the ninth floor, he would vomit in the hallway before reaching his room. There, he would pass out in his bed, unable to call his sister to tell her he was canceling dinner.
>
> Disgusted guests noticed the odor first, then the viscous, yellow stain on the brown carpet. Hotel staff moved quickly to clean up the mess, but by then, at least sixteen other guests had made their way past the pool of vomit on the floor. . . . [98]

In the book's endnotes, Greenfeld states that he reconstructed this day's events from interviews with Liu's "relatives, fellow physicians, and staff at the Metropole Hotel," with cross-references to several WHO and Hong Kong government reports.[99] Yet many of his tantalizing details, while they boost the book's overall reality effect, are not corroborated by or are outright inconsistent with the scientific archive on Liu. According to the medical records, Liu had taken two chest x-rays as well as treated himself with antibiotics before leaving Guangzhou.[100] Moreover, according to several epidemiological studies, the Metropole outbreak was due to "environmental contamination" rather than direct human-to-human transmission.[101] Not only did the other infected guests not have direct contact with Liu, none could even recall having seen him during their stay at the hotel, much less report their alarm at his "coughing fit" in the elevator.[102] In another context, Greenfeld avows, "One of the reasons I became a writer is because of a desire to entertain. Yet so much journalism and nonfiction is written to educate or inform, and the notion of entertainment is reduced to clever turns of phrase or similes. That's not really entertainment, that's verbiage."[103] To reinject entertainment into journalism, Greenfeld somehow saw fit to memorialize Liu as a careless physician who prioritized his pleasure-seeking over his health and the global public's, a determined shopper to boot who foolishly coughed and vomited his way to discount stores in a global city. As with other media accounts, there is an underlying censure here of Liu's bad judgment as a root cause for the global pandemic. Within the book's larger narrative of China's many secret cover-ups, Liu fits neatly.

At the extreme end of this blame-driven paradigm were certain conspiracy theories that circulated internationally, and not just in underground outlets. *La Repubblica*, one of Italy's main national newspapers, carried an article in April 2003 titled "From Super Scientist to Great Infector: Patient Zero of the Killer Virus."[104] This article was picked up the following week on the anglophone internet by various news sites and blogs. According to this story, Liu was a star microbiologist who had been promised "everything he wanted, money, fame" by the Chinese government to develop a vaccine for avian flu, and he allegedly became "obsessed" with this mission, engaging in "very risky" procedures of "virus manipulation" in his laboratory. In the process, he purportedly spawned a lethal new pathogen and accidentally infected himself with it, thereby becoming SARS's "patient zero." The family wedding in Hong Kong, so the story went, was a cover for a top-secret meeting with an operative from Beijing, and the Chinese government's delay in allowing WHO into Guangdong was due to its efforts to first destroy the evidence of Liu's research; and while few colleagues knew about Liu's clandestine work, none would talk to foreign reporters, pretending even not to have known the elderly doctor.[105] The overall message of this article seemed to be that, while Liu was guilty of personal greed and ambition as well as professional negligence, the Chinese state was the principal culprit for both the creation and cover-up of SARS, with a wider network of terrified Chinese doctors contributing to the mass censorship. This story later reappeared in Gits Ferrari's memoir *Not SARS Just Sex*, about an American expat in Taipei during SARS. Quoting the *La Repubblica* article at length, Ferrari further embellishes Liu's tale by imagining him wracked with guilt as he lay dying in the hospital.[106] Both accounts imagine Liu as possessing some originary guilt and moral failing, and both float one particularly salacious detail that exists in no other sources: that on his day of arrival in Hong Kong, Liu met up with his brother-in-law to visit a "zona a luci rosse" or red-light district—a detail that resurrects an AIDS-era association between bodily contagion and sexual depravity.[107]

This conspiracy tale represents a classic yellow peril narrative, if updated in the terms of global capital, international biosecurity, and emerging microbes. It recasts the significance of SARS and contemporary pandemics from a biological and environmental to a georacial problem. In this retelling, SARS was not the natural mutation of an animal virus or even the product of honest human error and a lab accident but the culmination of a set of distinctly Chinese actions and flaws. China's reckless drive for economic development and scientific power corrupted and killed one of its own top minds while endangering human health on a planetary scale. Meanwhile, the communist state's culture of secrecy and surveillance cowed even potential whistleblowers into complicity and silence. Without the temptation of money and fame, this story intimates, Liu would not have embarked on his deadly research, and, without cutting-edge technology at his disposal, he would not have had the means to conduct such research. Several scholars have argued that orientalist and racist discourses around SARS reflect a new formation tied to Western neoliberal anxieties about China's ascendency.[108] Yet new and old orientalisms clearly overlap and coexist here. With Pang, anglophone accounts produced and reproduced Chinese racial, cultural, and economic difference through a multitude of tropes both old and new, from the anachronistic primitivism of the dead farmer to the transhuman capitalist assemblage of "wet markets" and wild animal merchants. With Liu, the conspiracy narrative locates him within a heterogeneous nexus of viral birds and bioengineered microbes, high-tech labs and red-light districts, communist machinations and hypercapitalist leisure. Long-standing motifs of China as an ancient exotic culture of filth and decay linger alongside more modern tropes of a biotechnologized authoritarian regime, where old dangers persist even as new ones multiply. The recurrent avian allusion is perhaps especially telling, since many accounts of Pang also singled out birds as the animal life that index patients presumably intermixed with, with some commentators speculating that a bird vendor was the original source of the virus.[109] These reports subtly aligned SARS with avian flu, which up until COVID had been widely projected as the most likely catastrophic pandemic to come. During COVID too, as discussed earlier, we have witnessed the replay of conspiracy theories via rumors of a Wuhan lab leak; whatever the veracity of such claims, they carry conspicuous echoes of SARS-era espionage tales.

One final recurrent pattern in anglophone reporting on Liu warrants highlighting—the erasure of his family, especially his wife. Almost without exception, anglophone accounts describe Liu as making the journey to Hong Kong alone and staying at the Metropole Hotel alone.[110] But in reality, Liu's wife accompanied him on the bus from Guangzhou and was by his side throughout his time in Hong Kong. And crucially, she survived. By narratively isolating Liu even before he was physically isolated as an infectious patient, these accounts fuel the biohorror theme of a SARS "superspreader" who killed almost everyone in proximate range. The formulaic conventions of this genre seem unable to tolerate close-encounter survivors. If a story happens to mention Liu's brother-in-law, it will not fail to mention that he was infected by Liu and died soon after, hence reinforcing the idea of Liu's supreme deadliness. In effect, elements of Liu's life that fit the "patient zero" or "superspreader" template are preserved and amplified, while those that undermine it are excised and continually forgotten. In this pandemic bio-orientalist imagination, "patient zeroes" and "superspreaders" are narratively severed from the most commonplace ties of human and social life. Accordingly, Liu is portrayed as interacting with other people only if they were shady coconspirators or doomed unsuspecting strangers, part of networks that showcase the persistent otherness and ongoing perils of China and Chinese bodies. Surviving spouses and ordinary kin are too normalizing for this cartography, which insists on mapping Liu as a catastrophic global hub.

Reconstituting Liu's Last Days

To rehumanize Liu and reconstruct his last days, we cannot, unfortunately, turn to survivor interviews as with Pang, and in-depth sources on him are few. Yet we can turn to a substantial epidemiological and medical archive, since the Metropole Hotel outbreak was extensively studied by both local and international investigators. The Hong Kong Legislative Council too, after conducting its formal inquiries into local outbreaks, published a comprehensive report, the appendices of which include a trove of documents, testimonies, and summaries on local index patients and their traced contacts. These primary records are not only rich in disease data but also surprisingly suggestive in their extra-epidemiological human details. Their emphasis on empirical evidence and social linkages provides us with a valuable alternative vantage point from which to cut through the ossified scripts and biases of remote storytelling. Most vitally, they allow us to restore to Liu his familial connections, to reembed his life within the most basic, small-scale, and unexceptional of social ties and communal worlds, and to piece back together some semblance of a human story.[111]

At the beginning of 2003, Liu Jianlun was sixty-four years old and in good health, living in an apartment in Guangzhou with his wife. A nephrology specialist and medical professor, he had been working at the No. 2 Affiliated Hospital of Zhongshan Medical University, also called Sun Yat-sen University of Medical Sciences, for more than two decades. He had been eligible for retirement a few years prior to SARS, but the hospital retained his services because, according to one nurse, "Professor Liu was highly skilled, with many patients specifically registered under his care, so he would frequently see over a hundred patients per day and work overtime."[112] Guangzhou, being the provincial capital and "a premier medical centre," frequently absorbed medical transfers from surrounding cities, so it was only routine that, in January and February that year, it "received transfers of several patients with respiratory complications associated with SARS," including from Foshan.[113] By his own account, Liu treated two patients suspected of atypical pneumonia presenting "with high grade fever and chest symptoms" at an outpatient clinic from February 11 to 13.[114] These were the days immediately following the Guangdong press conference in which, as discussed in chapter 2, provincial health authorities announced that the local atypical pneumonia outbreak was under control. We do not know whether Liu believed this official story, but, when treating his own patients, he followed protocol and "wore a mask and gloves."[115] Despite these precautions, he fell ill on the evening of February 15 with "flu-like symptoms": a fever, chills, and "pleuritic chest pain." He felt concerned enough to request a chest x-ray two days later, which came back showing "left lower zone haziness" but nothing alarming, so he treated himself with antibiotics.[116] A second x-ray on February 20 showed "increasing haziness," but, by that point, Liu felt "fully recovered."[117] So, on February 21, he and his wife took a three-hour bus trip to Hong Kong, where they planned to attend the wedding banquet of his nephew, his youngest sister's son, the following day.[118]

Upon their arrival, the couple checked into the Metropole Hotel (Jing Hua) on Waterloo Road in Kowloon—not to be confused with the more centrally located Metropole Hotel on Lai Chi Kok Road in Mongkok. Despite its upscale-sounding name, this was at the time a three-star hotel that catered to budget-conscious travelers who did not mind its slightly out-of-the-way location (by Hong Kong standards), about a ten-minute walk from the nearest metro stations and shopping district. For this reason, it was often included in discount packages, a deal that some guests on the Lius' floor had also taken advantage of.[119] The Lius stayed in room 911, conveniently located at the intersection of two perpendicular hallways and almost directly across from the two elevators on that floor.[120] After checking in that afternoon, the couple met up with Liu's brother-in-law, his sister's husband and father of the groom, to do some shopping.[121] Afterward, they had dinner at the sister and brother-in-law's home.[122] Back at the hotel that night, Liu began to feel sick again, with an "increased cough, shortness of breath, fever and peripheral cyanosis."[123] A WHO investigative team later conjectured that, at some point that evening, Liu vomited in the hallway outside his room and in the elevator waiting area a few feet away, contaminating the carpet and lobby fan.[124] Viral particles were probably "protected for quite some time by the high level of humidity of the hotel environment (over 80% relative humidity)."[125] But there was no record of the hotel staff cleaning up a soiled carpet in that hallway that night, and if Liu's wife did it herself, she could no longer remember the incident afterward.[126] The next morning, the couple walked the half-mile to the emergency department at nearby Kwong Wah Hospital, where Liu was admitted.[127] Ten days later, on March 4, Liu died in isolation, but it was not until mid-April, when test kits became available, that he was posthumously diagnosed with SARS.[128]

A near-retirement nephrologist caring for patients at his university hospital and clinic, an untimely cross-border family wedding, a budget hotel with high interior humidity levels, a hotel room positioned at a hallway intersection across from the elevators, and an as-yet-unidentified microbe with fluctuating and delayed flu-like symptoms—these were some of the fortuitous elements composing the scene of the Metropole Hotel outbreak. In that partial day of the Lius' stay, up to twenty guests and visitors across thirteen different rooms were infected, but, since no one could recollect crossing paths with Liu, they most likely simply walked by the contaminated spots in the ninth-floor hallway.[129] As noted above, epidemiological studies postulate that this outbreak was due to "environmental contamination" rather than direct human-to-human transmission.[130] Contrary to the popular image of superspreaders as somehow biologically hardwired to be more contagious than the rest of the human population—"spewing germs out like teakettles" or "biological bombs," as some anglophone news stories would have it— medical records indicate that Liu "did not have an unusually high viral load when tested on days 9 and 11 of the illness," typically the height of the infectious period for SARS patients.[131] This key piece of data lends strong empirical, rather than just sociopolitical, support to the argument against the "superspreader" idea. As Lynteris points out, the discourse on "superspreaders" assumes that those like Liu are inherently hyperinfectious even before contracting any disease, as if "there is a particular human type who can be accurately described as a superspreader in the waiting . . . always already a superspreader, even if the 'chance' of infection never arises."[132] In this instance, however, what contributed most to the scope of the Metropole outbreak was not Liu's physiology but the building's damp interior, the hotel's fateful floor plan, and the "late recognition of the environmental contamination of hotel facilities and the failure of timely intervention on the hotel guests with close contact" with him.[133] Indeed, had Liu truly been the biotic germ bomb of popular stereotype, he would have infected not just guests on his floor but countless others in this 500-room hotel with a 285-person staff. Instead, not one hotel worker fell sick, not even the housekeepers who cleaned the Lius' room.[134] "A miracle!" exclaimed one employee—but only if we subscribe to the thesis that "superspreaders" are unique biological entities rather than ideologically fraught discursive constructs.[135]

If we approach the epidemiological and medical archive on the Metropole outbreak with an eye toward its counternarrative potential, we can begin to dispel some of the gross distortions about Liu. Against the many popular accounts that portray him as already highly symptomatic on arrival in Hong Kong, winded and hacking to the point of collapse, Kwong Wah Hospital's admissions records classified Liu's condition as "fair" rather than "poor" upon check-in.[136] The triage nurse who assessed him noted "mild shortness of breath" but considered him "alert"; in fact, she recalled perceiving him as "just an ordinary old man."[137] Liu's most concerning symptom, and the emergency department supervisor's main reason for admitting him into the ICU, was his "very low" oxygen level, which was at only 65 percent, though he could still "speak clearly."[138] After ordering a chest x-ray that showed a "ground glass" appearance, doctors worried "there was a possibility that intubation might be required if the patient's condition deteriorated."[139] In short, without these tests, Liu's outward symptoms were not extraordinarily alarming, so that neither the triage nurse nor the resident physician who first assessed him felt the need to don a face mask or other personal protective equipment.[140] Even the Hospital Authority's senior manager at the time, upon reviewing Liu's medical file with a team of infectious disease experts in a February 27 meeting, did not find anything unusual in it to suggest that Liu was not simply one of the city's seventy or so pneumonia cases requiring intensive care each month.[141]

Certainly, Liu himself believed he was stricken with nothing more than a relapse of regular pneumonia. He did not attempt to hide his contact history with patients in Guangzhou and voluntarily disclosed this to the Kwong Wah emergency staff.[142] Still, he insisted he did not suffer from "that kind of thing" (*m hai gwo D je*).[143] Incidentally, it is also through the medical archive that we learn that Liu spoke Cantonese rather than Mandarin to the hospital staff. Linguistically at least, he would not have necessarily presented as a mainlander, a city outsider. We do not know at what point he came to realize he had contracted SARS; according to the records, it might have been after he was shown his x-ray results or after his ICU admission.[144] In any case, it was partly due to his prompt self-disclosure that the consulting physician that day, who was already aware of a surveillance memorandum on the Guangdong atypical pneumonia outbreak, advised all workers in the emergency department to wear paper masks when treating Liu.[145] Once he was placed in isolation, ICU staff adopted full precautionary measures with N95 masks and protective gowns.[146] Again, had Liu been a "superspreader" who killed all those in close contact with him, there would have been a major outbreak at Kwong Wah. Instead, even with the delay in initiating infection protocol, only two healthcare workers at the hospital contracted SARS during the entire outbreak, and both recovered. One was an emergency department nurse who, according to the records, "did not have direct contact history" with Liu but "worked in the cubicle next to one where he stayed," and the other was a healthcare assistant who had worked in the isolation room of Liu's brother-in-law.[147] As at the Metropole Hotel, Liu directly infected zero staff.

It is also from the medical records and epidemiological literature that we start to regain a sense of Liu's extended clan and the intimacy of his family circle. We learn that, in 2003, Mrs. Liu was also sixty-four years old, her husband's exact contemporary. The couple had a daughter and a son, both in their thirties, both also living in Guangzhou at the time.[148] The two adult children arrived in Hong Kong the day after their parents, on February 22, a Saturday, possibly to attend their cousin's wedding banquet later that day, possibly in response to news of their father's relapse.[149] In any event, the triage nurse who first evaluated Liu at Kwong Wah remembered him being "accompanied by relatives (at least 2 female relatives)," so it was likely that the daughter and possibly the son were already in the emergency room with their parents.[150] After Liu was admitted later that day, Mrs. Liu checked out of the Metropole and, along with her daughter and son, moved into the home of Liu's sister.[151] This was the sister the older couple had dined with the previous night and mother of the groom. Liu had another sister who lived in Guangzhou, and her son was also in town that weekend for the family wedding.[152] This other nephew also stayed at the Metropole, though not on the ninth floor.[153] We do not know whether the wedding took place as scheduled, or, if it did, whether Mrs. Liu and her children attended the banquet, but we do know that Hong Kong had no reported outbreaks of SARS from a wedding-related gathering. The next day, a Sunday, Liu's son returned to Guangzhou, asymptomatic.[154] The following day, a Monday, Mrs. Liu herself developed a fever. She decided to seek treatment in Guangzhou rather than Hong Kong, so that evening, she, too, returned home with her daughter.[155] Once back in Guangzhou, both the daughter and the older nephew developed symptoms, but, along with Mrs. Liu, all three recovered.[156] In Hong Kong, both Liu's brother-in-law and then his sister fell ill a few days later, and both were admitted to Kwong Wah.[157] She was in stable condition and released with antibiotics a few days later, never receiving a confirmed SARS diagnosis, but her husband's condition deteriorated over the next two weeks, and he died on March 19.[158] Posthumously, he would play an important role in the epidemiological history of SARS, for it was a specimen from his lung tissue that led the Hong Kong University microbiology team to make its discovery that the disease's causal agent was a novel coronavirus.[159] In this instance, to follow through on the afterlife of Liu's brother-in-law is to resist premature narrative closure, to reframe the import of index clusters beyond their mere destructiveness. Even among Liu's handful of infected relatives, all but one survived—including his equally elderly wife, his constant and closest companion throughout the journey.

From the fragments of this archive, we can piece back together a fuller picture of Liu himself. We come to see him as not an imprudent doctor, mad scientist, or suspicious communist agent but a husband, father, brother, brother-in-law, and uncle. He was a husband who lived and traveled with his life partner, a father whose two adult children lived in the same city, and an older brother who would take time out of his work schedule to spend a weekend with his sister's family on the special occasion of her son's wedding. The older couple's choice of the Metropole Hotel in Yau Ma Tei, a modest establishment in a less busy area of the city rather than one of the numerous four- and five-star hotels in bustling Tsim Sha Tsui or Causeway Bay, also speaks volumes about their nonextravagant habits. We can also infer that Liu's clan was relatively close, at least close enough that a groom on the Hong Kong side of the family could expect an uncle and aunt as well as three cousins to make the journey from the mainland to attend his wedding, and close enough that his parents would host his uncle's family during a medical emergency. These are signs of a close-knit cross-border family. From the hospital records, we also learn that Liu's sister visited him in the ICU on the day she herself was admitted, dressed in her hospital gown, even as her husband was isolated in another ward.[160] And we learn that Liu's "son and nephew accompanied him when he succumbed," his son having returned to Hong Kong at some point to watch over Liu outside the isolation room, even as his sister and mother recuperated back home.[161] So, though isolated, Liu was not alone, not someone his family would have left utterly alone—not upon his arrival in Hong Kong, not upon his admission to the hospital, and not in his final moments.

In this revised light, the meanings of Liu's illness shift, resonating at smaller scales and refracting across the people for whom his passing was not merely the opening act of a global calamity. For his wife, it was the loss of her husband, and, for his children, the loss of their father. The tragedy was compounded for his sister, who within two weeks lost both her brother and husband. For her son, the wedding must have assumed an ambivalent quality, a joyous occasion that accidentally precipitated his father's death. Ultimately, the epidemiological archive cannot preserve the internal texture of these smaller meanings: what each family member thought about the misfortune of being part of a SARS index cluster, and what each felt about their mixture of loss and survival. Yet what we can come away concluding with relative certainty is that, contrary to rumors within Hong Kong as well as in the news abroad, Liu did not intentionally cross the border to seek medical attention for what he already knew to be a mysterious killer virus, whether as a solitary maverick or a spy sent by the Chinese government.[162] As the Hong Kong Legislative Council's investigative committee reasons, "If [Liu]'s purpose of coming to Hong Kong was to seek treatment here, he would have gone to a hospital as soon as he arrived instead of spending the first day of his arrival shopping and having dinner with his relatives."[163] Indeed, he would not have traveled with his wife at all or welcomed his children's arrival, nor would the family have checked out of the hotel to stay at his sister's home, risking infecting everyone, and then chosen to return to Guangzhou for treatment afterward. The story of the Lius, in the end, was that of an ordinary family's tragedy, not exceptional biology or nefarious geopolitics.

Unjust Memories

There are too many ordinary connections that drop out of or get excised from mainstream anglophone accounts of Liu. Ironically, for all that long-form creative nonfiction is supposed to humanize science, it has marshaled tropes that generate exactly the opposite effect of narratively segregating index patients, suppressing their closest relationships, and relegating them to a kind of social death. Even scholarly works tend to summon Liu's life and death primarily for purposes of ideological critique. So, although the Metropole outbreak has been covered and recapped countless times across the world, we are left with a humanly anemic story, with the greatest blanks around the people most intimately affected. The version that has Liu's family at its center and as its own telos remains untold, is perhaps now untellable. Unlike with Pang, no public records preserve the traces of what Liu thought or felt about SARS. Like Pang and Huang, the Liu family became intensely self-protective about their privacy, and Liu's sister even stopped answering medical surveillance phone calls from the Hong Kong health authorities after her personal data was leaked to the press.[164] This withdrawal from the public eye, too, might have contributed to the general dearth of information on the family and their experiences. Soon after SARS, even the physical landscape of the index site itself would change, effacing the trail of the past. Room 911 at the Metropole, according to one report, was "renumbered out of existence" and became room 913 a year later.[165] Another few years later still, the hotel was renamed the Metropark (Wei Jing) to erase any lingering association with SARS.[166] In an ironic twist, in December 2020, this very Metropark branch, now owned by an investor group from China, was designated by the Hong Kong government as one of the city's three dozen or so COVID quarantine hotels.[167] At the time of this chapter's writing, it was advertising hotel quarantine packages for nonmainland travelers.

Where other doctors and nurses were celebrated and commemorated as SARS heroes or martyrs, whether inside China or internationally, Liu has been memorialized with striking tepidness and ambivalence. We can contrast the anglophone treatment of Liu with the sinophone fictions analyzed earlier in this book. Instead of being mourned as an elder who died tragically in isolation, cut off from family and friends like Hu Fayun's Teacher Wei, and, instead of being venerated as a forerunner of courageous frontline medical workers who died in the line of duty like Chen Baozhen's Su Weiling or *Golden Chicken 2*'s Dr. Facemask, Liu has more often than not been depicted in varying shades of pandemic responsibility, hovering between unlucky victim and guilty instigator.

This unequal narrative treatment becomes even more pronounced when we compare Liu's skeletal obituaries with Carlo Urbani's. Urbani was an Italian physician and infectious disease specialist based in Vietnam at the time and the first WHO official to alert the organization to the gravity of SARS.

In Hanoi, he attended to Johnny Chen, the Chinese American businessman who had stayed in the hotel room across from the Lius' at the Metropole and who was one of the guests infected there.[168] Chen would become Vietnam's index case, triggering an outbreak among healthcare workers at Hanoi-French Hospital before being medically evacuated back to Hong Kong, where he died on March 13.[169] When Urbani saw the Hanoi hospital staff falling sick around Chen, he notified the Vietnam Ministry of Health and WHO about the possibility of a serious epidemic outbreak in the region, and he was instrumental in strengthening the hospital's infection controls and containing Vietnam's outbreak.[170] He himself, however, contracted the virus from Chen and died on March 29 in Bangkok. The global media quickly and uniformly eulogized him as a valiant and self-sacrificing medical hero, and his obituaries, in contrast to Liu's, never fail to mention his surviving wife and three children. One widely repeated anecdote recounts how, when Urbani's worried wife asked him at the time to limit his exposure to SARS patients, his gallant reply had been "If I can't work in such situations, what am I here for? Answering emails, going to cocktail parties and pushing paper?"[171] A recent WHO memorial envisages how, "if Dr. Urbani were alive today, he would have enjoyed spending much time with his lovely wife and going on vacations with the whole family. He would have seen how his three children had grown up to become beautiful human beings like him. He was an affectionate husband and a hands-on dad."[172] Another WHO publication highlights Urbani's family and community in his Italian hometown, quoting one colleague's words: "I met his wife, his children, and his mother. I now understand why this kind man was so selfless. The life there is simple, and the community is very close-knit. Everyone respects each other. And everyone seemed genuinely solid and warm-hearted. It's not a coincidence that Dr. Urbani, who was born and raised in this close-knit community, made such a great contribution to the battle against disease."[173] Numerous tributes supplement this portrait of the devoted family man with that of a dynamic renaissance man: Urbani was "a passionate photographer, an expert ultra-light airplane pilot, and a good organist"; "an avid hang glider, motorcycle rider, and musician"; and "an adventurer" who "looked so cool riding his motorcycle he could even give Clint Eastwood a run for his money."[174]

None of these humanizing gestures were ever conferred on Liu, despite the parallels in their circumstances. Both were physicians who caught SARS unwittingly, and both died from their medical labor caring for infected patients. In fact, Urbani, too, made a decision to take a cross-border trip on the heels of his exposure, when he was already symptomatic. On March 11, about a week after he had personally examined Chen, as the Hanoi hospital staff was falling ill at an alarming rate around him, Urbani boarded a flight from Vietnam to Thailand to attend a conference—even though he was experiencing symptoms prior to travel.[175] As a colleague of his recalls, Urbani had called her from the Hanoi airport with reports of feverishness: "He said he didn't feel well, and at first, I didn't think much of it," she relates, thinking it was mere fatigue. "I told him to go, that we could handle things in Viet Nam without him."[176] This same colleague then remembered Urbani "shivering when they had last met in her office," and it was partly due to her intervention that Urbani was met with a medical team upon his arrival at the Bangkok airport and then swiftly isolated.[177] As with Liu, it was perhaps a matter of good fortune that Urbani did not infect any fellow passengers, and early medical disclosure helped prevent a hospital outbreak, this time in Thailand.[178] Yet memories around the two men cannot be more different: on one side, innuendos of a pandemic originator; on the other, hagiographies of a pandemic hero. The loving family and community around Urbani gets enshrined while the supportive clan around Liu gets systematically erased, and Urbani's possible lapse in judgment becomes barely a footnote in SARS chronicles even as the same behavior attributed to Liu gets scripted as the key opening act of a global calamity. Here, we see perhaps the starkest illustration of a georacial disparity in Sara Ahmed's cultural politics of emotion, where one life is supremely loved and grieved while the other seems hardly "grievable," much less "imagined as loveable and liveable."[179]

Outbreaks That Never Were

One final observation merits mention. If global pandemic crisis discourse has fixated on SARS's explosive episodes and their terrifying aspects, whether couched in terms of "superspreaders" or "superspreading events," Liu's story, as reconstructed here, actually compels us to appreciate how few and infrequent those events were. We can scrutinize Liu's itinerary with an eye toward all the outbreaks that did not happen. Not only were no employees infected at the Metropole Hotel, and not only was there no major outbreak at Kwong Wah Hospital, but, as far as the records show, no one caught the virus from Liu on the bus from Guangzhou to Hong Kong, and no one caught the virus from Mrs. Liu and her daughter on their bus ride back to Guangzhou from Hong Kong, nor was there any report of an outbreak in the shops around the hotel or in the neighboring shopping districts. Indeed, the fact that at most twenty hotel guests and visitors became infected—out of the 1,730 guests from forty-three countries staying at the Metropole that night—and that out of those infected only four cities came to develop major outbreaks, puts the whole episode in a much more temperate perspective.[180] A follow-up study further reveals that other ninth-floor guests from Canada, England, Germany, and the United States were also infected and went on to travel home or to other international destinations within the week, but they averted triggering additional outbreaks in Vancouver, the Philippines, and Australia.[181] The case of Canada is especially illustrative.

On March 7, "within a three-hour period, two middle-aged men with undiagnosed SARS, one in Vancouver and the other in Toronto, were admitted to hospital."[182] One had been a guest at the Metropole who had stayed in room 909, right next to the Lius, before being switched to a room on the fourteenth floor; the other was the son of an elderly couple who had returned home after staying at the Metropole in room 904, down the hall from the Lius.[183] According to the Ontario government's SARS report, "Though outwardly similar events, the outcomes were poles apart," a dramatically divergent "tale of two cities," and "one key difference was the level of knowledge of front-line staff about events in China and Hong Kong."[184] In February that year, the British Columbia CDC, long on the lookout for pandemic influenza, had issued a pandemic plan warning hospitals of potential infectious diseases out of Southeast Asia, so the Vancouver emergency room crew that night was "actively looking for unexplained fevers and respiratory ailments in patients who had been in Asia."[185] By contrast, Ontario's system for communicating public health threats was "fragmented," so the Toronto hospital staff was not on guard for an infectious disease and did not think to isolate their patient until twenty-one hours later.[186] Beyond a centralized health surveillance system, diasporic linkages and information networks played a crucial role. Chinese newspapers in Canada had been reporting on the Guangdong outbreak since January, weeks before the virus actually spread into the country and entered into mainstream anglophone news in North America.[187] By the time Vancouver's first SARS patient walked into the city's biggest hospital in early March, many of its healthcare workers with ties to China and Hong Kong had already heard of the cases there, and combined with the provincial CDC alert, they were ready with infection protocol. By chance, the emergency department head physician on duty that day, Dr. Tom Lee, was a Chinese Canadian who had visited Hong Kong over the Christmas holiday and had

PANDEMIC FIRST PATIENTS   215

read in the local newspaper there about "all sorts of activity in southern China."[188] Hence, under his direction, Vancouver's index patient was isolated within five minutes of admission, and a provincial outbreak was "essentially headed off by that single act of an emergency room physician."[189]

While the above factors made all the difference in Vancouver, two analogous cases related to the Metropole remain more inexplicable. A German woman who also stayed on the hotel's ninth floor on the night of February 21 flew to Australia with a companion the next day, and a Filipino British couple who stayed down the hall from the Lius flew to the Philippines two days later. All had contracted SARS, all fell ill during their travels, all sought medical attention at local hospitals, and the British woman was even put on a nebulizer by the hospital staff, but in none of these cases was a single airline passenger or attendant, travel companion, or healthcare worker infected.[190] We might be tempted to call these outbreaks that never happened lucky near misses, perhaps even miracles. But as the Metropole outbreak demonstrates, SARS was a disease highly dependent on the right set of social and environmental conditions. It may be that, if we reviewed each possible index patient who never became one with the same level of care and fairness that we grant Liu here, we would likewise be left not with pandemic enigmas but with many more not-so-exceptional micro stories.

In this regard, the Ontario SARS Commission report is heartening in its fastidiously non-otherizing reconstruction of Toronto's index case, Kwan Sui-Chu, and her infected son, Tse Chi-Kwan. Drawing on testimonies by nurses and doctors, the report emphasizes the family's "dignity and cooperation in the face of fear and uncertainty," and it takes care to note that the family "lost Mrs. K., a mother, grandmother and wife, and Mr. T., a husband, son, father and brother."[191] Amid the morass of anglophone SARS literature, this report offers some hope that Chinese index patients can be portrayed with terms of ordinariness and community, even at a Western pandemic epicenter.

Singapore: Esther Mok

In many ways, the patterns of international reporting on Liu Jianlun, especially the framework of the "superspreader," apply also to Esther Mok, Singapore's index patient. Yet, in Mok's case, there was an additional gendered fascination with her as a unique combination of supreme toxicity and seemingly undeserved miraculous survival. Mok was one of three Singaporean women who stayed on the ninth floor of the Metropole Hotel the night of February 21, 2003. She and a friend stayed in room 938, while a third woman, the guide from their tour group, was in room 915, adjacent to the Lius.[192] All three came to be infected with SARS there. All three traveled back to Singapore on February 25, all three fell sick once back home, and all three were admitted to hospital from March 1 to March 3.[193] All three survived, but only Mok transmitted the virus to others, 21 directly and up to 195 indirectly, thus becoming the index case for a major outbreak in Singapore.[194]

"Superinfector" and "Typhoid Mary"

In April that year, the Associated Press released a news article on Mok that was later reprinted across anglophone outlets worldwide. Entitled "Singapore Woman Linked to 100 SARS Cases," this article adopted motifs similar to those about Liu. It marshaled, for instance, a mathematical idiom to emphasize Mok's destructive magnitude as a "superspreader," noting that "all but a handful of the 118 reported cases in Singapore have been traced to Mok." It also compared Mok to Typhoid Mary—the analogy now made gender appropriate—wryly adding that Mok "is living her own modern-day exile in a hospital room networked with televisions and telephones," thus evoking an image of technological privilege even amid medical isolation. Like many other accounts on the Singapore outbreak, and echoing tropes on Liu at the Metropole, this article further linked the danger of "superspreaders" to Asian capital, middle-class consumption, and transnational mobility by pointedly marking Mok as a "former flight attendant" who "went to Hong Kong to shop" but "came home carrying a deadly flu-like virus."[195] This profile created an impression of Mok as a pampered and materialistic young woman who quit her job to go luxury shopping at another Asian metropolis and who, even when quarantined with a lethal virus she had passed on to many compatriots, would keep herself entertained through assorted media, in a blending of bio-orientalism with techno-orientalism. "I feel sorry for her, but you might wonder whether Singapore would be so badly affected had she not been in the wrong place at the wrong time," said one "deliveryman" at the article's end, proxy for the Singaporean everyman, ambivalently caught between pity and blame.[196] A range of outlets soon reposted this article online, from Fox News to the UCLA School of Public Health, and one newspaper even glibly prefaced the original title with "Deadly Shopping Trip."[197] The article's content was also recycled, sometimes verbatim, across US, British, and Australian outlets, with headlines such as "Superspreaders May Hold SARS Clue" and "SARS Timebombs: Fatal Threat of the Super-Carriers."[198] Within the month, Mok became front-page news on both American coasts, with the *New York Times* and *Los Angeles Times* both naming her a "superspreader" and the latter, under the lurid headline "Outbreak in Asia: A Hotbed of SARS Warfare," dubbing her "a modern-day Typhoid Mary."[199] If reportage on Liu tended to target his Chineseness and tapped into specifically sinophobic sentiments, coverage on Mok tended to generalize the racially othering language to all of Asia, entwined now with a gendering of SARS through the hyperinfectious Asian female body.

For Mok, this discourse hit home in deeply personal ways that Liu did not have to contend with, at least not on this side of the veil. By the time the vocabulary of *patient zeroes* and *superspreaders* became prevalent, Liu had already passed on. He did not have to confront the stigma of these labels or endure the indignity of living with distorting stories about him. Also, these terms were never officially used by his medical teams during his illness and sprang up only posthumously around his case. For Mok, though, the situation was entirely different. She lived through SARS only to face being branded a "superspreader," not just colloquially by foreign journalists in foreign languages but officially by both her own government and WHO, and in one of her own native languages. At a press conference at the end of March, Singapore's health minister Lim Hng Kiang not only miscategorized all three women returning from Hong Kong as "superinfectors" but singled out Mok by name, even as she was still recovering in the hospital.[200] In a remark that went viral, he proclaimed to the local media that "Esther Mok infected the whole lot of us." While this comment was widely considered "tone-deaf" and was "not well-received" within Singapore, it was extensively requoted by anglophone news outlets worldwide.[201] By May, WHO's weekly epidemiological report on Singapore's outbreak had officially adopted the term *superspreaders* to refer to "persons who directly infected >10 other persons," and the Singapore government's website on SARS reproduced this usage.[202] Though neither source explicitly named Mok, it was by then no mystery to anyone who this Case 1 "superinfector" was.

As with Liu, it is worth highlighting that there exists no scientific evidence to suggest Mok was biologically more infectious than any other SARS patient. The outbreak around her, like the Metropole outbreak, was largely due to the fact that infection control measures were not adopted when she first checked in at Tan Tock Seng Hospital. According to medical records,

Mok was admitted to an open ward on March 1, then transferred to the ICU on March 4 due to "decreased blood oxygen saturation," and finally placed in isolation on March 6.[203] As one of her attending physicians later attested, "She had come in for pneumonia.... At that point in time, we had no idea what SARS was. SARS was still very much an unknown entity. In fact, the term *SARS* had not even been coined yet. So we treated Esther for what we thought was an ordinary pneumonia."[204] Another doctor at the hospital later echoed, "Our staff were in contact with her without knowing her illness and just how contagious it was."[205] And as Mok herself later recalled, the doctors at first suspected dengue fever, then bird flu, then Legionnaire's disease, but each theory was discounted in turn, and, in the end, "they didn't know what it was."[206] It was during her three-day stay in the open ward that Mok infected nine healthcare workers, including a nurse who was then admitted into another six-person ward for three days before she, too, was isolated. This ancillary delay triggered a second cluster of infections as this nurse transmitted the virus to twenty-some other people, including one of her wardmates, a diabetic and heart disease patient who was then transferred to the coronary ICU for eight days before being placed in isolation. This coronary patient in turn infected dozens of others before passing away at the end of the month, initiating a third cluster of cases at the hospital.[207] As at the Metropole Hotel, environmental factors and medical ignorance played a key role, as all three patients were not isolated promptly but were allowed to come into close contact with a host of family and visitors, hospital workers and fellow patients. Without knowledge of SARS as a novel infectious disease, Singapore's public health system simply did not know to respond with anything other than standard operating procedures.

With Mok as with Liu, we can retrace her itinerary with an eye toward all the outbreaks that did not happen. Had she truly been a biologically exceptional "superspreader," she would have sparked outbreaks all over Hong Kong, as she and her friend "spent days eating and shopping" in some of the most popular spots in the city, including Ladies' Market and Tsim Sha Tsui, and they even visited the Ocean Park theme park.[208] She would also have sparked outbreaks at the Metropole itself since she and her friend stayed an additional three nights, or at the Hong Kong airport while waiting for their flight back to Singapore, or on the airplane itself, or at the Singapore airport on arrival, or in whatever public transit she took around the city in the four days before her hospitalization. But none of these transmissions transpired. Instead, a series of understandable delays at the Tan Tock Seng Hospital led to three nosocomial clusters that then spread into the wider community. To chalk all the subsequent cases and fatalities in Singapore up to Mok alone is to erect a monstrous biotype in the place of an ordinary patient—one whose all-too-mundane set of circumstances turned almost unbearably tragic within that one month of her life.

While index cases out of China such as Pang Zuoyao were written off as dead or likely dead and "superspreaders" such as Liu Jianlun were themselves stricken down by the disease and hence somewhat exonerated by personal demise, Mok was represented in international media as having an extraordinarily fatal touch on those around her while she herself endured to infect more and more victims. If accounts of Liu erase his wife as well as his sister and two adult children, effectively suppressing references to all the family members who lived through SARS despite close contact with him, those of Mok by contrast almost unfailingly mention her family and especially her parents—in order not to humanize her, but to accentuate the unforgivingly destructive power of the virus she carried and her horrific lack of control over her own poisonous body. For, unbeknownst to her, Mok transmitted the virus to both her parents as well as her maternal grandmother, an uncle, and an aunt's pastor. On March 25, Esther's fifty-year-old father, Joseph Mok, died from SARS, becoming the disease's first fatality in Singapore. The next day, the pastor, thirty-nine-year-old Simon Loh, also died, Singapore's second fatality.[209] Twelve days later, on April 7, Esther's forty-two-year-old mother, Helen Mok, followed, Singapore's eighth victim.[210] Eight days later, on April 15, Esther's uncle also followed, Singapore's eleventh victim.[211] The next day, April 16, Esther herself was discharged from the hospital, and, bafflingly, her seventy-three-year-old grandmother, the oldest member of the family to be infected, likewise recovered and was later discharged.[212]

Local Shifts

In contrast to global anglophone news, the *Straits Times*, Singapore's main English-language and largest daily newspaper, underwent a noticeable shift in its reporting on Mok over the course of the local outbreak. Toward the end of March and into early April, after Lim Hng Kiang had revealed Mok's name to the public and identified her as Singapore's index case and a "superinfector," the paper's coverage on SARS at first repeatedly promoted these details.[213] By mid-April, however, as news of Mok's parents' passing spread throughout the island, the "superinfector" discourse on her began to fracture. Journalists and readers began to openly question the ethics of continually parading her story in the public eye and insinuating her culpability for the local outbreak.

One turning point was a searching and heartfelt April 13 editorial entitled "Try a Little Kindness." Here, Tracy Quek narrated how, two weeks earlier, Mok's younger brother had texted her with a plea: "Could you tell your paper to stop using my sister's name and the Health Ministry to stop calling her a 'super infector'?" He explained that the exposure socially stigmatized his sister and hurt her prospects for future employment. Quek admitted that she "couldn't think of a reply" and was "for the first time in a long while lost for words." She decided to schedule an interview with the brother so he could tell the family's side of the story, but, in the interval, Mok's mother passed away, so the interview never occurred. When Quek relayed the brother's request to her editors, one editor's response was perfunctory. "The paper's policy on naming . . . is to withhold only the names of the victims of sexual assault or children involved in court proceedings," she was told, and "every other case would be judged on its own merit." Mok, the editor reasoned, "didn't fall into any of those categories. She was a patient with atypical pneumonia. There was no question then of ever not using her name." In the paper's defense, Quek noted that the editors never pushed their reporters to "hunt down the Moks" or "hound . . . the families of the other SARS patients." It was simply the banality of professional habit that prevented journalists from considering the plight of SARS patients from their perspectives. But after hearing anecdotes of discrimination against hospital nurses by taxi drivers and of verbal abuse hurled at suspected patients by their neighbors, Quek wondered: "Gosh, if people react that way to nurses and their neighbors, how are they going to treat Esther Mok?" She ended her article with an exhortation: "So perhaps now, more than ever, is the time for journalists to tell these stories so that people don't write them off as 'SARS patients,' but realize that they are part of the same community and deserve our support and understanding."[214]

This sentiment also touched other journalists at the *Straits Times*. On the same day that Quek's piece appeared, Salma Khalik, a staff reporter who had penned several of the paper's earlier articles calling Mok a "superinfector," published a self-reflection on how, in her five weeks covering SARS, "the biggest medical story this decade" had transformed from "a rather exciting though somewhat scary news story" to "a very painful and very emotional experience" filled with "sorrow, as one after another, healthy people succumb to the mystery bug and die." Contemplating Mok's situation, Khalik came to adopt a much more empathetic tone: "How much loss can one person take? ... [While Mok] will always be plagued with ... guilt ... [it was] unwarranted guilt, for she herself is a victim. She had not done anything wrong or gone anywhere extraordinary. She went to Hongkong as hundreds of thousands of Singaporeans do every year. She went to hospital when she was sick. She did everything by the book."[215] While not retracting the term *superinfector*, Khalik attempted to deexceptionalize it, untangling feelings of guilt from actual moral responsibility and normalizing Mok's trip as part of an ordinary local pattern of behavior. In Singapore's anglophone discourse, Mok's family tragedy helped put into motion an alternative set of idioms and affects around index patients. Splitting from global tropes of pandemic fear and catastrophe, these narratives about Mok circulated epidemic sympathy and empathic identification with the infectious, where even first patients could be embraced as part of "the same community" rather than expelled as toxins.

From some of the newspaper's reader reactions, it would seem that at least a portion of the Singaporean public had been awaiting just such an opening to insert their dissenting views on the "superinfector" discourse. The day after Quek's and Khalik's articles appeared, one reader submitted a letter passionately imploring the paper to stop singling Mok out for "unfair labelling." Emphasizing again that the local outbreak "was no fault of hers," this reader beseeched everyone to "feel" alongside Mok rather than against her: "Can anyone even begin to imagine how Miss Mok feels, as she turns the pages of a newspaper or watches the news on the television, only to see or hear herself being called a super infector? We all run the risk of being infected by SARS, and of becoming super infectors ourselves. How would we feel if we were to see our names splashed in the media as examples of super infectors, or if we were connected to the deaths of family, friends and fellow citizens?"[216] This reader rejected the idea of exceptional "superinfectors" altogether and posited instead a universal disease vulnerability. Two days later, two other readers expressed their agreement. "With all this talk about ethics, I am deeply disturbed that I have yet to hear or read of anyone questioning the stand of those who deemed it necessary and acceptable to release Miss Mok's name," wrote one. Pointing to Quek's article, this reader commented, "It appears to me that the matter of ethics did not cross the minds of Ms. Quek's editors."[217] More acerbically, another reader remarked on the paper's seeming double standards as it singled out "an innocent victim" like Mok while treating with charity "those who, after the news on SARS broke, still took a cavalier attitude and continued with their travel arrangements," such as a local banker who voiced "hardly any remorse ... for putting so many others at risk!"[218] The newspaper thus became a site of public debate, registering people's diverse and shifting views toward the ethics of epidemic journalism and storytelling.

By the first week of May, these community sentiments had filtered back up the government ranks to become official state rhetoric. When asked at a public panel about Mok's lifestyle and whether it was linked to her infectiousness, then acting prime minister Lee Hsien Loong replied, in language that was at once paternalistic and jocular, "Please have some consideration for the poor girl . . . she lost her parents, her pastor. It is not her fault. She didn't do anything wrong. She has no special lifestyle, but it so happens that she went to Hongkong for holiday, like so many other Singaporeans, and she had the misfortune of being in the same hotel as this chap from Guangzhou. . . . And we had the misfortune not to understand and isolate her quickly enough."[219] The meaning of Mok's illness thus changed again. Beyond an object of national pity, she and her story were now co-opted by state authorities as a cautionary lesson about Singapore's epidemic unpreparedness. Her case was used to justify what Chua Beng Hua calls the "logic of a total surveillance" that the Singapore party-state could implement through strict quarantine measures and mass mobilization campaigns.[220] In Chua's analysis, SARS was the "crisis that the PAP [People's Action Party] government had been waiting for," the emergency event via which "new behaviors of self-discipline were reassembled and framed . . . under the metasignifier of the 'nation.'" With this official turn, "everyone was reframed as acting as 'Singaporeans' . . . oriented, individually and collectively, toward a unified nation" and its fight against infectious disease.[221] This use of a global pandemic for the local ideological production of postcolonial nationhood and a consensual citizenry entailed appropriating Mok's singular "misfortune," as well as the increasingly popular lingo of sympathy and compassion toward SARS patients, as the cohesion point for forging proper national feelings. In short, Mok came to be instrumentalized for a state biopoliticization of epidemic affect.

Mok's Own Story

State-affiliated discourse, however, even within a one-party authoritarian country, can produce heterogeneous offshoots. At the end of 2003, Singapore's Ministry of Information, Communications and the Arts commissioned a book on SARS and asked the local Institute of Policy Studies think tank to publish it. The institute director agreed but stipulated that there be no government restrictions on the book's content. Chua Mui Hoong, a senior political correspondent for *Straits Times*, was tasked with the research and writing. Along with two young interns at the paper—Maria Almenoar and Teh Joo Lin, both twenty-three years old at the time, the same age as Esther Mok—they interviewed over 120 people over the next two months.[222] *A Defining Moment: How Singapore Beat SARS* was published the following spring, with its first chapter's opening story devoted to Mok. Eschewing the trope of "patient zero," Chua chose the more delicate phrase "Patient Number 1" to introduce her.[223] This was the first public profile based on interviews with Mok and remains one of the few published sources to capture her voice, her own reflections on SARS, and her memories, however fragmentary, of her epidemic experience. The narrative that emerges highlights not just the heartbreaking ordinariness of Mok's pre-SARS family life but also the subtle distortions that international media accounts wrought on it.

In early 2003, the Moks were a tight-knit middle-income family. Esther lived with her parents and two brothers in a public housing flat, while three of her paternal aunts—whom she affectionately called her "aunties"—lived in an adjacent flat. (Esther has no sisters, despite the Associated Press article's reference to a sister named Rebecka.) Her father was an accountant, her older brother was a civil servant, her younger brother was still in school, and her mother was a homemaker and "a good cook." "Barely a month before this," Chua writes, "mother and daughter had been making pork floss mini-spring rolls for the Chinese New Year." Esther herself had worked in information technology before becoming a flight attendant. The reason she quit the airlines job, contrary to global media insinuations, was so she could spend more time at home with her family, especially her paternal grandmother, who had been diagnosed with lung cancer; in fact, this grandmother died about a week after Esther herself was admitted into the same hospital.[224] On her last day in Hong Kong, Esther started to feel sick, developing a fever and cough, but, as she explained to Chua's team, "I didn't see a doctor initially. I don't like seeing doctors." A few days after her return home, though, Esther's mother persuaded her to get checked out while they were visiting her paternal grandmother at the hospital anyway, and it was during this examination that Esther had a chest x-ray and was admitted for pneumonia.

"It was scary," Esther recalled, but, at first, she felt only "dull and lethargic but not very weak."[225] It was not until the next day, when she tried to take a shower, that she felt so dizzy and weak that she had to sit in the bathroom waiting for help. A few days later, she was "gasping for air" and was transferred to an ICU isolation room. She stayed in the hospital for a total of forty-six days.[226] In that period, she had frequent x-rays and daily injections and blood draws. "They draw from both arms and when they can't find any more veins to poke, then they will poke on the wrist," she recounted. "Anywhere they can find."[227] Even after discharge, the "medication caused her shoulder-length hair, always fine and dark brown, to fall out in clumps that littered the floor of her home," growing back only two months later. "All these she could bear," Chua relates. "But the loss of her family members wore her down." In those same weeks, even as Esther's condition improved, her family members fell sick and were hospitalized one by one: first her mother, then her aunt's pastor, then her father, then her maternal grandmother, and, finally, her uncle. (But not her brothers, neither of whom caught SARS, contrary to another error in the Associated Press article.) The Tan Tock Seng Hospital staff cared for many Moks that March and April. And within those months, two in the family circle would recover, but four would not.

The Esther Mok that comes through in Chua's portrait is someone of great emotional strength in the face of serial tragedies—a "very brave young woman," as Chua admiringly puts it.[228] "Stoic by nature, friends say they have never seen Miss Mok get angry or lose her cool," Chua writes. "She is the kind of person who will open up to friends but tries not to cry in front of strangers, even when the pain wells up in her." But when the doctor came to Esther's hospital room to inform her of her father's death, she broke down sobbing.[229] Her mother was unconscious by that point, kept alive by a ventilator and feeding tubes. "When I saw her, I cried," Esther recollected. "As days passed, she became very bloated. And they had to use all this scotch-tape to hold all the tubes in place, so her skin was dry and patchy, like with rashes." Yet Esther tried to stay steadfast. By then, she had recovered enough physical strength to walk on her own to her mother's room, so she did so every day, sitting by her mother's bedside, "holding her hand and stroking her, talking to her in Mandarin": "I'd tell her to be strong and to hang in there. I'd tell her what happened that day. I watched the news and then I'd tell her. Basically that. And then I would say I'd pray for her and that she must also pray for herself."[230] Contrary to the Associated Press article's faintly disparaging spin, television was not a medium of entertainment for a bored Esther but a desperate lifeline she extended to her comatose mother in those weeks, a channel by which she could feel connected to the outside world and in turn sustain her mother's connection to the world of the living. She watched the news so she could anchor herself and her mother in a present social reality and its daily happenings, as every day of disease survival was a struggle and a victory. And she continued to watch the news despite its blatant aggression toward her as Singapore's "superinfector."

In retrospect, "the whole period remains shrouded in a kind of darkness" for Esther. What she remembered was trying "not to think too much" and keeping herself "busy and active" with correspondence. Someone gave her a laptop so she could receive encouraging emails from her wide circle of friends. These emails, combined with a constant stream of supportive phone calls and text messages from friends and family, became "her main sources of contact with the outside world" on a personal level.[231] If Huiling Ding spotlights these new communication technologies as performing the function of "guerilla media" during SARS, as discussed in chapter 2, for Esther these technologies were nothing short of survival devices. Serving as countermeasures to the mainstream media and its stigmatizing discourse about her, they made possible an alternative mental health support network, one whose countermessages helped her combat the psychic stresses of illness, loss, grief, and guilt. In this sense, they may be considered technologies of epidemic resilience—all the more vital for Esther as verifiable communications with her parents disappeared. She never discovered if her comatose mother ever heard what she said during those final weeks, for, though her mother blinked once or twice, she never woke up. On the day her mother died, Esther rushed to the ICU as doctors tried unsuccessfully to revive her, and, afterward, Esther sat alone by her mother's body a long time, until the rest of her family arrived. "My family is not a hugging family," she told Chua's team. "It was the first time I hugged my brother."[232] Surrounded by her two brothers and three aunts for the first time since her isolation, Esther hugged and wept. Nine days later, she was discharged. It was a sign of the hospital staff's confidence in her emotional toughness that they asked her to come back and relay the news of her parents' passing to her maternal grandmother, who was still hospitalized at Tan Tock Seng. Flanked by social workers, nurses, and a doctor, Esther broke the news to her grandmother in Cantonese. They cried and embraced, and, this time, in addition to being a fellow griever, Esther assumed the role of consoling caregiver.[233]

Spirituality after SARS

A decade later, Esther's voice resurfaces in Singapore's anglophone media, in Norhaya Fong's documentary *A Tale of Two Esthers*. This film tracks the religious journeys of two Singaporean women named Esther: Mok in the first part, and Esther Tan in the second, also age twenty-three, a copyeditor who trained to become part of Singapore's first women's team to reach the top of Mount Everest despite a congenital heart condition. Both are tales of overcoming, of extraordinary adversities faced and conquered. The segment on Mok, similar to the profile in Chua's book, works to offset the criminal-izing rhetoric of "superinfector" and showcases instead Mok's emotional arc through the epidemic experience. Here, too, the language of ordinariness is adopted to describe her pre-SARS life: "Esther Mok, at age 23, was just an ordinary girl," the film's promotional material asserts. "What really hap-pened? What was her journey?"[234] The documentary strives to construct the meaning of this journey through a Christian framework of unfathomable human suffering culminating in redemptive faith. As a capstone of this les-son, it ends with a sermon delivered by a local church leader, Rick Yamamoto. Speaking directly at the camera to viewers and analogizing Mok to the bibli-cal Job, Yamamoto offers an exegesis of her SARS encounter in the scriptural terms of moral trial and divine salvation: "She did not allow adverse cir-cumstances to overcome her. She could easily have moved toward anger and bitterness, and instead she drew closer to God. She did not allow the family's tragedy or circumstances to overcome her, but what she did is she connected to God, and she found power and energy and meaning in this life." Yamamoto then concludes on a note of recruitment: "I invite you, join God's movement, join the two Esthers, and move with God."[235] The metaphysical compass of religion, for which earthly life and death do not constitute the ultimate ends of human meaning, opens up an alternative frame for resig-nifying disease mortality and survival. Here, it counters bio-orientalist and infrahumanist ontologies that cast Chinese index cases as unworthy life, celebrating them instead as unabandoned children of God and potential paragons of spiritual strength. At the same time, this religious discourse also attempts to control the meaning of Mok's story, and, tellingly, it does not give her the last word.

Still, among anglophone accounts of Mok, this film comes closest to re-turning narrative agency to the first patient herself. It is also one of the few archival sites to preserve audio traces of Mok's voice at length. Most impor-tantly, the film anchors its reconstruction of events in *her* recollections and reflections, with SARS as much as God coming to the fore or receding into the background in faithful accordance with her self-narration. What shines through, then, is not an externally imposed script but the shape of one life as it seeks to narrate and heal itself after a traumatic watershed episode. And what we are bequeathed is a story of pandemic resilience and prosociality on more-than-ordinary scales.

"I was born and raised in Singapore," Esther says in English in her opening line in the film. "I lived with my parents and my older brother and my younger brother. We were, in a sense, quite a close-knit family. My father would take us out to the beach during the weekends to have picnic and we would swim there. My mom was a very good cook, and we would have special dinner on Friday nights every week. My brother is two years older than me. We are quite close." Reiterating some of the information she had shared with Chua's team a decade earlier but filling in additional details about that period, Esther here goes on to relate how she quit her airlines job to spend more time at home with her sick grandmother, and how the trip to Hong Kong was "a small break" from that eldercare situation. In Chua's book, Esther had appeared as the filial granddaughter who provided occasional elder support within the family, but, in the film, her caregiver role comes across more distinctly, with the Hong Kong "holiday" more explicitly tied to her need for a reprieve from the daily stress of elder caregiving. And while the Esther in Chua's book attributed her delay in seeking medical help to a personal aversion to doctors, the Esther in this film repeatedly declares of her own symptoms: "I didn't really think much of it because I thought it was a normal fever and it would just go away . . . [and] recover on its own." This tendency to neglect self-care, to downplay one's own unwellness, is a refrain in narratives of and by caregivers, especially among Asian women. What can get minimized or taken for granted as proper daughterly behavior and labor within the Confucian family emerges here within a more spiritual framework of mutual care and attentive listening.

The film also paints a more precarious picture of Esther's time at the hospital. "When I was in the ICU, I was semi-conscious," she narrates. "I didn't know what was really happening. And the people I came across in the hospital were the doctors, the nurses, and they were all dressed in a gown and gloves and with a mask on." When she improved and was transferred back to an open ward, she spent two nights there with her mother, who had been admitted to the same ward. "She was there, and she looked quite all right," Esther recalls. Even after her mother's condition worsened and she was transferred to the ICU, where her father was already isolated, Esther did not feel overly concerned: "I felt pretty confident that they would recover because I recovered. I recovered, I got better from the ICU, and I didn't think it was very serious." Drawing from her own disease trajectory, Esther had faith in medicine's capacity to treat and cure. She was also counseled to have faith in God, and she did. One of her aunts gave her a Bible and pointed her to Psalm 91: "He that dwelleth in the secret place of the most High shall abide under the shadow of the Almighty. I will say of the Lord, He is my refuge and my fortress: my God; in him will I trust. Surely he shall deliver thee from the snare of the fowler, and from the noisome pestilence...." So she visited her parents in the ICU every day, relaying to them the daily news while praying for their deliverance from noisome pestilence.

"But things didn't get better," she continues, her voice soft. When her father died, she prayed harder for her mother, retaining her conviction in the power of faith and prayer. "I prayed very hard to God because that was the only hope I could cling on to," she narrates. But when her mother died too, she had a crisis of faith:

> I remember I was kneeling in front of her bed and crying for a long time, and asking why did this have to happen to my parents, why did this have to happen to me. I was very sorry that I had spread the disease to them and caused them to die.... I made this pact with God that if my parents recover I would go to church, I would be more fervent. But things didn't happen that way. I was very angry with God. I was bitter with God. I even didn't know whether God is real or not. I just wanted to do away with him and control my own life. Just stop all contact with God.

The media labeling of her as a "superinfector" complicated these feelings of rage and bitterness and prompted her to internalize a sense of responsibility for Singapore's many SARS deaths: "There were a lot of news going on about this disease, and they labeled me as a 'superspreader' and how I spread it to a lot of other people. This disease was really very fatal, and I felt... guilty. I blamed myself. I felt guilty that I had to pass on the disease to them. I felt guilty that I recovered but that they didn't make it." And in language of not just survivor's guilt but suicidal ideation, she recalls, "I felt really angry and bitter with God for allowing this to happen, my parents to die, and why not me since I brought the disease to Singapore, since I went on holiday." Had the mental health of first patients been taken into consideration earlier by the media and the state, Esther could have been spared this lacerating self-blame that exacerbated the helplessness and despair she already felt.

Beneath these layers of religious anger and epidemic guilt was a deeper self-blame about her own failure as a daughter. When she first saw her father in the ICU, "lying on a bed, motionless and unconscious," she berated herself for having judged him harshly as an inadequate father and husband who periodically quit his job and saddled her mother with work. "Though we were a close-knit family, I had a lot of expectations on him to provide for the family," she professes. "I didn't really talk to my father about this. It was just like a silent defiance. I knew he loved me, but he didn't live up to my expectations." But in the ICU, her reproach turned inward: "It was the first time I really see him up close after a long time, and from there I really saw, like he has really aged a lot. But I didn't take notice of that before. I cried for a long time there, and I repeated, apologizing, I kept saying sorry to him." After her mother too passed away, Esther began to censure herself for having been an ungrateful daughter: "I really missed them at that point in time. I thought that I didn't cherish the time I had with them. I couldn't accept the fact that they were gone so soon." In her book, Chua mentions a phase when Esther was haunted by nightmares: "Twice, she woke up frightened and sobbing in the middle of the night."[236] Although her brothers and aunts were "very supportive" and never blamed her for anyone's death, even going out of their way to never mention SARS in her presence and to shield her from both estate matters and intrusive reporters, Esther nonetheless felt adrift and hounded in Singapore. As she narrates in the film, "They showed their love and their concern for me through just being normal, just life carries on as usual." But this feeling of normality was no longer accessible to her: "I didn't know what to do, what to live for. I felt that I lost all aim or purpose in life. I didn't want to find a job as well. I was afraid that people would recognize and shun me." While in the hospital, she had felt that the Singaporean public was "quite supportive" of her, sending her "a lot of cards and soft toys" with messages telling her "to be strong, to persevere on ... that [she] wasn't to blame for this disease." But in the posthospital months, even after the pandemic's end, though having lived through SARS itself, she no longer had the same home to inhabit, the same life to resume, or a future she could imagine.

From Esther's complex self-narration, we can detect more than just one story arc or one register of epidemic significance. Her memories and reflections unfold over multiple terrains and scales, from the unit of the nuclear family to the larger contexts of the state media and national public to an international anglophone disease discourse and a suprahuman realm of prayer and faith. Accordingly, the affective scope of her self-narrative encompasses personal reckonings not only with the Christian God but also with her parents, her brothers and aunts, other Singaporeans and SARS patients, and, above all, herself. As much as the film may construct Esther's story as possessing a unified lesson and spiritual journey, Esther's voice actually delivers a much more heterogeneous and multistranded narrative. At the same time, the film's religious crescendo is precisely what allows Esther's post-SARS life to surface as no other work has done. It is this latter portion of the film that most endows her not just with survival but with dignity and self-reclamation.

About five months after her release from the hospital, Esther needed to have her wisdom teeth extracted, so she visited a dentist a friend had recommended. She was still unemployed, mostly staying at home and hiding from the outside world. In retrospect, she considered this visit a kind of divine intervention, for it was during her appointment that the dentist, a stranger to her until then, suggested that she join his church youth group's upcoming expedition to the Philippines to refurbish a student center. "For my character," she recounts, "I wouldn't go any place with a group of strangers, and this was a trip to the Philippines with a group of people I've never met before." But then: "I thought, why not? At that point in time, I just wanted to get out of Singapore, do something different. I didn't want to face the media. I just wanted to get out and not think of anything else." So she joined the youth group and traveled to the Philippines at year's end. During one Sunday church service there, she saw a pamphlet with the sentence "For God to explain a trial would be to destroy its purpose, calling forth simple faith and implicit obedience." Esther herself stages this moment as one of divine communion and spiritual restoration, the turning point in her post-SARS life:

> That sort of jumped out and spoke to me. Because I was asking God, "Why does this have to happen, why me and why my parents? I already made a pact with you, but it didn't work out this way. Why does this have to happen to me? I had a happy family, and all these are taken away from me." Something really was stirring in my heart. I could feel that God was speaking to me, and it was very real. For the first time I experienced this feeling. I remember him telling me to return to him, and at first I rejected. I was struggling. I didn't want to return to him. But his voice grew stronger and louder, and I couldn't fight it anymore and said, "Okay God, I will return to you." And at that point when I made that decision, I felt that I was at peace. There was this sense of peace that I have never felt before that just came over me and this serenity that I experienced. And from

then, just at that instant, I thought I could get over my parents' deaths and move on with life. . . . It was the very first time I truly had a personal encounter with God, over there in the Philippines. After the Philippines trip, I told God that I was ready to start life anew, to get a job.

From there, the film brings Esther's story to a rapid, happy closure. She returned to Singapore and was soon connected through a friend to a job as a youth worker at a Christian organization. The pastor there was at first reluctant to hire Esther, and his voice in the film highlights the degree to which even religious groups and their leaders were not immune to resentment and anger toward Esther as the national index case for SARS. "When I first heard that it was Esther Mok," the pastor admits on camera, "the Esther Mok who brought SARS into Singapore, who was trying to get this job that we had, I hesitated a bit because we lost a good friend, a doctor in our church. I was his pastor for six years, and we grappled with that quite a bit. Why? Why him? And then suddenly hearing that Esther Mok, the one who brought SARS to Singapore, was coming in for this interview, it just stirred my heart a bit." Affected by personal loss, the pastor, too, echoing Esther after her parents' deaths, asked, "Why?" In his case, rather than rejecting God, he felt inclined to spurn Esther, the available public target of disease blame. After listening to her story at the interview, though, he realized "she really had a lot to offer young people going through difficulties, both youths at risk and those who have challenges." In the pastor's narration, he was the one who took a leap of faith in hiring Esther. But between the lines, we can discern the persuasive power of Esther's own storytelling, her crafting the narrative of her disease experiences into a form that, for once, would facilitate her own healing and reentry into postcrisis social life.

In fact, she told her story so well that the sympathetic pastor went on to "play cupid," introducing Esther to another volunteer, Kendrick Teo, who would soon become her husband. After marrying, the two continued their work with the organization together while also starting and coaching a tchoukball club, eventually joining Singapore's national teams. In her closing speech in the film, Esther describes her ongoing work with youths and conveys her message more broadly to those facing personal loss: "The youths that I work with, whenever I tell my story, I hope that they will cherish their parents, will cherish their loved ones. . . . My advice to those who have lost their loved ones is that it's inevitable that people die, but what we can do is not to dwell in the past, not to ask why did this happen to me, why does this have to happen, but rather, what can I learn from this and how can God use me to help others who are also experiencing similar difficulties." Going beyond resilience and prosociality, Esther converts disease survival into healing service.

From disease pariah and bereaved daughter to youth worker, national athlete, and spiritual counselor, the Esther Mok of this film models a tale of such superlative SARS transcendence—of such epidemic overcoming and survivor success, and with such decisive validation by institutional powers—that a skeptical, secular viewer might be tempted to simply scoff it away as a case of doctrinal hyperbole. Yet this is the very parable that emerges through Esther's own voice. Instead of reading this personal narrative of found faith as a de facto metanarrative of Christian propaganda, we might attend to its seriality and reversals, the ways Esther spotlights her micro choices as well as life-changing decisions along the way, from conditional bargaining with God to vehement rejection of him to belated affirmation of her belief. This genre of spiritual recovery and awakening—so in alignment with Esther's own storytelling, and so empowering and healing for her posttraumatic life—has been largely suppressed and dismissed by the secularizing tendencies of global reporting on SARS. With Mok, we leave the realm of first patient microagency as primarily pandemic ordinariness and smallness, though these elements persist. With her, we see ordinariness channeled into the extraordinary, a category now reclaimed from the zone of disease catastrophe into the space of the transformative, the spiritual, the personal divine.

Coda: Ghostly Returns and Folk Prayers

During COVID-19, reports of ghost sightings and other paranormal activities have soared across the Anglo-American world.[237] For the most part, these are not titillating tales driven by age-old gothic tropes of death and decay. Unlike "CoronaGothic" fiction that, according to Victoria Harrison, serves as "a device to deal with horror," to put our collective dread of pandemic annihilation "in its place," the recurrent affect in these more mundane real-life reports is comfort.[238] "The hallway ghost . . . brings me comfort," relates one Chicago woman. "It feels like even in the loneliest of times during the pandemic, especially living alone, I have a friend who checks in on me. Even though this friend is a ghost who lives in my hallways, I am never scared when I feel its presence."[239] Another woman echoes this sentiment: "As a New Yorker, it's been impossible for me to navigate life in the city without feeling incredibly devastated by all we've lost this year," so ghostly returns are "comforting," "one of the best ways to honor the dead."[240] Particularly for those who have lost loved ones to the coronavirus, visitations and signs—from "hyper-real dreams" to "a sudden whiff of fragrance," from "a touch on the shoulder at night" to the sighting of a "full-bodied form"—can feel like "a second chance to say goodbye."[241] As one former hospice worker attests, "These kinds of reports are normal in my world. It would make sense that in a pandemic or other event that leads to mass deaths that there will be numerical increase in reports and experiences, given the shared grief and trauma."[242] These Western anecdotes of supernatural solace may constitute a more minor and eccentric archive than Esther Mok's deeply spiritual story, but they, too, have a precursor in SARS-era Singapore.

If *A Defining Moment* and *A Tale of Two Esthers* record some of Singapore's most official SARS memories, Russell Lee's *The Almost Complete Collection of True Singapore Ghost Stories* delivers a more heterodox account of epidemic experience. A massively popular book series that purportedly compiles "true" indigenous strange tales relayed by readers, *True Singapore Ghost Stories*—or TSGS as it is known to beloved fans—encapsulates, in Lee's words, "the collective psychic experience of the peoples of Singapore and Malaysia," representing "a store of our supernatural heritage and a shared experience that bonds us."[243] Launched in 1989, the series comprises twenty-six volumes and counting as of 2020. In the 25th Year Special Edition, the ever-enigmatic Lee (whose name is a nom de plume and whose true identity remains literally under wraps, as they never appear in public without their whole body covered from head to toe in black) notes at the end of one contributor's story, "I shall never forget the dreaded SARS that broke out in 2003. Doctors and nurses sacrificed their lives to bring the deadly scourge under control. Book 11 was launched during the outbreak."[244] Book 12, published one year later, contains a story entitled "Sisters in SARS," credited to a thirty-one-year-old nurse under the alias Natalie Wong.

"When the SARS outbreak hit Singapore," she recounts through Lee's ghostwritten voice, "it was tragic to see one's colleagues fall ill and lose their lives in the line of duty. One day a fellow nurse would be healthy, the next he or she would be feverish. The doctors were not spared either." Ruth, one of her closest friends and a fellow nurse, also died from SARS, and later that same week, Natalie herself contracted the virus from a patient. As she lay in the isolation ward at 3 a.m. one night, Natalie "had the feeling that [she] was

234 CHAPTER 4

going to die" when suddenly "two figures clad in white" materialized by her bedside. One was Ruth, and the other was Natalie's long-dead grandmother, the role model who had originally inspired her to become a nurse. The grandmother, brought along by Ruth from the other side to save Natalie, promptly shared a story and a prayer:

> "Well, a long, long time before you were born, and long before I gave birth to your mother, we had a terrible outbreak of flu in Singapore. Hundreds of people died. In those days there were none of the modern drugs they have now. I contracted the flu when I was on duty, just like you have SARS now.
>
> "I nearly died except for the fact that an old lady, a missionary, taught me a prayer. It saved my life. I've come along tonight to teach you that prayer. . . ."
>
> She told me it was a very special prayer, and swore me to secrecy.
>
> "The prayer can only be used when you are at death's door, and you can only share it with one other person. . . ."
>
> I learned the prayer and repeated it over and over again throughout the early hours of the morning.[245]

When the doctors came at daybreak, expecting Natalie to have perished in the night, they found instead her fever broken, her condition much improved—and, mysteriously, "a little photo of [her] grandmother, in an antique silver frame," by her bed.[246]

True Singapore Ghost Stories is often credited with inaugurating a Singaporean popular literature as well as a Singapore-identified mass readership. As one local journalist and publisher observes, "This series marked the start of Singaporeans reading Singapore originals. Prior to that, the tendency was to reach for foreign titles on the bookshelves, while local publishers—entrenched in the British literary mode, a legacy of our colonial past—did not have the know-how to publish lighthearted and mass market titles."[247] The series's "long-running popularity" further attests to "a reading public . . . hungry for locally written and produced books," and not surprisingly, it has spawned numerous local imitators.[248] Analyzing this popular genre in relation to Singapore's collective memory of World War II, Carole Faucher explores the ways ghost tales can interact with official history to "creat[e] platforms where memories . . . may be experienced over and over again outside the unequivocal space of commemoration." Figurative spirits anchored in indigenous belief systems help to mediate "emotion-laden memories that produce an alternative mode of dealing with official historical accounts," and they constitute "propitious sites for breeding public awareness on the need for unity and solidarity against impending and hidden threats."[249]

One contemporary threat to indigenous traditions is the Singapore government's urban demolition and redevelopment policy. Since the 1960s, the state has razed and landscaped over much of the island's historic buildings and sites, aiming to remodel the country into a "crypto-ecological fantasy" sanitized of unruly elements.[250] Under this modernizing agenda, even the dead are not safe, as common graveyards across the city have been mandatorily excavated, with bones and bodies cremated and relocated to remote columbaria. Yet "attachments to places die hard, and attachments to places of dying die harder," notes Joshua Comaroff. So it is precisely due to people's lingering attachments to the departed and their places of rest that acts of micropolitical resistance have blossomed, as the populace carries out small guerilla funerals with paper offerings to the dead at former burial grounds around the city every Hungry Ghost Festival. "The effect is extraordinarily moving to the observer," Comaroff writes. "As darkness falls, it is as if a second map, a ghostly historical topography, appears on top of the familiar one, a radical disjuncture of memory and topography that is violently, temporarily conflated within the hyper-controlled surfaces of the contemporary city. The new landscapes are thus infiltrated by the ghosts of history, by familiar entreaties for memory within the unending flood of the new."[251] In this battle over everyday necropower as much as its embrace of fabulous ghost tales, Singapore might just live up to its reputation as the most haunted city on earth.

With these perspectives in mind, we can read "Sisters in SARS" contrapuntally on at least two levels. Tapping into premodern reservoirs of folk spirit beliefs and resuscitating haunting experiences buried by the modernizing authoritarian state, the story may be viewed as a subversive and decolonizing text vis-à-vis local power. At the same time, read in relation to global pandemic discourse, it raises another microepisteme against pandemic crisis epistemologies. The story constellates many of the themes explored in this book: female community and sentimental kinship ties as the enduring ethos of epidemic life; near-death sickness and eleventh-hour recovery without the looming menace of planetary apocalypse; the infected hospital as a space for heterogeneous and dissonant styles of epidemic narration; and the disease epicenter at the global periphery as a site of crisis resilience, local memory, and overwritten affects. Even the form of the entertaining apocryphal ghost yarn, relayed from and shared with an anonymous public, recalls those digi-

236 CHAPTER 4

tal SARS jokes with prosocial small humor. Here specifically, the forgotten past of the grandmother's brush with death during what must have been the local outbreak of the 1918 influenza pandemic gets revived through her apparitional voice during SARS, connecting the two pandemics for local readers through a lineage of preternatural healing, care work, and survival, across the very border of life and death. In this plebeian rendering of the gothic genre, death, whether by disease or other means, is decidedly not final or even scary, whether for the dead or the loved ones left behind. The secret lifesaving prayer may not get transmitted to readers, but the telling of its singular miraculous power puts into circulation another mode of folk knowledge amid and between pandemic disasters, part of a crowdsourced lore to live on and believe in.

As Russell Lee sums up in their author's note in the special edition: "I do hope that the supernatural and the intangible will always be an important part of our lives. As we make progress, we may become deluded into thinking that all we need is a healthy bank balance. Please don't worship money. Reality is more than what we can see and touch, and our timeline is not merely our lifespan but eternity."[252] In this invocation of a suprahuman temporality and order of meaning that both precedes and transcends secular capitalist modernity, we are reminded that our mortal lives as much as our current epoch are neither the beginning nor the end, sharing as we do a common cosmos with countless beings beyond our purview. But exactly so, wisdom may come from the most unforeseen quarters if we keep the right things at heart.

Afterword

When I started researching SARS for this book, I began by looking at literature and culture, at novels and then, more adventurously, digital media and film and music, partly because these realms constitute my relative comfort zone as a literary scholar, but mostly because I assumed the history and real-life stories would have been told by others before me. This was over a decade after SARS's end, so I took it on faith that the facts were well documented in the voluminous body of writing already published on the topic, and that even early infection cases in China would have been properly archived by then. Moreover, since English, as WHO itself acknowledges, remains the dominant language of global public health information and "the lingua franca of scientists—including those working in public health," I took it on faith that knowledge about specialized epidemiological matters, such as index cases and early outbreak clusters, would be firmly in place in the anglophone public record.[1] In short, I took the pandemic first patients and their stories for granted, as things already told and known, things I did not have to bother investigating for myself. I was content to stay in my disciplinary lane and focus on fictional texts and fictional lives, venturing into empirical sources only for context and self-education. It took several years of writing and reading, until the book's last chapter, for me to fully realize my misplaced faith.

What I discovered with shock, when I started digging into accounts of Pang Zuoyao, was that much had been written on his death but not on his life, even though he did not die, as chapter 4 details. The emotions that predominated my writing of this final chapter's beginning were incredulity and fury: Why hadn't more people cared enough about Chinese index patients to research their lives? Why had such rampant misinformation been allowed to stand, not just in popular media but in official history? Yet there was also self-disappointment: Why did it take me so long to look into this archive myself? Elsewhere, I have written about the need for a critical reckoning— of the anglophonization of SARS, of English as the language of global public health knowledge and power, and of its production and reproduction of the narrative silences, oversights, blunders, and disfigurements around pandemic first patients.[2] But, three years into COVID-19, the story that lingers, that gifts strength, is Esther Mok's. If anger precipitated the beginning of this book's end, the emotions that close it are sadness but also hope.

Throughout this book, I have highlighted similarities between SARS and COVID. Perhaps most salient is the resurgence of bio-orientalism in global pandemic discourse, such as zoonotic origin stories involving Chinese "wet markets" that fuel sinophobic fear, disgust, and violence. These disheartening echoes can trigger a sense of déjà vu, as if we are simply repeating the same mistakes and hatreds of pandemic history. But, less commonly recognized, and what I have attempted most to retrieve here, are the positive reanimations: the tremendous vibrancy of prosocial practices despite contagion threats, the enduring desire for resilience models amid mass infections, and the communal faith in ordinary peopleness and everyday small acts of caring. Within my SARS archive, these have been exemplified by Ru Yan's return to dog-walking at the end of Hu Fayun's novel as much as Aunty Hong and Yue E's shopping adventures in Chen Baozhen's novella; Ah Kum's many crisis comebacks in *Golden Chicken 2* as much as the Hong Kong media industry's rallying for the 2003 film awards ceremony and *Project 1:99*; Pang's postsickness shift toward healthier living as much as Mok's return to spiritual belief and turn to youth work; and, not least, the innumerable acts of digital good humor by anonymous texters and netizens who told and relayed epidemic jokes and microaffirmations during SARS.

Indeed, it was the realm of digital media that first restored my equilibrium and crystallized this book in COVID's early months. Amid evergrimmer accounts of escalating illnesses and deaths within China but before international news began reporting on the coronavirus in earnest, a slew of homemade videos emerged out of Wuhan on Chinese social media, rapidly going viral as people shared and reshared them to deliver communal recognition, concern, and cheer. In that period, even a ten-second clip could move me to tears or laughter—from the January 27, 2020, "Wuhan jiayou!" videos of residents under city lockdown shouting encouragements out their apartment windows in spontaneous bursts of solidarity to the quarantine boredom videos of people amusing themselves with ingenious and silly antics, such as fishing out of home aquariums or playing mahjong with plastic bags over their heads.[3] These mundane acts and their recording helped me feel, on a gut level, what I had grasped only cerebrally up until that point: that life at pandemic epicenters does not have to be defined apocalyptically or grandiosely—as horror scenarios of collapse or epic struggles of heroes and villains—but can be and is being lived through with heart and humor, creativity and prosociality, and sheer human ordinariness and humaneness. Guobin Yang captures this epiphanic insight poignantly in his preface to *The Wuhan Lockdown*: "[COVID-19] upset the lives of a nation overnight. The certainty of everyday life dissolved into quicksand. Little was known about this virus in January 2020. No one knew how long the lockdown would last. Yet as the lockdown passed from days to weeks, the city endured.... Ordinary residents ... lived through COVID-19 and the lockdown with a silent courage that filled me with awe.... Their extraordinary experiences cannot be distilled into a few propositions without losing their sheer wealth and human touch. Their concreteness defies abstraction." As Yang puts it, in the face of this awe-inspiring endurance, "mere attempts to theorize look rather pale."[4]

So I offer this book with humility, as a modest attempt at concretizing abstraction for a much more settled archive, not to gain authority over SARS stories and lives but to remember them for strength and wisdom in our COVID present. While there is no one template for how pandemics will unfold—SARS's relatively short duration seems so remote now from COVID's protracted temporality—the abiding sense of affirmative peopleness is what I hope will last.

NOTES

Introduction

1 Leung P., "Feidian shiqi," 101 (my translation).

2 Ngai, *Ugly Feelings*, 4; Ngai is paraphrasing Paolo Virno's "sentiments of disenchantment."

3 KPIX, "Anti-Asian Hate Crimes."

4 See, for example, "Elderly Asian Woman"; Brooks, "Elderly Asian Woman"; and Jaclyn Peiser, "Asian Woman, 75, Beats Back Man Who Punched Her in San Francisco," *Washington Post*, March 19, 2021.

5 Li Meiyan, "Huayi popo yuxi hou fenqi fanji, benbao manhuajia zuohua zhengqi shuaping" [Overseas Chinese grandma suffers attack but strikes back with vigor, our newspaper cartoonist's picture floods the internet with righteousness], *Yangcheng wanbao*, March 22, 2021, https://ep.ycwb.com/epaper/ycwb/html/2021-03/22/content_108_369664.htm; "Apo Meiguo."

6 Chappell, "Asian Grandmother."

7 Liu X., "Yingyong huanji."

8 See John Chen, "Help My Grandmother Recover from This Trauma," *GoFundMe*, June 7, 2021, https://www.gofundme.com/f/2b8zh292uo.

9 KPIX, "Anti-Asian Hate Crimes."

10 See, respectively, comments by Brenda Weber, 980ssb Bearcat, J, AzNstat, and Paolo García in KPIX, "Anti-Asian Hate Crimes."

11 Li M., "Huayi popo."

12 Lah and Kravarik, "Family of Thai Immigrant"; Nielsen, "Suspect Arrested."

13 Jeung et al., *Stop AAPI Hate*, 1.

14 See video uploaded by the San Francisco Public Defender Office on April 8, 2021, https://drive.google.com/file/d/1baU _5h8BlqpfMgdmR5Q7JAUToy5v164A/view.

15 McBurney, "Deputy Public Defender."

16 Qtd. in JTSF Television, "Zuotian."

17 California has one of the worst rates of affordable housing for extremely low-income renters out of the fifty US states, due to zoning laws as well as local homeowners' protests against low-income housing projects; see German Lopez, "The Morning," *New York Times*, July 15, 2022.

18 McBurney, "Deputy Public Defender."

19 Qtd. in Thomas Fuller, "The Complex Case Emerging of the Attack of an Asian Woman in San Francisco," *New York Times*, June 10, 2021.

20 Atkins, Wilson, and Hayes, *Prosocial*, 207.

21 Atkins, Wilson, and Hayes, *Prosocial*, 1.

22 Fuller, "Complex Case."

23 Whyte, "Against Crisis Epistemology," 52–53.

24 Whyte, "Against Crisis Epistemology," 53–55.

25 Whyte, "Against Crisis Epistemology," 57.

26 See, for example, WHO, "Impact of COVID-19"; World Bank, "World Bank/ IMF"; and FEMA, *COVID-19 Pandemic*.

27 *Dictionary.com*, "8 Pandemic Words and Phrases People Absolutely Never Want to Hear Again," April 22, 2020, https://www.dictionary.com/e /pandemic-words-people-hate/.

28 Agamben, "Invention of an Epidemic."

29 See, respectively, Allen, "Death by Sneezing"; Omi, "Overview"; J.-W. Lee, "Speech"; Fidler, *SARS*; Duffy, "Anatomy of an Epidemic"; and LeDuc and Barry, "SARS, the First Pandemic."

30 Fidler, *SARS*, 3, 7, 53.

31 WHO, "Update 17."

32 WHO, *International Health Regulations*.

33 John M. Broder, "The SARS Epidemic: The American Response," *New York Times*, May 5, 2003.

34 Anderson et al., "Epidemiology," 80.

35 Ahmed, *Cultural Politics of Emotion*, 2.

36 See Kong, "Pandemic as Method" and "Totalitarian Ordinariness."

37 Zhan, "Civet Cats," 37–38.

38 Berlant, *Cruel Optimism*, 7.

39 Young, "New Plague."

40 Wald, *Contagious*, 44–45.

41 Anthony Spaeth, "The Revenge of the Birds," *Time*, February 9, 2004.

42 Heinrich, "Future Repeats Itself," 168.

43 Heinrich, "Future Repeats Itself," 172–74, 176.

44 See R. G. Lee, *Orientals*; N. Shah, *Contagious Divides*; Craddock, *City of Plagues*; Molina, *Fit to Be Citizens?*

45 Qtd. in N. Shah, *Contagious Divides*, 1; qtd. in Molina, *Fit to Be Citizens?*, 15, 27.

46 See my "Pandemic as Method" for points summarized in this discussion.

47 National Intelligence Council, *SARS*.

48 K.-H. Chen, *Asia as Method*, vii.

49 For one example of his thesis on a planetary state of exception, see Agamben, *Homo Sacer*.

50 According to WHO data, on February 26, 2020, the day Agamben published his initial article on "Invention of an Epidemic" on the Italian website *Quodlibet*, China had 78,191 confirmed cases and 2,718 deaths from COVID; see WHO, "Coronavirus Disease 2019," table 1.

51 Marco della Cava, "Asian Americans in San Francisco Are Dying at Alarming Rates from COVID-19: Racism Is to Blame," *USA Today*, October 21, 2020.

52 Pike, "Why 15 US States."

53 Qtd. in Maria Cramer and Knvul Sheikh, "Surgeon General Urges the Public to Stop Buying Face Masks," *New York Times*, February 29, 2020.

54 Leetaru, "Mask-Wearing Guidance."

55 S. Feng et al., "Rational Use," 435.

56 See, for example, MacIntyre et al., "Face Mask Use."

57 S. Feng et al., "Rational Use," 436.

58 Y. Zhang and Xu, "Ignorance, Orientalism and Sinophobia," 211.

59 Y. Zhang and Xu, "Ignorance, Orientalism and Sinophobia," 220–21.

60 Meinhof, "Othering the Virus."

61 Ahmed, *Cultural Politics of Emotion*, 28, 31.

62 Ahmed, *Cultural Politics of Emotion*, 191.

63 Ahmed, *Cultural Politics of Emotion*, 130.

64 Hayot, *Hypothetical Mandarin*, 10–11, 15.

65 Berlant, *Cruel Optimism*, 10.

66 Berlant, *Cruel Optimism*, 3.

67 Berlant, *Cruel Optimism*, 10.

68 Berlant, *Cruel Optimism*, 101.

69 Berlant, *Cruel Optimism*, 10.

70 Berlant, *Cruel Optimism*, 8.

71 Berlant, *Cruel Optimism*, 262.

72 Berlant, *Cruel Optimism*, 98–99.

73 Berlant, "Without Exception."

74 B. Davis and Catlin, "Theses for Theory."

75 Lin, "Archives of the Future."

76 Tang, *Visual Culture*, 178, 7.

77 J. Lau, "Besides Fists and Blood," 162.

78 Laughlin, "Why Critics."

79 Evasdottir, *Obedient Autonomy*, x–xi.

80 Hillenbrand, *Negative Exposures*, 12.

81 Hillenbrand, *Negative Exposures*, 2–3.

82 Yapp, *Minor China*, 2–3, 13.

83 Guo, *Evolution of the Chinese Internet*, 1–2.

84 Guo, *Evolution of the Chinese Internet*, 3.

85 Sedgwick, *Touching Feeling*, 145; Sedgwick, *Epistemology of the Closet*, 23.

86 Sedgwick, *Touching Feeling*, 124–44.

87 My method of cultural archaeology is akin to Jenny Sharpe's reclamation of Black enslaved women's agency in *Ghosts of Slavery*.

88 Y. Lee, *Modern Minority*, 4.

89 Ngai, *Ugly Feelings*, 6–7.

90 Ahmed, *Cultural Politics of Emotion*, 201.

91 Ahmed, *Cultural Politics of Emotion*, 202, 191.

92 Sedgwick, *Touching Feeling*, 143.

93 Sedgwick, *Touching Feeling*, 149–50.

94 Whyte, "Against Crisis Epistemology," 58.

95 Whyte, "Against Crisis Epistemology," 62.

96 Whyte, "Against Crisis Epistemology," 53.

97 Thornber, *Global Healing*, 28.

98 Piepzna-Samarasinha, *Care Work*, 15, 17.

99 Piepzna-Samarasinha, *Care Work*, 19, 24–25.

100 For analyses of these genres, see Mayer, "Virus Discourse"; and Schweitzer, *Going Viral*.

101 Wald, *Contagious*, 2; Berlant, *Cruel Optimism* , 20.

Chapter 1: Pandemic Ordinariness

1   Chang, "From the Ashes," 47.

2   Chang, "From the Ashes," 39–40.

3   Chang, "Writing of One's Own," 18; Chang, "From the Ashes," 40–41.

4   L. Lee, *Shanghai Modern*, 302; N. Huang, introduction, xii.

5   Aside from the works analyzed in this chapter, SARS romances include Ni Houyu's novel *Love in the Time of SARS* (*Feidian shiqi de aiqing*) (2003), Tai Yang's short story of the same name (2007), and Mo Bao Fei Bao's novel *Together Forever* (*Zhi ci zhong nian*) (2013).

6   Haiyan Lee, *Revolution of the Heart*, 2–3.

7   Ahmed, *Cultural Politics of Emotion*, 191.

8   Chang, "From the Ashes," 48–49.

9   Berlant, *Cruel Optimism*, 98–99.

10 Ngai, *Ugly Feelings*, 6.

11 Ngai, *Ugly Feelings*, 33, 207–8.

12 Berlant, "Without Exception."

13 Chang, "From the Ashes," 48.

14 Qtd. in Stein, "Joan Chen's Ode."

15 The name Xiu Xiu invokes the eponymous protagonist in Joan Chen's 1998 directorial debut film, *Xiu Xiu: The Sent Down Girl*, based on Geling Yan's short story "Celestial Bath." Though *Shanghai Strangers* is clearly not reprising the same character, the intertextual echo of Xiu Xiu's name implies a thematic continuity between the two films for Chen.

16 Bernards, review.

17 Clark, preface, i–ii.

18 Link, "China: The Anaconda."

19 Mirsky, "Banned in China."

20 Kong, "Totalitarian Ordinariness."

21 Throughout this chapter, I give in-text citations to both the English edition of Hu's novel (*STW*), translated by A. E. Clark and based on the author's full original manuscript, as well as the 2006 abridged Beijing edition (*RY*), for the purpose of tracking censorship practices. Unless otherwise noted, my quotations are taken from Clark's translation. As Clark points out, the blogger Shi Yan Wu Tian has compiled an online synopsis of the novel's excisions by comparing the Beijing edition with an unabridged online version. For a discussion of Shi Yan Wu Tian's restorative work, see T. Chen, "Workshop," 25–27, 31–33, and *Made in Censorship*, 154–56, 160–63. As Chen details, Shi Yan Wu Tian's

original posts were repeatedly deleted by state censors, replicating the digital censorship Hu himself both depicted and experienced.

22 Hu Fayun, afterword to *Ruyan@sars.come*, 271–72.

23 Haiyan Lee, "Déjà Vu."

24 Hu Fayun, "Xie SARS 'jinshu.'"

25 Hu Fayun, "Xie SARS 'jinshu.'"

26 Lieberthal and Oksenberg, *Policy Making in China*, 3.

27 Lieberthal, introduction, 8.

28 Agamben, *Homo Sacer*, 8.

29 See Arendt's last chapter "Ideology of Terror" in *Origins of Totalitarianism.*

30 My translation; I depart from Clark's translation here to bring out Hu's language of disappearance.

31 Haiyan Lee, *Stranger*, 90–92.

32 Haiyan Lee, *Stranger*, 113.

33 Barthes, "Reality Effect," 141.

34 My translation; I depart from Clark's translation here to highlight Hu's language of ordinary living.

35 Berlant, *Cruel Optimism*, 261–62, 95–96.

36 To highlight the distinctiveness of Hu's understated ending, we can contrast *Such Is This World* with another Chinese epidemic novel, Yan Lianke's *Dream of Ding Village*, which dramatizes the plight of one AIDS-stricken Henan village in the 1990s. While Yan's novel also contains a central story line on second-chance romance, the lovers there die tragically, with extravagant acts of self-sacrifice and devotion. In the final chapter, the grandfather protagonist returns home to his village after being arrested for murdering his son, only to find a ghost town utterly decimated by disease and human greed. The torrential rainstorm that ensues conjures up at once planetary apocalypse, the world's renewal, and Nu Wa's (re)creation of humans, images that showcase Yan's much more eschatological and mythic aesthetic.

37 Link, "From Famine," 54–56.

38 Bai Hua, comment on Hu Fayun's *Ruyan, Jinshu wang*, August 10, 2011, https://www.bannedbook.org/forum2/topic171.html.

39 Xiao, *Family Revolution*, 22–23.

40 Veg, *Minjian*, 29–30.

41 Veg, *Minjian*, 7, 10.

42 Veg, *Minjian*, 246.

43 Qtd. in Johnson, "Inside and Outside."

44 Johnson, "Inside and Outside."

45   Feng, Y., "Wei pingfan zhe."

46   Feng, Y., "Wei pingfan zhe."

47   For links to Chen Baozhen's poetry and essays, see *Xun sheng shi she* (Shyun-Sheng poetic club), 2005, http://shyun-sheng.com/author.php?id=65#.

48   "Chen Baozhen," *Baike*, 2022, https://www.baike.com/wikiid /798212889000695561l?view_id=2bzcxxvnkd2k8w.

49   All translations to Chen Baozhen's *SARS Bride* are mine, hereafter cited in the text.

50   Xiao, *Family Revolution*, 9.

51   H. Zhang, "Making Light," 156–57.

52   Chen B., preface to *SARS Bride*.

53   Ding, *Rhetoric of Global Epidemic*, 92.

54   Zhang M. et al., *Ji feng jing cao*, 182–88.

55   Zhang M., foreword, 8.

56   Wang, "Young Feminist Activists," 60–62.

57   Ahmed, *Cultural Politics of Emotion*, 170–71.

58   Ahmed, *Cultural Politics of Emotion*, 180–82.

59   Berry, translator's afterword, 361–62.

60   Qtd. in Fedtke, Ibahrine, and Wang, "Corona Crisis," 806.

61   Nie and Elliott, "Humiliating Whistle-Blowers," 544.

62   Xiong, Alam, and Gan, "Wuhan Hospital."

63   Qtd. in Y. Zhang and Xu, "Ignorance, Orientalism and Sinophobia," 213.

64   Fang Fang, *Wuhan Diary*, 56–58.

65   Fang Fang, *Wuhan Diary*, 60.

66   Fedtke, Ibahrine, and Wang, "Corona Crisis," 796.

67   Fedtke, Ibahrine, and Wang, "Corona Crisis," 806, 800.

68   Fedtke, Ibahrine, and Wang, "Corona Crisis," 799, 795.

69   Fang Fang, *Wuhan Diary*, 111–12.

70   Qtd. in Fedtke, Ibahrine, and Wang, "Corona Crisis," 804.

Chapter 2: Pandemic Humor

1   Rea, *Age of Irreverence*, 7.

2   "China Information and Sources."

3   Ding, *Rhetoric of Global Epidemic*, 107.

4   H. Zhang, "SARS Humor," 141n2.

5 Ding, *Rhetoric of Global Epidemic*, 47.

6 Guo, *Evolution of the Chinese Internet*, 4.

7 Guo, *Evolution of the Chinese Internet*, ix.

8 H. Zhang, "SARS Humor," 121; see also her "Making Light," 148–49.

9 Berlant, *Cruel Optimism*, 262.

10 Deleuze and Guattari, *Thousand Plateaus*, 25, 7.

11 X. Zhang, *Postsocialism and Cultural Politics*, 15.

12 H. Zhang, "SARS Humor," 120, 130.

13 Ding, *Rhetoric of Global Epidemic*, 106–7.

14 See, for example, Marcus and Singer, "Loving Ebola-chan"; Dundes, "At Ease, Disease"; Morrow, "Those Sick Challenger Jokes"; and Kuipers, "'Where Was King Kong.'"

15 H. Zhang, "SARS Humor," 122–30; an earlier version of this taxonomy appears in her "Making Light."

16 H. Zhang, "SARS Humor," 126.

17 Qtd. in H. Zhang, "SARS Humor," 119.

18 H. Zhang, "SARS Humor," 133.

19 Link and Zhou, "*Shunkouliu*," 89.

20 Link and Zhou, "*Shunkouliu*," 107–8.

21 Tao, "Making Fun," 209.

22 Tao, "Making Fun," 214, 217.

23 Liu X., "From Wang Shuo's," 185, 187.

24 Hall, "Notes," 443.

25 Rea, "Spooling (*e'gao*) Culture," 151.

26 Zhu, introduction, 1–4.

27 Qtd. in Zhu, introduction, 4.

28 Zhu, introduction, 4–6.

29 H. Zhang, "SARS Humor," 136–37.

30 Li Yaguang, "'Feidian' shiqi zhi 'feichang' youmo" ['Atypical' humor for 'atypical pneumonia' times], *Renminwang*, May 21, 2003, http://www.people.cn/GB/guandian/30/20030521/997007.html.

31 Xu Xinghan, ed., "Tebie cehua: Feidian shiqi de feidianxing youmo" [Special production: Atypical humor in the times of SARS], *Renminwang*, June 12, 2003, http://www.people.com.cn/GB/news/9719/9720/20030509/987752.html.

32 "'Feidian' shiqi."

33 Qtd. in Xu X., "Tebie cehua" and "'Feidian' shiqi.'" These two websites have slightly different versions of the same joke, so I have amalgamated them here.

34 H. Zhang, "Making Light," 154; H. Zhang, "SARS Humor," 123.

35 "'Feidian' shiqi."

36 H. Zhang, "SARS Humor," 136–39.

37 J. Davis, "Humour," 3–4; Chey, "*Youmo*," 4.

38 Rea, *Age of Irreverence*, 4–5.

39 Chey, "*Youmo*," 7, 25.

40 Qtd. in H. Zhang, "SARS Humor," 125–26.

41 H. Zhang, "SARS Humor," 126.

42 H. Zhang, "Making Light," 166–67.

43 All translations of pieces in *Laughing at SARS* are mine, hereafter cited in the text.

44 See Y. Huang, "SARS Epidemic," 117–23; and Ding, *Rhetoric of Global Epidemic*, 70–98.

45 Ding, *Rhetoric of Global Epidemic*, 72.

46 Y. Huang, "SARS Epidemic," 121; see also his *Governing Health*, 91.

47 Qtd. in Ding, *Rhetoric of Global Epidemic*, 72.

48 Y. Huang, "SARS Epidemic," 118.

49 Y. Huang, "SARS Epidemic," 122.

50 Qtd. in Y. Huang, "SARS Epidemic," 122.

51 Ding, *Rhetoric of Global Epidemic*, 79–81.

52 H. Zhang, "SARS Humor," 122.

53 E. Ma and Chan, "Global Connectivity," 27–28. Ma and Chan also point out that, just one year later, "SARS reporting in the mainland had returned to a very restrictive media environment" and "untamed journalists who reported new SARS cases in early 2004 were prosecuted" (30).

54 H. Zhang, "Making Light," 170.

55 Ding, *Rhetoric of Global Epidemic*, 91, 274n3.

56 Ding, *Rhetoric of Global Epidemic*, 67.

57 Ding, *Rhetoric of Global Epidemic*, 106.

58 Ding, *Rhetoric of Global Epidemic*, 116.

59 Jiang, afterword, 358.

60 Hong Z., foreword.

61 Provine, *Curious Behavior*, 56–57.

62 Ding, *Rhetoric of Global Epidemic*, 111–15.

63 From the consistent use of *feidian* for SARS, we can infer that these jokes circulated primarily among mainland users since in Taiwan the virus was customarily called by its English acronym and sometimes shortened to the loan

word *sha* to rhyme with "fiend," whereas in Hong Kong SARS was typically called *saasi*, the Cantonese transliteration of "SARS."

64   Chey, "*Youmo*," 4.

65   Chey, "*Youmo*," 6.

66   Chey, "*Youmo*," 15–17.

67   G.-H. Chen, "Chinese Concepts of Humour," 194.

68   Rea, *Age of Irreverence*, 107.

69   Rea, *Age of Irreverence*, 124, 128.

70   Gan, *Comic China*, 13–14.

71   This ditty was also posted on the Wuhan Centers for Disease Prevention and Control website; see Qin, "'Feidian' yufang ge."

72   "Gaochang 'Feidian yufang ge'" [Loudly singing 'SARS prevention song'], *Sohu News*, May 1, 2003, http://news.sohu.com/38/79/news208957938.shtml.

73   Ding, *Rhetoric of Global Epidemic*, 93.

74   For TCM discourse during SARS, see Hanson, *Speaking of Epidemics*, 160–68.

75   Rea, *Age of Irreverence*, 130.

76   Hellekson and Busse, introduction, 8–10.

77   Hellekson and Busse, introduction, 12.

78   Li Weitao and Wang Xing, "CNNIC: China Had 298 Million Netizens by Dec 2008," *China Daily*, January 13, 2009, https://www.chinadaily.com.cn/business/2009-01/13/content_7392547.htm; C. Chiu, Ip, and Silverman, "Understanding Social Media."

79   China Internet Network Information Center, *47th Statistical Report*, 12.

80   Lin, "Archives of the Future."

81   Lin, "CUT!"

82   G. Yang, *Wuhan Lockdown*, 135, 138.

83   G. Yang, *Wuhan Lockdown*, 139–41.

84   For hyperlinks to the examples cited in this coda, see Kong, "How Chinese People."

85   Koetse, "Coronavirus."

Chapter 3: Pandemic Resilience

1   B. Davis and Catlin, "Theses for Theory."

2   "Covid Resilience Ranking."

3   See Martinelli, Oksanen, and Siipi, "Deextinction," 424.

4   Novak, "Deextinction," 548.

5   Lee S. H., "SARS Epidemic in Hong Kong," 374.

6   Stella Lee, "Amoy Residents Sent to Isolation Camps," *South China Morning Post*, April 2, 2003; Leung et al., "Public Health Viewpoint," 60–61.

7   Clifford Lo and Heike Phillips, "Hoaxer Sparks Panic Buying," *South China Morning Post*, April 2, 2003; Alex Lo, "'Infected City' Hoaxer Likely to Escape with a Police Warning," *South China Morning Post*, April 3, 2003.

8   C. Lo and Phillips, "Hoaxer Sparks Panic"; Seno and Reyes, "Unmasking SARS," 11; Loh and Welker, "SARS and Hong Kong," 217.

9   Ritter, "Mystery Illness"; McHugh, "Hong Kong's Darkest Hour."

10   WHO, "Update 17."

11   Mary Ann Benitez, "First HK Doctor Dies After Being Infected by Patient," *South China Morning Post*, April 4, 2003.

12   Clifford Lo and Niki Law, "Leslie Cheung Had Last Drink Before Leaping to His Death," *South China Morning Post*, April 3, 2003.

13   Ke, "Chuanmei."

14   Yip et al., "Effects of a Celebrity Suicide," 247–48.

15   Qtd. in Yip et al., "Effects of a Celebrity Suicide," 250–51.

16   Qtd. in "Hong Kong Scholars: Report Suicides Objectively," *Xinhua News Agency*, April 2, 2003.

17   MimiFanmi, "ATV."

18   "A Survival Guide for Hong Kong's Spirits," *South China Morning Post*, April 3, 2003.

19   Winnie Chung, "Leslie Cheung Fans Unite to Mourn Their Idol," *South China Morning Post*, April 8, 2003.

20   Winnie Chung, "Hong Kong Bids a Tearful Farewell to Leslie Cheung," *South China Morning Post*, April 9, 2003.

21   Qtd. in MimiFanmi, "ATV."

22   Teo, "*Promise* and *Perhaps Love*," 342.

23   Law and Bren, *Hong Kong Cinema*, 281, 293.

24   Lii, "Colonized Empire," 107–8.

25   Bordwell, *Planet Hong Kong*, 1.

26   Teo, *Hong Kong Cinema*, vii–viii; Law and Bren, *Hong Kong Cinema*, 294.

27   Bordwell, *Planet Hong Kong*, 75.

28   Teo, "*Promise* and *Perhaps Love*," 341–42.

29   Siu and Chan, "Eulogy and Practice," 77.

30   Teo, "*Promise* and *Perhaps Love*," 345.

31   Teo, "*Promise* and *Perhaps Love*," 343; Bordwell, *Planet Hong Kong*, 78–79.

32   Winnie Chung, "Film Industry Unable to Screen Out SARS' Impact," *South China Morning Post*, April 7, 2003, 3.

33   Qtd. in Helen Katherine, "2003 di ershi'er jie" (my translation).

34   Siu and Chan, "Eulogy and Practice," 77–78.

35   Abbas, *Hong Kong.*

36   Li C., "Journal," 10.

37   J. Lau, "Besides Fists and Blood," 162.

38   Sedgwick, *Touching Feeling*, 145.

39   All translations to these films in this chapter are mine.

40   J. Lau, "Besides Fists and Blood," 162.

41   W. Leung, "Multi-Media Stardom," 41.

42   Choi, "From Dependence," 161.

43   See Tam, "Death of Cantonese?"; V. Yu, "Can Cantonese Survive?"

44   Shih, *Visuality and Identity*, 4.

45   Shih, *Visuality and Identity*, 30. According to Eric Kit-wai Ma and Joseph Man Chan, Hong Kong's print and radio journalism, unlike the popular media industry, tends to carry a stronger "social advocacy" and "surrogate democracy function," especially in the posthandover era. During SARS, talk radio provided a channel for delivering epidemic-related commentary and a space for facilitating discussions and debates between experts and listeners, enabling the public to call in with concerns and anecdotes, including those that went beyond or contradicted the local government's version of the outbreak. Albert Cheng's *Tea Cup in a Storm*, for example, had "nurses and doctors [ringing] the show, speaking in trembling voices about unprotected medical workers being 'sent to die' at the front line." See E. Ma and Chan, "Global Connectivity," 24, 34–35.

46   W. Leung, "Multi-Media Stardom."

47   Corliss, "Cantopop Kingdom," 58.

48   Shih, *Visuality and Identity*, 31.

49   K. Chen, "Imperialist Eye," 15.

50   Lii, "Colonized Empire," 109–10.

51   Choi, "From Dependence," 161.

52   Teo, "*Promise* and *Perhaps Love*," 342.

53   Abbas, *Hong Kong*, 21.

54   Law and Bren, *Hong Kong Cinema*, 293.

55   Abbas, *Hong Kong*, 7.

56   Abbas, *Hong Kong*, 16.

57   J. Lau, "Besides Fists and Blood," 162.

58 Choi, "From Dependence," 169.

59 Choi, "From Dependence," 169.

60 Bordwell, *Planet Hong Kong*, 66–67, 64.

61 Bordwell, *Planet Hong Kong*, 65, 79.

62 J. Yang, *Once Upon a Time*, 45.

63 Bordwell, *Planet Hong Kong*, 65–66.

64 Choi, "From Dependence," 169.

65 Teo, *Hong Kong Cinema*, 59; see also his "The 1970s."

66 Arendt, *Origins of Totalitarianism*, 293.

67 Nixon, *Slow Violence*, 2.

68 Berlant, *Cruel Optimism*, 95, 97.

69 Bordwell, *Planet Hong Kong*, 75.

70 J. Yang, *Once Upon a Time*, 46.

71 Heise, *Imagining Extinction*, 12.

72 Qtd. in Podvin and Vivier, "Interview Gordon Chan."

73 Qtd. in Mathew Scott, "A Series of 11 Short Films by Hong Kong's Finest Directors Take a Look at the Fighting Spirit of the City and Its People during the SARS Crisis," *South China Morning Post*, September 9, 2003.

74 Qtd. in Tom Hilditch, "The Mask of Sorrow: Hong Kong Is Hitting Back," *South China Morning Post*, June 8, 2003.

75 Hilditch, "Mask of Sorrow."

76 Qtd. in Scott, "Series of 11 Short Films."

77 Podvin and Vivier, "Interview Gordon Chan."

78 For Hong Kong comedy films' popularity with local audiences, see J. Lau, "Besides Fists and Blood," 162.

79 J. Yang, *Once Upon a Time*, 58, 153.

80 Kam and Berlinger, "Alfonso Wong."

81 Qtd. in Hilditch, "Mask of Sorrow."

82 J. Lau, "Besides Fists and Blood," 167; James Wong, "Yueyu liuxing," 118.

83 Qtd. in Hilditch, "Mask of Sorrow."

84 Lam, *Chopsticks and Gambling*, 85.

85 All translations to song lyrics in this chapter are mine.

86 2sizuku, "Hua fu."

87 Hilditch, "Mask of Sorrow."

88 Qtd. in Hilditch, "Mask of Sorrow."

89 A Hong Kong native, Steve Cheng started out as a production assistant on local television in the 1980s before turning to film in the late 1990s, mostly along the lines of horror comedy, cop thriller, and soft erotica, sometimes all rolled into one. By 2003 he had directed some fifteen low-budget movies.

90 S. Ng, "Mystery of Amoy Gardens," 101–3, 108–10; Abraham, *Twenty-First Century*, 71–75.

91 Qtd. in HK Movie Extras, "Golden Chicken 2 (2003)."

92 Qtd. in HK Movie Extras, "Golden Chicken (2002)."

93 Kan dianying, "Zuo ji."

94 Qtd. in HK Movie Extras, "Golden Chicken (2002)."

95 V. Lee, *Hong Kong Cinema*, 170–71.

96 Qtd. in Jun Pang, "Thinking beyond the Stereotypes: The Diverse Experiences of Hong Kong's Sex Workers," *Hong Kong Free Press*, October 22, 2017, https://hongkongfp.com/2017/10/22/thinking-beyond-stereotypes-diverse -experiences-hong-kongs-sex-workers/.

97 V. Lee, *Hong Kong Cinema*, 170–71.

98 Teo, "*Promise* and *Perhaps Love*," 344.

99 Curtain, "Renationalizing Hong Kong Cinema," 255.

100 Erni, "SARS, Avian Flu," 51–54.

101 Lai, "Film and Enigmatization," 232.

102 Grace Woo, Facebook post, "Lang chumo zhuyi: Pandian Xianggang liu da selang" [Beware of stalking wolves: Taking stock of Hong Kong's six major lechers], May 8, 2017, https://www.facebook.com/groups/400493963620504 /posts/448831012120132/?mibextid=6NoCDW.

103 Qtd. in HK Movie Extras, "Golden Chicken (2002)."

104 Vaudine England, "Hong Kong's Lavish Nightclubs Lose Their Appeal," *Guardian*, December 12, 2012.

105 Sylvia Yu, "'I Trafficked Women at a Famous Hong Kong Nightclub,'" *South China Morning Post*, June 11, 2017.

106 Zeng, *Xianggang yueyu*, 51.

107 Gren Manuel, "PCCW-Exchange Pact Is Cleared," *Asian Wall Street Journal*, April 9, 2001.

108 Lai, "Film and Enigmatization," 238–39.

109 Chu and Chan, "Policing One-Woman Brothels," 6.

110 Qtd. in HK Movie Extras, "Golden Chicken (2002)."

111 Gary Cheung, "Musician, Eye Surgeon and a Politician Who Married an Actress: Patrick Ho Led a Varied, Eventful Life Before Bribery Scandal," *South China Morning Post*, December 6, 2018.

112 Stephen Chow's *Kung Fu Hustle*, released the following year in 2004, is often seen as inspired by *The House of 72 Tenants*, but the latter's influence on the *Golden Chicken* films is rarely recognized.

113 J. Yang, *Once Upon a Time*, 57–58.

114 McMillin, "House of 72 Tenants."

115 Teo, *Hong Kong Cinema*, 145.

116 Appadurai, *Modernity at Large*, 181.

117 Teo, *Hong Kong Cinema*, 144–45.

118 McMillin, "House of 72 Tenants."

119 Qtd. in Curtain, "Renationalizing Hong Kong Cinema," 254.

120 Qtd. in HK Movie Extras, "Golden Chicken (2002)."

121 Merianos and Plant, "Epidemiology," 191; A. Lau, "Numbers Trail," 92.

122 Siu and Chan, "Eulogy and Practice," 94; Kleinman and Lee, "SARS and the Problem," 175.

123 Qtd. in Siu and Chan, "Eulogy and Practice," 92.

124 Scott, "Series of 11 Short Films."

125 Lai, "Film and Enigmatization," 247.

126 McLeod, "Psychology of Forgetting."

127 Yang X., *Huang Zhan*, 129–30.

128 Wong, "Yueyu liuxing," 135n92.

129 Wong, "Yueyu liuxing," 7.

130 Wong, "Yueyu liuxing," 133.

131 Wong, "Yueyu liuxing," 145.

132 Wong, "Yueyu liuxing," 182.

133 W. Leung, "Multi-Media Stardom," 49.

134 R. Chen, "Golden Chicken 2."

135 Choy, "Xianggang dianying," 65.

136 K. Chan, "Crossing the Transnational," 33; Li C., "Journal," 10.

137 K. Chan, "Crossing the Transnational," 33–34.

138 Hong Kong Trade Development Council, "Film Entertainment Industry."

139 Curtain, "Renationalizing Hong Kong Cinema," 255.

140 Qtd. in "Chen Guanxi."

141 Qtd. in Pat C., "Sandra Ng."

142 "Chen Guanxi."

143 Jason Chen, "Musical Characteristics," 15.

144 Sam Hui, Instagram, April 9, 2020, https://www.instagram.com/p/B-vidCiA9SN/.

145 Kang-chung Ng, "Coronavirus: 2.5 Million Watch Livestream of Canto-Pop Legend Sam Hui Tell Hong Kong to 'Stay United' in Free Concert," *South China Morning Post*, April 12, 2020.

Chapter 4: Pandemic First Patients

1 Bill Gertz, "Coronavirus Link to China Biowarfare Program Possible, Analyst Says," *Washington Times*, January 26, 2020; Glenn Kessler, "Timeline: How the Wuhan Lab-Leak Theory Suddenly Became Credible," *Washington Post*, May 25, 2021.

2 "Petition Urges US Gov't to Clarify Army Lab Shutdown as Doubts Grow Over COVID-19's Origin," *Renminwang*, March 21, 2020, http://en.people.cn/n3/2020/0321/c90000-9670852.html.

3 Worobey et al., "Huanan Seafood," 1; Pekar et al., "Molecular Epidemiology," 5.

4 Worobey et al., "Huanan Seafood," 3–4.

5 Worobey et al., "Huanan Seafood," 15.

6 Zhan, "Civet Cats," 37–38.

7 Zhan, "Civet Cats," 40n10.

8 Yeoh C. Y., foreword, 1.

9 Lynteris, "Prophetic Faculty," 121–22.

10 Lynteris and Fearnley, "Why Shutting Down."

11 Y. Zhang and Xu, "Ignorance, Orientalism and Sinophobia," 217.

12 Wikipedia, "SARS," last modified December 12, 2022, https://en.wikipedia.org/wiki/SARS.

13 Wikipedia, "2002–2004 SARS Outbreak," last modified December 22, 2022, https://en.wikipedia.org/wiki/2002%E2%80%932004_SARS_outbreak.

14 See Kong, "Recovering First Patients."

15 See Kong, "Recovering First Patients."

16 Khan and Patrick, *Next Pandemic*, 165.

17 Qtd. in Wu and Li, "Bu xiang."

18 Wu and Li, "Bu xiang."

19 Hu, Shi, and Ma, "Tanfang woguo."

20 Leu Siew Ying, "On the Trail of SARS' Ground Zero Patient," *South China Morning Post*, April 30, 2003.

21 Zheng, Wang, and Chen, "Foshan Bitang."

22 Zheng, Wang, and Chen, "Foshan Bitang"; Hu N., Shi, and Ma, "Tanfang woguo"; Wu and Li, "Bu xiang."

23 Zhou et al., "Guangdong sheng," 599; R.-H. Xu et al., "Epidemiologic Clues," 1033; Zheng, Wang, and Chen, "Foshan Bitang"; Hu N., Shi, and Ma, "Tanfang woguo."

24 Zhou et al., "Guangdong sheng," 598; R.-H. Xu et al., "Epidemiologic Clues," 1033; see also Zhong et al., "Epidemiology and Cause," 1357.

25 Qtd. in Zheng, Wang, and Chen, "Foshan Bitang."

26 Qtd. in Hu N., Shi, and Ma, "Tanfang woguo."

27 Leu, "On the Trail."

28 Giesecke, "Primary and Index Cases," 2024.

29 Qtd. in Ching-Ching Ni, "Tracing the Path of SARS: A Tale of Deadly Infection," *Los Angeles Times*, April 22, 2003.

30 Qtd. in Leu, "On the Trail."

31 Qtd. in Zheng, Wang, and Chen, "Foshan Bitang."

32 Qtd. in Leu Siew Ying, "One Year On, the Spectre of SARS Has Returned," *South China Morning Post*, November 14, 2003.

33 Qtd. in Hu N., Shi, and Ma, "Tanfang woguo."

34 Qtd. in Yang L., "Feidian shi nian," and Hu N., Shi, and Ma, "Tanfang woguo."

35 Wu and Li, "Bu xiang."

36 Tom Blackwell, "All Quiet at SARS Ground Zero," *National Post* (Canada), June 23, 2003.

37 Qtd. in Hu N., Shi, and Ma, "Tanfang woguo."

38 Hu N., Shi, and Ma, "Tanfang woguo."

39 Yang L., "Feidian shi nian."

40 Qtd. in Yang L., "Feidian shi nian."

41 Wu and Li, "Bu xiang."

42 D. Lee and Wing, "Psychological Responses," 144.

43 Qtd. in Audra Ang, "Earliest Known SARS Case Stays Anonymous," *Edwardsville (IL) Intelligencer*, April 10, 2003.

44 Qtd. in Blackwell, "All Quiet."

45 Yang L., "Feidian shi nian."

46 Qtd. in Wu and Li, "Bu xiang."

47 Yang L., "Feidian shi nian."

48 Zhou et al., "Guangdong sheng," 598; Wu and Li, "Bu xiang."

49 Zhou et al., "Guangdong sheng," 598; Hu N., Shi, and Ma, "Tanfang woguo."

50   R.-H. Xu et al., "Epidemiologic Clues," 1033.

51   Zhou et al., "Guangdong sheng," 598; Wu and Li, "Bu xiang"; Hu N., Shi, and Ma, "Tanfang woguo."

52   Qtd. in Leu, "On the Trail."

53   Farquhar, *Appetites*, 122.

54   Yang L., "Feidian shi nian."

55   Tsing, *Mushroom*, 2.

56   Tsing, *Mushroom*, 2, 5.

57   Abraham, *Twenty-First Century*, 30.

58   Quammen, *Spillover*, 170–71.

59   Adam Luck, "Hell That Is the Source of SARS," *Mail on Sunday* (London), May 4, 2003.

60   Jan Wong, "How China Failed the World," *Globe and Mail* (Toronto), April 5, 2003.

61   R.-H. Xu et al., "Epidemiologic Clues," 1032, 1035.

62   See Kong, "Recovering First Patients."

63   See, for example, Elisabeth Rosenthal, "From China's Provinces, a Crafty Germ Breaks Out," *New York Times*, April 27, 2003; Laurie Garrett, "A Breeding Ground? Markets in China That Sell Live Animals Could Be Link to SARS," *Newsday*, April 23, 2003; Ann Perry, "China Admits Wider Spread of SARS," *Toronto Star*, April 3, 2003; Jeremy Laurance, "Something in the Food," *Independent* (London), April 6, 2003; and Luck, "Hell."

64   Zhong et al., "Epidemiology and Cause," 1355; R.-H. Xu et al., "Epidemiologic Clues," 1033.

65   R.-H. Xu et al. "Epidemiologic Clues," 1033.

66   Huang X., "China's SARS."

67   R.-H. Xu et al., "Epidemiologic Clues," 1033–34.

68   Qtd. in Xia, "Feidian 'duwang.'"

69   Zhong et al., "Epidemiology and Cause," 1355; R.-H. Xu et al., "Epidemiologic Clues," 1033, table 6 on 1036.

70   Qtd. in Huang X., "China's SARS."

71   Duffy, "Anatomy of an Epidemic."

72   Huang X., "China's SARS"; Xia, "Feidian 'duwang.'"

73   Huang X., "China's SARS."

74   Qtd. in He Huifeng, "A Decade on from SARS: Torment of the First Patient," *South China Morning Post*, April 1, 2013.

75   Huang X., "China's SARS"; He, "Decade on."

76 Kraut, *Silent Travelers*, 2–3.

77 Glick, *Infrahumanisms*, 197.

78 See Leong, "Chaos, SARS, Yellow Peril"; H. Hung, "Politics of SARS"; Loh and Welker, "SARS and Hong Kong"; Kleinman and Lee, "SARS and the Problem"; and Keil and Ali, "Racism"; Lynteris, "Yellow Peril."

79 "SARS Fast Facts."

80 Gaby Hinsliff, Mark Townsend, and John Aglionby, "The Day the World Caught a Cold," *Guardian*, April 26, 2003.

81 Huddleston, "This Hotel."

82 McKay, "Patient Zero: Why."

83 McKay, "Patient Zero and the Early North American."

84 Wald, *Contagious*, 3–4.

85 Wald, *Contagious*, 215–16.

86 Wolfe, *Viral Storm*, 159.

87 Qtd. in "WHO Points."

88 Qtd. in "Rush to Develop."

89 WHO, "Severe Acute Respiratory Syndrome (SARS)"; Balasegaram, "First Super-Spreading Event," 136. For examples of this usage in anglophone media, see Donald G. McNeil Jr. and Lawrence K. Altman, "How One Person Can Fuel an Epidemic," *New York Times*, April 15, 2003; Rosenthal, "From China's Provinces"; Philip P. Pan, "A 'Superspreader' of SARS: How One Woman Touched Off Beijing's Outbreak," *Washington Post*, May 29, 2003; Jerome Groopman, "The SARS Epidemic," *Wall Street Journal*, April 23, 2003; Michael D. Lemonick, "Will SARS Strike Here?," *Time*, April 14, 2003; Shute, "SARS Hit Home"; Normile, "Battling SARS"; "Solid Response"; "Rush to Develop"; and "Effect of SARS."

90 McNeil and Altman, "How One Person."

91 Donald G. McNeil Jr. and Lawrence K. Altman, "Doctors Worry That 'Superspreaders' Are Dotting the Map with SARS," *International Herald Tribune* (Paris), April 16, 2003; Donald G. McNeil Jr. and Lawrence K. Altman, "Tracking Typhoid Marys," *Edmonton Journal* (Alberta, Canada), April 20, 2003.

92 Rosenthal, "From China's Provinces."

93 Estok, "Theorizing," 207–9.

94 See, for example, Nikiforuk, "Modern Plagues"; Lague, Lawrence, and Murthy, "China Virus"; and Chris Taylor, "The Chinese Plague," *Age* (Melbourne, Australia), May 4, 2003.

95 *Silent Killer.*

96 Greenfeld, *China Syndrome*, 151–52.

97   Greenfeld, *China Syndrome*, 231.

98   Greenfeld, *China Syndrome*, 153.

99   Greenfeld, *China Syndrome*, 414–15.

100   Legislative Council, *Report of the Select Committee*, A67, A80; SARS Expert Committee, *SARS in Hong Kong*, 18.

101   Braden et al., "Progress in Global Surveillance," 865.

102   Braden et al., "Progress in Global Surveillance," 865–66; Abraham, *Twenty-First Century*, 60.

103   Greenfeld, "Wild Flavor," 247.

104   Marco Lupis, "Da super scienziato a grande untore: Il paziente zero del virus killer," *La Repubblica* (Italy), April 4 2003, https://www.repubblica.it/online /cronaca/virusdue/zero/zero.html?refresh_ce.

105   Lupis, "SARS Patient Zero."

106   Ferrari, *Not SARS*, chap. 5.

107   Lupis, "Da super scienziato"; Lupis, "SARS Patient Zero"; Ferrari, *Not SARS*, chap. 5.

108   Zhan, "Civet Cats"; H. Hung, "Politics of SARS"; Keil and Ali, "Racism"; Lynteris, "Yellow Peril."

109   See, for example, Rosenthal, "From China's Provinces"; Perry, "China Admits"; Laurance, "Something"; and Luck, "Hell."

110   See, for example, Lupis, "Da super scienziato"; Lupis, "SARS Patient Zero"; Ferrari, *Not SARS*, chap. 5; Greenfeld, *China Syndrome*, 152–53; *Silent Killer*; Khan and Patrick, *Next Pandemic*, 167–68; Goudsmit, *Viral Fitness*, 140; Wolfe, *Viral Storm*, 159–60; S. Shah, *Pandemic*, 50–51; and National Intelligence Council, *SARS*, 10.

111   For my reconstruction of the Metropole Hotel outbreak and Liu Jianlun's last days, I cite below a number of epidemiological studies, WHO publications, and summary reports by the Hong Kong government. In particular, I draw on a primary archive of medical records, papers, testimonies, letters, presentations, and other supporting documents submitted by various bureaus, hospital staff and medical workers, and other witnesses for the Hong Kong Government and Hospital Authority Select Committee's investigative report on SARS; these sources appear under the section on "Lists of written evidence/ documents" in Legislative Council, *Report of the Select Committee*, and are cited by their reference numbers (letter followed by number, i.e., A67).

112   Qtd. in Wei, "Xianggang feidian."

113   Zhong et al., "Epidemiology and Cause," 1357.

114   Legislative Council, *Report of the Select Committee*, 17–18, A67, A80, A86; SARS Expert Committee, *SARS in Hong Kong*, 18.

115 Whaley, "Solving," 141.

116 Legislative Council, *Report of the Select Committee*, A67, A80, A86.

117 Legislative Council, *Report of the Select Committee*, A67 and A80; SARS Expert Committee, *SARS in Hong Kong*, 18.

118 Legislative Council, *Report of the Select Committee*, A67, A86; Whaley, "Solving," 141.

119 Jan Wong, "Family Hit by SARS Speaks Out," *Globe and Mail* (Toronto), April 8, 2003; Abraham, *Twenty-First Century*, 60.

120 Legislative Council, *Report of the Select Committee*, A49; Braden et al., "Progress in Global Surveillance," 864, figure 1; Whaley, "Solving," 143, figure 14.1.

121 Legislative Council, *Report of the Select Committee*, A80; SARS Expert Committee, *SARS in Hong Kong*, 19; Whaley, "Solving," 141.

122 Legislative Council, *Report of the Select Committee*, 38.

123 Legislative Council, *Report of the Select Committee*, A86.

124 WHO, "Consensus Document," 23; Braden et al., "Progress in Global Surveillance," 866; Whaley, "Solving," 147; Legislative Council, *Report of the Select Committee*, A49.

125 Qtd. in Whaley, "Solving," 147.

126 Whaley, "Solving," 147; Abraham, *Twenty-First Century*, 62.

127 Whaley, "Solving," 141.

128 SARS Expert Committee, *SARS in Hong Kong*, 18.

129 Braden et al., "Progress in Global Surveillance," 865–66; Whaley, "Solving," 142; Abraham, *Twenty-First Century*, 60.

130 Braden et al., "Progress in Global Surveillance," 865.

131 WHO, "Consensus Document," 23.

132 Lynteris, *Human Extinction*, 83.

133 K. Hung et al., "Role of the Hotel Industry," 6.

134 Legislative Council, *Report of the Select Committee*, A49; Whaley, "Solving," 143.

135 Qtd. in Whaley, "Solving," 143.

136 Legislative Council, *Report of the Select Committee*, H10 appendix I and attachment B (p. 4).

137 Legislative Council, *Report of the Select Committee*, W1(C).

138 Legislative Council, *Report of the Select Committee*, W1(C), W2(C), W3(C).

139 Legislative Council, *Report of the Select Committee*, W3(C).

140 Legislative Council, *Report of the Select Committee*, 18.

141 Dr. Liu Shao-haei, qtd. in Legislative Council, *Report of the Select Committee*, Verbatim Transcript of the Fourth Public Hearing, 136–37.

142 Legislative Council, *Report of the Select Committee*, 17–18, W3(C), A80; SARS Expert Committee, *SARS in Hong Kong*, 18.

143 Qtd. in Legislative Council, *Report of the Select Committee*, W3(C).

144 Legislative Council, *Report of the Select Committee*, X1.

145 Legislative Council, *Report of the Select Committee*, 18–19, W3(C).

146 Legislative Council, *Report of the Select Committee*, 19, A80; SARS Expert Committee, *SARS in Hong Kong*, 19.

147 Legislative Council, *Report of the Select Committee*, A80, A86.

148 Legislative Council, *Report of the Select Committee*, A67.

149 SARS Expert Committee, *SARS in Hong Kong*, 19.

150 Legislative Council, *Report of the Select Committee*, 18, W1(C).

151 SARS Expert Committee, *SARS in Hong Kong*, 19.

152 Legislative Council, *Report of the Select Committee*, A67.

153 Legislative Council, *Report of the Select Committee*, A49, A67.

154 Legislative Council, *Report of the Select Committee*, 22; SARS Expert Committee, *SARS in Hong Kong*, 19.

155 Legislative Council, *Report of the Select Committee*, A67; SARS Expert Committee, *SARS in Hong Kong*, 19.

156 Legislative Council, *Report of the Select Committee*, 22, A67; SARS Expert Committee, *SARS in Hong Kong*, 20.

157 Legislative Council, *Report of the Select Committee*, A67, H10 attachments C and D.

158 SARS Expert Committee, *SARS in Hong Kong*, 20–21.

159 SARS Expert Committee, *SARS in Hong Kong*, 21.

160 Legislative Council, *Report of the Select Committee*, 20.

161 Legislative Council, *Report of the Select Committee*, H17.

162 Hinsliff, Townsend, and Aglionby, "Day"; MIHK.tv_Youtube, "Da wan you luo"; Legislative Council, *Report of the Select Committee*, 24–25.

163 Legislative Council, *Report of the Select Committee*, 24.

164 Legislative Council, *Report of the Select Committee*, 22.

165 "Hong Kong Hotel Is Eliminating Memories of SARS," *Taipei Times*, February 23, 2005.

166 Voigt, "Outbreak Bad Luck"; K. Hung et al., "Role of the Hotel Industry," 4.

167 Government of Hong Kong, "Designated Quarantine Hotels," 4.

168 Whaley, "Solving," 143–46; Abraham, *Twenty-First Century*, 60.

169 Whaley and Mansoor, "SARS Chronology," 8–11; Ellen Nakashima, "Vietnam Took Lead in Containing SARS," *Washington Post*, May 5, 2003.

170 Brudon and Cheng, "Viet Nam," 94–95.

262 NOTES TO CHAPTER 4

171 Qtd. in Annemarie Evans, "Six Degrees," *South China Morning Post*, January 13, 2013; Donald G. McNeil Jr., "Disease's Pioneer Is Mourned as a Victim," *New York Times*, April 8, 2003; Medecins Sans Frontières, "In Memoriam"; Oransky, "Carlo Urbani (Obituary)"; Lorenzo Savioli, "Carlo Urbani," *Guardian*, April 21, 2003; Whaley, "Hanoi-French Hospital," 168; WHO, "If Dr. Carlo Urbani."

172 WHO, "If Dr. Carlo Urbani."

173 Whaley, "Hanoi-French Hospital," 171.

174 Savioli, "Carlo Urbani"; Whaley, "Hanoi-French Hospital," 169; WHO, "If Dr. Carlo Urbani."

175 Whaley and Mansoor, "SARS Chronology," 12–13; Whaley, "Hanoi-French Hospital," 169.

176 Qtd. in Brudon and Cheng, "Viet Nam," 98; Nakashima, "Vietnam."

177 Brudon and Cheng, "Viet Nam," 98.

178 Whaley, "Hanoi-French Hospital," 169; Whaley and Mansoor, "SARS Chronology," 13.

179 Ahmed, *Cultural Politics of Emotion*, 130.

180 Legislative Council, *Report of the Select Committee*, A49.

181 Braden et al., "Progress in Global Surveillance," 865.

182 Campbell, *SARS Commission*, 245.

183 Campbell, *SARS Commission*, 43n79.

184 Campbell, *SARS Commission*, 245, 102–3.

185 Campbell, *SARS Commission*, 247, 251.

186 Campbell, *SARS Commission*, 248, 50.

187 Campbell, *SARS Commission*, 41.

188 Qtd. in Campbell, *SARS Commission*, 247.

189 David Patrick, director of British Columbia CDC, qtd. in Campbell, *SARS Commission*, 250.

190 Whaley, "Solving," 145.

191 Campbell, *SARS Commission*, 80.

192 Whaley, "Solving," 143, figure 14.1, and 144, table 14.1; Abraham, *Twenty-First Century*, 60.

193 Whaley, "Solving," 144, table 14.1; Lambert, "Singapore," 101.

194 Whaley and Mansoor, "SARS Chronology," 9; Lambert, "Singapore," 101; Whaley, "Solving," 145; WHO, "Severe Acute Respiratory Syndrome—Singapore," 159; Chee, "SARS at TTSH," 24.

195 Yeoh E., "Singapore Woman."

196 Qtd. in Yeoh E., "Singapore Woman."

197 "Singapore Woman"; Yeoh E., "Singapore Woman"; Yeoh En-lai, "Deadly Shopping Trip—Woman Linked to More Than 100 SARS Cases After Hong Kong Visit," *Grand Rapids (MI) Press*, April 9, 2003.

198 See, for example, Philipkoski, "Superspreaders"; Julie Robotham, "SARS Timebombs: Fatal Threat of the Super-Carriers," *Sydney Morning Herald*, April 26, 2003; Julie Robotham, "On the Trail of the Super-Spreaders," *Age* (Melbourne, Australia), April 26, 2003; Audrey Hudson and Amy Fagan, "Victim Spread SARS to 100," *Washington Times*, April 10, 2003; and Jeremy Laurance, "SARS Victim Who Infected 133 Will Remain in Quarantine," *Independent* (London), April 11, 2003.

199 Rosenthal, "From China's Provinces"; Richard C. Paddock, "Outbreak in Asia: A Hotbed of SARS Warfare," *Los Angeles Times*, May 8, 2003.

200 "91 Cases."

201 Lim, "Singapore's Most Underrated Minister." For examples in the anglophone media, see "Singapore Woman"; Yeoh E., "Singapore Woman"; Ang, "Earliest Known"; Laurance, "SARS Victim"; Robotham, "On the Trail"; Robotham, "SARS Timebombs"; and Philipkoski, "Superspreaders."

202 WHO, "Severe Acute Respiratory Syndrome—Singapore," 157n2; Chew, "Severe Acute."

203 WHO, "Severe Acute Respiratory Syndrome—Singapore," 159; Lambert, "Singapore," 101.

204 Qtd. in Fong, *Tale of Two Esthers*.

205 Chee, "SARS at TTSH," 20.

206 Qtd. in Chua M. H., *Defining Moment*, 27.

207 WHO, "Severe Acute Respiratory Syndrome—Singapore," 159; Lambert, "Singapore," 102.

208 Chua M. H., *Defining Moment*, 27.

209 Salma Khalik, "Two Die in S'pore—Pastor and Father of Ex–Flight Stewardess Die," *Straits Times* (Singapore), March 27, 2003.

210 Bertha Henson, "Two Die, Infections Up Sharply," *Straits Times* (Singapore), April 8, 2003; Tracy Quek, "Try a Little Kindness," *Straits Times* (Singapore), April 13, 2003.

211 Salma Khalik, "Two Seriously Ill Patients Die—4 More People Linked to SGH Found to Have Virus," *Straits Times* (Singapore), April 16, 2003; Chua M. H., *Defining Moment*, 32.

212 "Living in the Shadow of Death," *Straits Times* (Singapore), July 18, 2004.

213 Salma Khalik, "Most Victims Here Infected by 3 Women," *Straits Times* (Singapore), March 31, 2003; "91 Cases Traced to Just One Woman Here," *Straits Times* (Singapore), April 3, 2003.

214 Quek, "Try a Little Kindness."

215 Salma Khalik, "In the Hazard Zone," *Straits Times* (Singapore), April 13, 2003.

216 Jonathan Goh, "Don't Single Patients Out for Unfair Labelling," *Straits Times* (Singapore), April 14, 2003.

217 Alvin Chan Chee Hoi, in "Was There a Need to Publicly Name 'Super-Infector'?," *Straits Times* (Singapore), April 16, 2003.

218 Tan Swee Kim, in "Was There a Need to Publicly Name 'Super-Infector'?," *Straits Times* (Singapore), April 16, 2003.

219 Qtd. in Krist Boo, "SARS: Biggest Danger Is to Relax Now," *Straits Times* (Singapore), May 5, 2003.

220 Chua B. H., "SARS Epidemic," 85.

221 Chua B. H., "SARS Epidemic," 93.

222 Lee Hui Chieh, "The Battle against SARS—Warts and All," *Straits Times* (Singapore), July 16, 2004.

223 Chua M. H., *Defining Moment*, 26.

224 Chua M. H., *Defining Moment*, 27–32.

225 Qtd. in Chua M. H., *Defining Moment*, 27.

226 Chua M. H., *Defining Moment*, 28–29.

227 Qtd. in Chua M. H., *Defining Moment*, 32.

228 Chua M. H., *Defining Moment*, 32.

229 Chua M. H., *Defining Moment*, 28.

230 Qtd. in Chua M. H., *Defining Moment*, 29.

231 Chua M. H., *Defining Moment*, 29.

232 Qtd. in Chua M. H., *Defining Moment*, 31.

233 Chua M. H., *Defining Moment*, 32.

234 *Tale of Two Esthers*, *Christian Cinema*, 2019, http://www.christiancinema.com/digital/movie/tale-of-two-esthers.

235 Qtd. in Fong, *Tale of Two Esthers*; all of Mok's quotations in this section are from the film.

236 Chua M. H., *Defining Moment*, 31.

237 Molly Fitzpatrick, "Quarantining with a Ghost? It's Scary," *New York Times*, May 14, 2020; Sarah Knapton, "'Ghost' Sightings Soar as Covid Spooks More into Believing the Paranormal," *Telegraph* (London), February 12, 2022.

238 Harrison, "CoronaGothic," 75.

239 Qtd. in McNamara, "Ghosts of COVID."

240 Qtd. in McNamara, "Ghosts of COVID."

241 Blake, "They Lost."

242   Qtd. in Blake, "They Lost."

243   R. Lee, author's notes to *True Singapore Ghost Stories: Book 12* and *25th Year*.

244   R. Lee, *True Singapore Ghost Stories: 25th Year*. Theories abound concerning the identity of Russell Lee. Some speculate that they are a collective of ghostwriters, others that they are native Chinese Singaporean, still others that they are white, perhaps another alter ego of Jim Aitchinson aka James Lee, the Australia-born author of the local children's horror series *Mr. Midnight*, published by the same press that publishes TSGS. The 2005 Routledge *Encyclopedia of Post-Colonial Literatures in English* gives an unconfirmed biography of Lee as Harjeet Kaur, a Malaysia-born woman with an arts degree from Monash University who supposedly writes under the pen names of both Russell Lee and H. Sidhu; see Veloo, "Lee, Russell," 834. In one recent interview, Lee maintains, "I am a faceless man. When I am in public, nobody knows me other than my friends. And even they don't know who Russell Lee is. Even my parents don't know"; see Nazren, "'Even My Parents.'"

245   R. Lee, *True Singapore Ghost Stories: Book 12*, 111.

246   R. Lee, *True Singapore Ghost Stories: Book 12*, 112.

247   Qtd. in Tan, "Booking Their Space," S8.

248   Koh, "Malaysia and Singapore," 76; Wagner, "Singapore's New Thrillers," 71–72.

249   Faucher, "As the Wind Blows," 192–93.

250   Comaroff, "Ghostly Topographies," 61.

251   Comaroff, "Ghostly Topographies," 63.

252   R. Lee, author's note to *True Singapore Ghost Stories: 25th Year*.

Afterword

1   Adams and Fleck, "Bridging the Language Divide," 365.

2   Kong, "Recovering First Patients."

3   See Kong, "How Chinese People."

4   G. Yang, *Wuhan Lockdown*, xi–xii.

BIBLIOGRAPHY

1:99 din jeng haang dung/1:99 dianying xingdong [*Project 1:99*]. Panorama, 2003.

2sizuku. "Hua fu xin shijie Huang Zhan fangwen Zhou Xingchi" [What a Glamorous World interview with Stephen Chow by Wong Jim]. YouTube video, April 14, 2017. https://youtu.be/y6gwmooyVRc.

Abbas, Ackbar. *Hong Kong: Culture and the Politics of Disappearance*. Minneapolis: University of Minnesota Press, 1997.

Abraham, Thomas. *Twenty-First Century Plague: The Story of SARS*. Baltimore: Johns Hopkins University Press, 2007.

Adams, Patrick, and Fiona Fleck. "Bridging the Language Divide in Health." *Bulletin of the World Health Organization* 93, no. 6 (2015): 365–66. https://doi:10.2471/blt .15.020615.

Agamben, Giorgio. *Homo Sacer: Sovereign Power and Bare Life*. Translated by Daniel Heller-Roazen. Stanford, CA: Stanford University Press, 1998.

Agamben, Giorgio. "The Invention of an Epidemic." *European Journal of Psychoanalysis*, February 26, 2020.

Ahmed, Sara. *The Cultural Politics of Emotion*. Edinburgh: Edinburgh University Press, 2014.

Allen, Arthur. "Death by Sneezing." *Salon*, April 2, 2003.

Anderson, Roy M., Christophe Fraser, Azra C. Ghani, Christl A. Donnelly, Steven Riley, Neil M. Ferguson, Gabriel M. Leung, Tai H. Lam, and Anthony J. Hedley. "Epidemiology, Transmission Dynamics, and Control of SARS: The 2002–2003 Epidemic." In *SARS: A Case Study in Emerging Infections*, edited by Angela R. McLean, Robert M. May, John Pattison, and Robin A. Weiss, 61–80. New York: Oxford University Press, 2005.

"Apo Meiguo yuxi fenli fanji!" [Granny attacked in US counterstrikes with all her might!]. *Sohu*, March 23, 2021. https://www.sohu.com/a/456969655_120209873.

Appadurai, Arjun. *Modernity at Large: Cultural Dimensions of Globalization*. Minneapolis: University of Minnesota Press, 1996.

Arendt, Hannah. *The Origins of Totalitarianism*. New York: Harcourt, 1976.

Atkins, Paul W. B., David Sloan Wilson, and Steven C. Hayes. *Prosocial: Using Evolutionary Science to Build Productive, Equitable, and Collaborative Groups*. Oakland, CA: Context, 2019.

Balasegaram, Mangai. "The First Super-Spreading Event." In World Health Organization, *SARS*, 135–40.

Barthes, Roland. "The Reality Effect." In *The Rustle of Language*, translated by Richard Howard, 141–48. Berkeley: University of California Press, 1989.

Berlant, Lauren. *Cruel Optimism*. Durham, NC: Duke University Press, 2011.

Berlant, Lauren. "Without Exception: On the Ordinariness of Violence." Interview by Brad Evans. *Los Angeles Review of Books*, July 30, 2018.

Bernards, Brian. Review of *Such Is This World@sars.come*, by Hu Fayun. *MCLC Resource Center*, August 2011. https://u.osu.edu/mclc/book-reviews/such-is-this/.

Berry, Michael. Translator's afterword to *Wuhan Diary: Dispatches from a Quarantined City*, by Fang Fang, 361–71. New York: HarperCollins, 2020.

Blake, John. "They Lost Their Loved Ones to Covid. Then They Heard from Them Again." CNN, June 20, 2021.

Bordwell, David. *Planet Hong Kong: Popular Cinema and the Art of Entertainment*. Cambridge, MA: Harvard University Press, 2000.

Braden, Christopher R., Scott F. Dowell, Daniel B. Jernigan, and James M. Hughes. "Progress in Global Surveillance and Response Capacity 10 Years After Severe Acute Respiratory Syndrome." *Emerging Infectious Diseases* 19, no. 6 (2013): 864–69. https://doi:10.3201/eid1906.130192.

Brooks, Eric. "Elderly Asian Woman Turns Tables, Sends Attacker to Hospital in Unprovoked SF Attack." MSN, March 17, 2021.

Brudon, Pascale, and Maria Cheng. "Viet Nam: Tough Decisions Pay Off." In World Health Organization, *SARS*, 94–100.

Campbell, Archie. *The SARS Commission Final Report*. Ontario SARS Commission, December 2006. http://www.archives.gov.on.ca/en/e_records/sars/report/index.html.

Chan, Gordon Ka-seung, and Dante Lam Chiu-yin, dirs. "Dang wan dou"/"Deng yun dao" [Waiting for luck]. In *Project 1:99*. Panorama, 2003.

Chan, Ka Ming. "Crossing the Transnational Hong Kong Cinema Co-Production: Production Culture, Policy, Business, and Individual Practitioners." PhD diss., Chinese University of Hong Kong, 2011.

Chang, Eileen. "From the Ashes." In *Written on Water*, translated by Andrew F. Jones, 39–52. New York: Columbia University Press, 2005.

Chang, Eileen. "Writing of One's Own." In *Written on Water*, translated by Andrew F. Jones, 15–22. New York: Columbia University Press, 2005.

Chappell, Bill. "Asian Grandmother Who Smacked Her Attacker with a Board Donates Nearly $1 Million." NPR, March 24, 2021.

Chee Yam Cheng. "SARS at TTSH (Part 4)." *SMA News* 35, no. 6 (2003): 20–27.

Chen, Guo-Hai. "Chinese Concepts of Humour and the Role of Humour in Teaching." In Davis and Chey, *Humour in Chinese Life and Culture*, 193–213.

Chen, Jason Chi Wai. "The Musical Characteristics of Sam Hui." Education Bureau of the Government of the Hong Kong Special Administration Region, 2009. https://www.edb.gov.hk/attachment/en/curriculum-development/kla/arts-edu/resources/mus-curri/mus-characteristics-sam-hui-e.pdf.

Chen, Joan, dir. *Feidian qingren* [Shanghai strangers]. Youku Originals, 2012.

Chen, Kuan-Hsing. *Asia as Method: Toward Deimperialization*. Durham, NC: Duke University Press, 2010.

Chen, Kuan-Hsing. "The Imperialist Eye: The Cultural Imaginary of a Subempire and a Nation-State." Translated by Yiman Wang. *positions* 8, no. 1 (2000): 9–76.

Chen, Ross. "Golden Chicken 2." *Love HK Film*, 2004. http://www.lovehkfilm.com/reviews/golden_chicken_2.htm.

Chen, Thomas. *Made in Censorship: The Tiananmen Movement in Chinese Literature and Film*. New York: Columbia University Press, 2022.

Chen, Thomas. "The Workshop of the World: Censorship and the Internet Novel 'Such Is This World.'" In *China's Contested Internet*, edited by Guobin Yang, 19–43. Copenhagen: Nordic Institute of Asian Studies Press, 2015.

Chen Baozhen. *SARS xinniang* [SARS bride]. New York: Cosy House, 2003.

"Chen Guanxi da nian chuyi fuchu" [Edison Chen's New Year's comeback]. *Sohu*, January 23, 2014. https://yule.sohu.com/20140123/n394018905.shtml.

Cheng, Steve Wai-man, dir. *Fei din yan sang/Feidian rensheng* [City of SARS]. Tai Seng, 2003.

Chew, Valerie. "Severe Acute Respiratory Syndrome (SARS) Outbreak, 2003." *Singapore Infopedia*, June 3, 2009. https://eresources.nlb.gov.sg/infopedia/articles/SIP_1529_2009-06-03.html?%20Singapore,%202003.

Chey, Jocelyn. "*Youmo* and the Chinese Sense of Humour." In Davis and Chey, *Humour in Chinese Life and Letters*, 1–29.

"China Information and Sources: China Statistics." *China Today*. Accessed December 23, 2022. http://www.chinatoday.com/data/data.htm.

China Internet Network Information Center. *The 47th Statistical Report on China's Internet Development*. February 2021. http://www.cnnic.com.cn/IDR/ReportDownloads/202104/P020210420557302172744.pdf.

Chiu, Cindy, Chris Ip, and Ari Silverman. "Understanding Social Media in China." *McKinsey Quarterly*, April 1, 2012.

Chiu, Samson Leung-chun, dir. *Gam gai/Jin ji* [Golden chicken]. Applause, 2002.

Chiu, Samson Leung-chun, dir. *Gam gai/Jin ji 2* [Golden chicken 2]. Applause, 2003.

Choi, Po-King. "From Dependence to Self-Sufficiency: Rise of the Indigenous Culture of Hong Kong, 1945–1989." *Asian Culture* 14 (1990): 161–77.

Chor Yuen, dir. *Cat sap ji gaa fong haak/Qishier jia fangke* [The house of 72 tenants]. Shaw Brothers, 1973.

Chow, Matt Hoi-kwong, dir. *Gam gai SSS/Jin ji SSS* [Golden chicken SSS]. Edko, 2014.

Chow, Stephen Sing-chi, dir. "Hoeng gong bit sing"/"Xianggang bisheng" [Hong Kong will sure win]. In *Project 1:99*. Panorama, 2003.

Choy, Samuel (Cai Zhongliang). "Xianggang dianying" [Hong Kong cinema]. *Wenhua yanjiu@lingnan* 29 (2012): 64–80.

Chu, Yiu Kong, and Carlie C. Y. Chan. "Policing One-Woman Brothels in Hong Kong: Alternative Strategies." *Journal of Asian Association of Police Studies* 5, no. 1 (2007): 3–14.

Chua Beng Huat. "SARS Epidemic and the Disclosure of Singapore Nation." *Cultural Politics* 2, no. 1 (2006): 77–96.

Chua Mui Hoong. *A Defining Moment: How Singapore Beat SARS*. Singapore: Institute of Policy Studies, 2004.

Clark, A. E. Preface to *Such Is This World@sars.come*, by Hu Fayun, i–iii. Dobbs Ferry, NY: Ragged Banner, 2011.

Comaroff, Joshua. "Ghostly Topographies: Landscape and Biopower in Modern Singapore." *Cultural Geographies* 14, no. 1 (2007): 56–73.

Corliss, Richard. "Cantopop Kingdom." *Time*, January 1, 2001.

"The Covid Resilience Ranking." *Bloomberg*, November 24, 2020. https://www.bloomberg.com/graphics/covid-resilience-ranking/.

Craddock, Susan. *City of Plagues: Disease, Poverty, and Deviance in San Francisco*. Minneapolis: University of Minnesota Press, 2000.

Curtain, Michael. "Renationalizing Hong Kong Cinema: The Gathering Force of the Mainland Market." In *Asian Popular Culture: The Global (Dis)continuity*, edited by Anthony Y. H. Fung, 250–66. New York: Routledge, 2013.

Davis, Benjamin P., and Jonathan Catlin. "Theses for Theory in a Time of Crisis." *Public Seminar*, March 30, 2020. https://publicseminar.org/essays/theses-for-theory-in-a-time-of-crisis/.

Davis, Jessica Milner. "Humour and Its Cultural Context: Introduction and Overview." In Davis and Chey, *Humour in Chinese Life and Culture*, 1–21.

Davis, Jessica Milner, and Jocelyn Chey, eds. *Humour in Chinese Life and Culture: Resistance and Control in Modern Times*. Hong Kong: Hong Kong University Press, 2013.

Deleuze, Gilles, and Félix Guattari. *A Thousand Plateaus: Capitalism and Schizophrenia*. Translated by Brian Massumi. Minneapolis: University of Minnesota Press, 1987.

Ding, Huiling. *Rhetoric of a Global Epidemic: Transcultural Communication about SARS*. Carbondale: Southern Illinois University Press, 2014.

Duffy, Jim. "Anatomy of an Epidemic: School Faculty Share Five Lessons from SARS." *Johns Hopkins Public Health*, Fall 2003. https://magazine.jhsph.edu/2003/fall/SARS/index.html.

Dundes, Alan. "At Ease, Disease—AIDS Jokes as Sick Humor." *American Behavioral Scientist* 30, no. 1 (1987): 72–81.

"Effect of SARS Epidemic on Affected Countries." *Talk of the Nation*, NPR, April 21, 2003.

"Elderly Asian Woman Attacked in San Francisco Fights Back, Sends Alleged Attacker to Hospital." CBS News, March 18, 2021.

Erni, John Nguyet. "SARS, Avian Flu, and the Urban Double Take." In *SARS: Reception and Interpretations in Three Chinese Cities*, edited by Deborah Davis and Helen Siu, 45–73. New York: Routledge, 2007.

Estok, Simon C. "Theorizing in a Space of Ambivalent Openness: Ecocriticism and Ecophobia." *Interdisciplinary Studies in Literature and Environment* 16, no. 2 (2009): 203–25.

Evasdottir, Erika E. S. *Obedient Autonomy: Chinese Intellectuals and the Achievement of Orderly Life*. Vancouver: University of British Columbia Press, 2004.

Fang Fang. *Wuhan Diary: Dispatches from a Quarantined City*. Translated by Michael Berry. New York: HarperVia, 2020.

Farquhar, Judith. *Appetites: Food and Sex in Post-Socialist China*. Durham, NC: Duke University Press, 2002.

Faucher, Carole. "As the Wind Blows and Dew Came Down: Ghost Stories and Collective Memory in Singapore." In *Beyond Description: Singapore Space Historicity*, edited by Ryan Bishop, John Phillips, and Wei-Wei Yeo, 190–203. New York: Routledge, 2004.

Federal Emergency Management Agency (FEMA). *COVID-19 Pandemic Operational Guidance: All-Hazards Incident Response and Recovery*. May 2021. https://www.fema.gov/sites/default/files/documents/fema_covid-19-pandemic-operational-guidance_5-17-2021.pdf.

Fedtke, Jana, Mohammed Ibahrine, and Yuting Wang. "Corona Crisis Chronicle: Fang Fang's *Wuhan Diary* (2020) as an Act of Sousveillance." *Online Information Review* 45, no. 4 (2021): 795–809.

"'Feidian' shiqi de shi da duanxin wenhouyu zhengji ji cui" [Essential collection of top ten text message greetings during SARS]. *CCTV*, May 31, 2003. http://www.cctv.com/program/zgzk/0005/02/index.shtml.

Feng, Shuo, Chen Shen, Nan Xia, Wei Song, Mengzhen Fan, and Benjamin J. Cowling. "Rational Use of Face Masks in the COVID-19 Pandemic." *Lancet Respiratory Medicine* 8, no. 5 (2020): 434–36.

Feng Yu. "Wei pingfan zhe lichuang—Fang Meiguo kejie chubanshe fuzeren Chen Wenqiao, Zeng Bihua fufu" [To record the achievements of common folks—Interview with US Cosy Publishing House head couple Chen Wenqiao and Zeng Bihua]. *Wenxinshe*, October 31, 2005. https://wxs.hi2net.com/home/news_read.asp?NewsID=7523.

Ferrari, Gits. *Not SARS Just Sex: Life in Taipei during SARS*. White Monkey, 2007. Kindle.

Fidler, David P. *SARS, Governance and the Globalization of Disease*. New York: Palgrave Macmillan, 2004.

Fong, Norhaya A., dir. *A Tale of Two Esthers*. Cru Asia, 2014.

Fu, Poshek, and David Desser, eds. *The Cinema of Hong Kong: History, Arts, Identity*. Cambridge: Cambridge University Press, 2000.

Gan, Wendy. *Comic China: Representing Common Ground, 1890–1945*. Philadelphia: Temple University Press, 2018.

Giesecke, Johan. "Primary and Index Cases." *Lancet* 384 no. 9959 (2014): 2024.

Glick, Megan. *Infrahumanisms: Science, Culture, and the Making of Modern Non/personhood*. Durham, NC: Duke University Press, 2018.

Goudsmit, Jaap. *Viral Fitness: The Next SARS and West Nile in the Making*. New York: Oxford University Press, 2004.

Government of the Hong Kong Special Administrative Region. "Designated Quarantine Hotels." January 29, 2021. http://www.coronavirus.gov.hk/pdf/designated-hotel-list-v2_en.pdf.

Greenfeld, Karl Taro. *China Syndrome: The True Story of the 21st Century's First Great Epidemic*. New York: Harper Perennial, 2006.

Greenfeld, Karl Taro. "Wild Flavor." In *The Best Creative Nonfiction*, vol. 1, edited by Lee Gutkind, 247–70. New York: Norton, 2007.

Guo, Shaohua. *The Evolution of the Chinese Internet: Creative Visibility in the Digital Public*. Stanford, CA: Stanford University Press, 2020.

Hall, Stuart. "Notes on Deconstructing the Popular." In *Cultural Theory and Popular Culture: A Reader*, edited by John Storey, 442–53. New York: Pearson, 2007.

Hanson, Marta E. *Speaking of Epidemics in Chinese Medicine: Disease and the Geographic Imagination in Late Imperial China*. New York: Routledge, 2011.

Harrison, Victoria S. "CoronaGothic: A Post-Mortem." *Critical Quarterly* 62, no. 4 (2020): 74–76.

Hayot, Eric. *The Hypothetical Mandarin: Sympathy, Modernity, and Chinese Pain*. New York: Oxford University Press, 2009.

Heinrich, Ari Larissa. "The Future Repeats Itself: COVID-19 and Its Historical Comorbidities." In *China Story Yearbook: Crisis*, edited by Jane Golley and Linda Jaivin with Sharon Strange, 166–77. Acton: Australian National University Press, 2021.

Heise, Ursula K. *Imagining Extinction: The Cultural Meanings of Endangered Species*. Chicago: University of Chicago Press, 2016.

Helen Katherine. "2003 di ershi'er jie Xianggang dianying jin xiang jiang" [2003 22nd Hong Kong film awards]. YouTube video, February 19, 2016. https://youtu.be/21YyAfosIAE.

Hellekson, Karen, and Kristina Busse. "Introduction: Why a Fan Fiction Studies Reader Now?" In *The Fan Fiction Studies Reader*, edited by Karen Hellekson and Kristina Busse, 1–17. Iowa City: University of Iowa Press, 2014.

Hillenbrand, Margaret. *Negative Exposures: Knowing What Not to Know in Contemporary China*. Durham, NC: Duke University Press, 2020.

HK Movie Extras. "Golden Chicken (2002) Making of *Jin ji*." YouTube video, February 17, 2018. https://youtu.be/dv-N2q2Xeoc.

HK Movie Extras. "Golden Chicken 2 (2003) Making of *Jin ji 2*." YouTube video, February 20, 2018. https://youtu.be/qBuVmKi2Hgs.

Hong Kong Trade Development Council. "Film Entertainment Industry in Hong Kong." *Hong Kong Means Business*, March 19, 2019. https://research.hktdc.com/en/article/MzExMjc4NDIz.

Hong Zhaoguan. Foreword to *Xiao dui SARS* [Laughing at SARS], edited by Jiang Zuohao et al., n.p. Beijing: Shiyou gongye, 2003.

Huang, Nicole. Introduction to *Written on Water*, by Eileen Chang, ix–xxvii. New York: Columbia University Press, 2005.

Huang, Yanzhong. *Governing Health in Contemporary China*. New York: Routledge, 2013.

Huang, Yanzhong. "The SARS Epidemic and Its Aftermath in China: A Political Perspective." In *Learning from SARS: Preparing for the Next Disease Outbreak*, edited by Stacey Knobler, Adel Mahmoud, Stanley Lemon, Alison Mack, Laura Sivitz, and Katherine Oberholtzer, 116–36. Washington, DC: National Academies Press, 2004.

Huang Xingchu. "China's SARS Patient Zero?" Interview by Li Xiao. *China.org*, June 9, 2003. http://www.china.org.cn/english/2003/Jun/66507.htm.

Huddleston, Tom, Jr. "This Hotel Is Infamous as Ground Zero for a SARS 'Super Spreader' in the 2003 Outbreak." CNBC, February 16, 2020. https://www.cnbc.com/2020/02/14/hong-kong-hotel-hosted-super-spreader-in-the-2003-sars-outbreak.html.

Hu Fayun. *Ruyan@sars.come*. Beijing: Zhongguo guoji guangbo, 2006.

Hu Fayun. *Such Is This World@sars.come*. Translated by A. E. Clark. Dobbs Ferry, NY: Ragged Banner, 2011.

Hu Fayun. "Xie SARS 'jinshu' de Wuhan zuojia Hu Fayun" [Wuhan writer Hu Fayun, author of SARS "banned book"]. Interview by Ding Yuanyuan. *Baodao zhe*, May 2, 2020. https://www.twreporter.org/a/2019-ncov-interview-china-writer-hu-fayun.

Hui, Michael Koon-man, dir. *Gwai maa soeng sing/Gui ma shuangxing* [Games gamblers play]. Golden Harvest, 1974.

Hung, Ho-fun. "The Politics of SARS: Containing the Perils of Globalization by More Globalization." *Asian Perspective* 28, no. 1 (2004): 19–44.

Hung, Kevin K. C., Carman K. M. Mark, May P. S. Yeung, Emily Y. Y. Chan, and Colin A. Graham. "The Role of the Hotel Industry in the Response to Emerging Epidemics: A Case Study of SARS in 2003 and H1N1 Swine Flu in 2009 in Hong Kong." *Globalization and Health* 14, no. 117 (2018). https://doi:10.1186/s12992-018-0438-6.

Hu Nianfei, Shi Xisheng, and Ma Xiaolu. "Tanfang woguo shouli SARS huanzhe" [Visiting our country's SARS index patient]. Sina, January 12, 2006. http://news.sina.com.cn/c/2006-01-12/10388845907.shtml.

Jeung, Russell, Aggie Yellow Horse, Tara Popovic, and Richard Lim. *Stop AAPI Hate National Report*. March 16, 2021. https://stopaapihate.org/wp-content/uploads/2021/05/Stop-AAPI-Hate-Report-National-210316.pdf.

Jiang Zuohao. Afterword to *Xiao dui SARS* [Laughing at SARS], edited by Jiang Zuohao et al., 358. Beijing: Shiyou gongye, 2003.

Jiang Zuohao et al., eds. *Xiao dui SARS: Zhansheng "feidian" youmo shouce* [Laughing at SARS: Defeating "feidian" humor manual]. Beijing: Shiyou gongye, 2003.

Johnson, Ian. "Inside and Outside the System: Chinese Writer Hu Fayun." *New York Review of Books*, November 28, 2016.

JTSF Television. "Zuotian zai Sanfanshi bei ren wugu gongji de Xie popo fangwen wanzheng ban" [Interview with Grandma Xie from yesterday's unprovoked attack in San Francisco]. Facebook, March 18, 2021. https://www.facebook.com/ktsf26/videos/560153134898906/.

Kam, Vivian, and Joshua Berlinger. "Alfonso Wong, 'Old Master Q' Cartoonist, Dies at 93." CNN, January 3, 2017. https://www.cnn.com/style/article/alfonso-wong-death-old-master-q/index.html.

Kan dianying le mei. "Zuo ji ye shi you lixiang de: *Jinji*" [Even a sex worker must have dreams: *Golden Chicken*]. YouTube video, August 17, 2017. https://youtu.be/wVdyaVWq9qo.

Ke Daqun. "Chuanmei you fangzhi zisha de nengliang" [The media has the ability to prevent suicides]. Radio Television Hong Kong, May 20, 2016. https://app3.rthk.hk/mediadigest/content.php?aid=2067.

Keil, Roger, and S. Harris Ali. "'Racism Is a Weapon of Mass Destruction': SARS and the Social Fabric of Urban Multiculturalism." In *Networked Disease: Emerging Infections in the Global City*, edited by S. Harris Ali and Roger Keil, 152–66. Malden, MA: Wiley-Blackwell, 2008.

Khan, Ali S., with William Patrick. *The Next Pandemic: On the Front Lines against Humankind's Gravest Dangers*. New York: PublicAffairs, 2016.

Kleinman, Arthur, and Sing Lee. "SARS and the Problem of Social Stigma." In Kleinman and Watson, *SARS in China*, 173–95.

Kleinman, Arthur, and James L. Watson, eds. *SARS in China: Prelude to Pandemic?* Stanford, CA: Stanford University Press, 2006.

Koetse, Manya. "Coronavirus on Chinese Social Media: The 8 Major Trends in Times of the 2019-nCoV Crisis." *What's on Weibo*, February 6, 2020.

Koh Tai Ann. "Malaysia and Singapore 1990–1993." *Journal of Commonwealth Literature* 30, no. 3 (1995): 71–107.

Kong, Belinda. "How Chinese People Came Together When Separated by Quarantine, Creating Hope, Humor, and Art." *Conversation*, March 18, 2020.

Kong, Belinda. "Pandemic as Method." *Prism: Theory and Modern Chinese Literature* 16, no. 2 (2019): 368–89.

Kong, Belinda. "Recovering First Patients." *b2o*, August 27, 2020. https://www.boundary2.org/2020/08/belinda-kong-recovering-first-patients/.

Kong, Belinda. "Totalitarian Ordinariness: The Chinese Epidemic Novel as World Literature." *Modern Chinese Literature and Culture* 30, no. 1 (2018): 136–62.

KPIX CBS SF Bay Area. "Anti-Asian Hate Crimes: Witnesses Say Elderly Asian Woman Beats Up Attacker." YouTube video, March 17, 2021. https://youtu.be/W_bayF4_dmE.

Kraut, Alan M. *Silent Travelers: Germs, Genes, and the Immigrant Menace*. Baltimore: Johns Hopkins University Press, 1994.

Kuipers, Giselinde. "'Where Was King Kong When We Needed Him?' Public Discourse, Digital Disaster Jokes, and the Functions of Laughter After 9/11." *Journal of American Culture* 28, no. 1 (2005): 70–84.

Lague, David, Susan V. Lawrence, and David Murphy. "The China Virus." *Far Eastern Economic Review*, April 10, 2003.

Lah, Kyung, and Jason Kravarik. "Family of Thai Immigrant, 84, Says Fatal Attack 'Was Driven by Hate.'" CNN, February 16, 2021. https://edition.cnn.com/2021/02/16/us/san-francisco-vicha-ratanapakdee-asian-american-attacks/index.html.

Lai, Linda Chiu-han. "Film and Enigmatization: Nostalgia, Nonsense, and Remembering." In *At Full Speed: Hong Kong Cinema in a Borderless World*, edited by Esther C. M. Yau, 231–50. Minneapolis: University of Minnesota Press, 2001.

Lam, Desmond. *Chopsticks and Gambling*. New Brunswick, NJ: Transaction, 2014.

Lambert, Stephen. "Singapore: Waves of Transmission." In World Health Organization, *SARS*, 100–108.

Lau, Alexis. "The Numbers Trail: What the Data Tells Us." In Loh and Civic Exchange, *At the Epicentre*, 81–94.

Lau, Jenny. "Besides Fists and Blood: Michael Hui and Cantonese Cinema." In Poshek and Desser, *Cinema of Hong Kong: History*, 158–75.

Laughlin, Charles A. "Why Critics of Chinese Nobel Prize-Winner Mo Yan Are Just Plain Wrong." *Asia Society*, December 12, 2012. https://asiasociety.org/blog/asia/why-critics-chinese-nobel-prize-winner-mo-yan-are-just-plain-wrong.

Law Kar and Frank Bren, with Sam Ho. *Hong Kong Cinema: A Cross-Cultural View*. Lanham, MD: Scarecrow, 2004.

LeDuc, James W., and M. Anita Barry. "SARS, the First Pandemic of the 21st Century." *Emerging Infectious Diseases* 10, no. 11 (2004). https://doi:10.3201/eid1011.040797_02.

Lee, Dominic T. S., and Yun Kwok Wing. "Psychological Responses to SARS in Hong Kong—Report from the Front Line." In Kleinman and Watson, *SARS in China*, 133–47.

Lee, Haiyan. "Déjà Vu: Revisiting Hu Fayun's SARS Novel during the 2020 Coronavirus Pandemic." *MCLC Resource Center*, May 2020. https://u.osu.edu/mclc/online-series/haiyan-lee/.

Lee, Haiyan. *Revolution of the Heart: A Genealogy of Love in China, 1900–1950*. Stanford, CA: Stanford University Press, 2007.

Lee, Haiyan. *The Stranger and the Chinese Moral Imagination*. Stanford, CA: Stanford University Press, 2014.

Lee, Jon D. *An Epidemic of Rumors: How Stories Shape Our Perceptions of Disease*. Logan: Utah State University Press, 2014.

Lee, Jung-Wook. "Speech to the Fifty-Sixth World Health Assembly." World Health Organization, May 21, 2003. https://apps.who.int/iris/handle/10665/78361.

Lee, Leo Ou-fan. *Shanghai Modern: The Flowering of a New Urban Culture in China, 1930–1945*. Cambridge, MA: Harvard University Press, 1999.

Lee, Robert G. *Orientals: Asian Americans in Popular Culture*. Philadelphia: Temple University Press, 1999.

Lee, Russell. *The Almost Complete Collection of True Singapore Ghost Stories: 25th Year Special Edition*. Singapore: Angsana, 2018. Kindle.

Lee, Russell. *The Almost Complete Collection of True Singapore Ghost Stories: Book 12*. Singapore: Angsana, 2004.

Lee, Vivian P. Y. *Hong Kong Cinema since 1997: The Post-Nostalgic Imagination.* New York: Palgrave Macmillan, 2009.

Lee, Yoon Sun. *Modern Minority: Asian American Literature and Everyday Life.* New York: Oxford University Press, 2013.

Lee Shiu Hung. "The SARS Epidemic in Hong Kong: What Lessons Have We Learned?" *Journal of the Royal Society of Medicine* 96, no. 8 (2003): 374–78. https://doi:10.1177/014107680309600803.

Leetaru, Kalev. "Mask-Wearing Guidance: A Timeline of Slow-to-Shift Messaging." *Real Clear Politics,* May 22, 2020.

Legislative Council of the Hong Kong Special Administrative Region (LegCo). *Report of the Select Committee to Inquire into the Handling of the Severe Acute Respiratory Syndrome Outbreak by the Government and the Hospital Authority.* July 2004. https://www.legco.gov.hk/yr03-04/english/sc/sc_sars/reports/sars_rpt.htm.

Leong, Russell. "Chaos, SARS, Yellow Peril: Virulent Metaphors for the Asian American Experience?" *Amerasia Journal* 29, no. 1 (2003): v–viii.

Leung, Gabriel M., Anthony J. Hedley, Edith M. C. Lau, and Tai-Hing Lam. "The Public Health Viewpoint." In Loh and Civic Exchange, *At the Epicentre,* 55–80.

Leung, Wing-Fai. "Multi-Media Stardom, Performance and Theme Songs in Hong Kong Cinema." *Canadian Journal of Film Studies* 20, no. 1 (2011): 41–60.

Leung Ping-kwan. "Feidian shiqi de qingshi" [Love poem in the time of SARS]. In *Bianhua de bianjie: Liang Bingjun shiji* [Shifting borders: Poems by Leung Ping-kwan], translated by Chris Zijiang Song, Kit Kelen, and Debby Vai Keng, 97–101. Macao: Association of Stories in Macao, 2009.

Li Cheuk-to. "Journal: Hong Kong." *Film Comment,* September/October 2004, 10–12.

Lieberthal, Kenneth. "Introduction: The 'Fragmented Authoritarianism' Model and Its Limitations." In *Bureaucracy, Politics, and Decision Making in Post-Mao China,* edited by Kenneth G. Lieberthal and David M. Lampton, 1–30. Berkeley: University of California Press, 1992.

Lieberthal, Kenneth, and Michel Oksenberg. *Policy Making in China: Leaders, Structures, and Processes.* Princeton, NJ: Princeton University Press, 1988.

Lii, Ding-Tzann. "A Colonized Empire: Reflections on the Expansion of Asian Countries." In *Trajectories: Inter-Asia Cultural Studies,* edited by Chen Kuan-Hsing, 107–26. New York: Routledge, 1998.

Lim, Benjamin. "Singapore's Most Underrated Minister Is the Minister It Needs the Most." *Rice,* April 30, 2018. http://www.ricemedia.co/current-affairs-commentary-singapores-underrated-minister-minister-needs/.

Lin, Shiqi. "Archives of the Future: Documentary Impulse in a Time of Crisis." *positions politics,* May 2020. https://positionspolitics.org/episteme-2-lin/.

Lin, Shiqi. "CUT! Community, Immunity, Vulnerability in the Time of Coronavirus." *UCHRI Foundry,* March 2020. https://uchri.org/foundry/cut-community-immunity-vulnerability-in-the-time-of-coronavirus/.

Link, Perry. "China: The Anaconda in the Chandelier." *New York Review of Books,* April 11, 2002.

Link, Perry. "China: From Famine to Oslo." *New York Review of Books*, January 13, 2011.

Link, Perry, and Kate Zhou. "*Shunkouliu*: Popular Satirical Sayings and Popular Thought." In *Popular China: Unofficial Culture in a Globalizing Society*, edited by Perry Link, Richard P. Madsen, and Paul G. Pickowicz, 89–109. Lanham, MD: Rowman and Littlefield, 2002.

Liu Xianjin. "Yingyong huanji feitu Jinshan huayi popo jiang juan shengyu zhongchou kuan" [Heroically fighting back against bandit, San Francisco overseas Chinese grandma to donate crowdfunding proceeds]. *Shijie xinwen wang*, March 23, 2021. https://www.worldjournal.com/wj/story/121472/5337343.

Liu Xiaobo. "From Wang Shuo's Wicked Satire to Hu Ge's *Egao*: Political Humor in a Post-Totalitarian Dictatorship." Translated by Teresa Zimmerman-Liu. In *No Enemies, No Hatred: Selected Essays and Poems*, edited by Perry Link, Tienchi Martin-Liao, and Liu Xia, 177–87. Cambridge, MA: Harvard University Press, 2012.

Loh, Christine, and Civic Exchange, eds. *At the Epicentre: Hong Kong and the SARS Outbreak*. Hong Kong: Hong Kong University Press, 2004.

Loh, Christine, and Jennifer Welker. "SARS and the Hong Kong Community." In Loh and Civic Exchange, *At the Epicentre*, 215–34.

Lupis, Marco. "SARS Patient Zero: Chinese Doctor's Research Causes Epidemic." Translated by Robin Good. *Master New Media*, April 12, 2003. https://www.masternewmedia.org/2003/04/12/sars_patient_zero_chinese_doctors.htm.

Lynteris, Christos. *Human Extinction and the Pandemic Imaginary*. New York: Routledge, 2020.

Lynteris, Christos. "The Prophetic Faculty of Epidemic Photography: Chinese Wet Markets and the Imagination of the Next Pandemic." *Visual Anthropology* 29, no. 2 (2016): 118–32.

Lynteris, Christos. "Yellow Peril Epidemics: The Political Ontology of Degeneration and Emergence." In *Yellow Perils: China Narratives in the Contemporary World*, edited by Franck Billé and Sören Urbansky, 35–59. Honolulu: University of Hawai'i Press, 2018.

Lynteris, Christos, and Lyle Fearnley. "Why Shutting Down Chinese 'Wet Markets' Could Be a Terrible Mistake." *Conversation*, January 31, 2020.

Ma, Eric Kit-wai, and Joseph Man Chan. "Global Connectivity and Local Politics: SARS, Talk Radio, and Public Opinion." In *SARS: Reception and Interpretations in Three Chinese Cities*, edited by Deborah Davis and Helen Siu, 19–43. New York: Routledge, 2007.

Ma, Joe Wai-ho, dir. "Seoi si hoeng gong siu ze"/"Shei shi Xianggang xiaojie" [Who's Miss Hong Kong?]. In *Project 1:99*. Panorama, 2003.

MacIntyre, C. Raina, Simon Cauchemez, Dominic E. Dwyer, et al. "Face Mask Use and Control of Respiratory Virus Transmission in Households." *Emerging Infectious Diseases* 15, no. 2 (2009): 233–41. https://doi:10.3201/eid1502.081167.

Marcus, Olivia Rose, and Merrill Singer. "Loving Ebola-chan: Internet Memes in an Epidemic." *Media, Culture and Society* 39, no. 3 (2017): 341–56.

Martinelli, Lucia, Markku Oksanen, and Helena Siipi. "Deextinction: A Novel and Remarkable Case of Bio-Objectification." *Croatian Medical Journal* 55, no. 4 (2014): 423–27. https://doi:10.3325/cmj.2014.55.423.

Mayer, Ruth. "Virus Discourse: The Rhetoric of Threat and Terrorism in the Biothriller." *Cultural Critique* 66 (Spring 2007): 1–20.

McBurney, Eric. "Deputy Public Defender Eric McBurney's Statement on Case Involving His Client Steven Jenkins + Video Surveillance." San Francisco Public Defender Office, April 8, 2021. https://sfpublicdefender.org/news/2021/04/deputy-public-defender-eric-mcburneys-statement-on-case-involving-his-client-steven-jenkins/.

McHugh, Fionualla. "Hong Kong's Darkest Hour: SARS and the Suicide of an Icon." *South China Morning Post Magazine*, March 31, 2013.

McKay, Richard A. "Patient Zero and the Early North American HIV/AIDS Epidemic—Lesson 3: AIDS and Infectious Disease Epidemiology." National Library of Medicine, December 16, 2013. https://www.nlm.nih.gov/exhibition/surviving-and-thriving/lesson-details12.html.

McKay, Richard A. "Patient Zero: Why It's Such a Toxic Term." *Conversation*, April 1, 2020.

McLeod, Saul. "The Psychology of Forgetting and Why Memory Fails." *Simply Psychology*, December 14, 2008.

McMillin, Calvin. "The House of 72 Tenants." *Love HK Film*, 2005. http://www.lovehkfilm.com/reviews_2/house_of_72_tenants.htm.

McNamara, Brittney. "The Ghosts of COVID: Why People Are Finding Comfort in the Paranormal." *Teen Vogue*, October 28, 2021.

Medecins Sans Frontières. "In Memoriam: Carlo Urbani." April 26, 2003. https://www.msf.org/obituary-carlo-urbani.

Meinhof, Marius. "Othering the Virus." *Discover Society*, March 21, 2020. https://archive.discoversociety.org/2020/03/21/othering-the-virus/.

Merianos, Angela, and Aileen Plant. "Epidemiology." In World Health Organization, *SARS*, 185–98.

MIHK.tv_Youtube Hong Kong Hotel di 229 ji a: Jianhua ba nian zhi luan zhi shashi shiwu nian [Lowjoke episode 229a: Eight years of chaos at Jianhua fifteen years after SARS]. YouTube video, March 2, 2018. https://youtu.be/LFXGXGpggb8.

MimiFanmi. "ATV—Xing dong yazhou@huainian gege—Yanxu Zhang Guorong chuanqi" [ATV Asian stars @ in memory of big brother—Continuing the legend of Leslie Cheung]. YouTube video, May 5, 2013. https://youtu.be/ev_E6d1pkGY.

Mirsky, Jonathan. "Banned in China." *New York Review of Books*, January 9, 2012.

Molina, Natalia. *Fit to Be Citizens? Public Health and Race in Los Angeles, 1879–1939.* Berkeley: University of California Press, 2006.

Morrow, Patrick D. "Those Sick Challenger Jokes." *Journal of Popular Culture* 20, no. 4 (1987): 175–84.

National Intelligence Council. *SARS: Down but Still a Threat.* August 2003. https://www.dni.gov/files/documents/Special%20Report_SARS%20Down%20But%20Still%20a%20Threat.pdf.

Nazren, Fasiha. "'Even My Parents Don't Know Who Russell Lee Is': True S'pore Ghost Stories Writer Shares More About Himself After 32 Years." *Mothership*, February 6, 2021. https://mothership.sg/2021/02/russell-lee-true-singapore-ghost-stories-interview/.

Ng, Stephen. "The Mystery of the Amoy Gardens." In Loh and Civic Exchange, *At the Epicentre*, 95–115.

Ngai, Sianne. *Ugly Feelings*. Cambridge, MA: Harvard University Press, 2005.

Nie, Jing-Bao, and Carl Elliott. "Humiliating Whistle-Blowers: Li Wenliang, the Response to Covid-19, and the Call for a Decent Society." *Bioethical Inquiry* 17, no. 4 (2020): 543–47. https://doi:10.1007/s11673-020-09990-x.

Nielsen, Katie. "Suspect Arrested in Oakland Robbery, Assault That Left 75-Year-Old Asian Man Brain Dead." CBS SF Bay, March 9, 2021. https://www.cbsnews.com/sanfrancisco/news/75-year-old-asian-man-left-brain-dead-from-injuries-in-latest-oakland-assault/.

Nikiforuk, Andrew. "Modern Plagues." *Canadian Business*, October 14, 2003.

Nixon, Rob. *Slow Violence and the Environmentalism of the Poor*. Cambridge, MA: Harvard University Press, 2011.

Normile, Dennis. "Battling SARS on the Frontlines." *Science*, May 2, 2003.

Novak, Ben Jacob. "Deextinction." *Genes* 9, no. 11 (2018): 548.

Omi, Shigeru. "Overview." In World Health Organization, *SARS*, vii–x.

Oransky, Ivan. "Carlo Urbani (Obituary)." *Lancet* 361, no. 9367 (2003): 1481.

Pat C. "Sandra Ng—Interview by Grady Hendrix Golden Chickensss—NY Asian Film Festival 2014." YouTube video, July 1, 2014. https://youtu.be/UfM4p39OvC4.

Pekar, Jonathan E., Andrew Magee, Edyth Parker, et al. "The Molecular Epidemiology of Multiple Zoonotic Origins of SARS-CoV-2." *Science*, July 26, 2022.

Philipkoski, Kristen. "Superspreaders May Hold SARS Clue." *Wired*, May 21, 2003.

Piepzna-Samarasinha, Leah Lakshmi. *Care Work: Dreaming Disability Justice*. Vancouver: Arsenal Pulp, 2018.

Pike, Lili. "Why 15 US States Suddenly Made Masks Mandatory." *Vox*, May 29, 2020.

Podvin, Thomas, and David Vivier. "Interview Gordon Chan, from *The Big Heat* to *A-1*." *Hong Kong Cinemagic*, January 13, 2005. http://www.hkcinemagic.com/en/page.asp?aid=319&page=0.

Provine, Robert R. *Curious Behavior: Yawning, Laughing, Hiccupping, and Beyond*. Cambridge, MA: Harvard University Press, 2012.

Qin Yingyun. "'Feidian' yufang ge" [SARS prevention song]. Wuhan Centers for Disease Prevention and Control, April 15, 2003. https://whcdc.org/view/902.html.

Quammen, David. *Spillover: Animal Infections and the Next Human Pandemic*. New York: Norton, 2012.

Rea, Christopher. *The Age of Irreverence: A New History of Laughter in China*. Berkeley: University of California Press, 2015.

Rea, Christopher. "Spooling (*e'gao*) Culture on the Chinese Internet." In Davis and Chey, *Humour in Chinese Life and Culture*, 149–91.

Ritter, Malcolm. "Mystery Illness Raises Concerns in US." *Access World News*, April 2, 2003.

"Rush to Develop Test for Detecting SARS." *All Things Considered*, NPR, April 15, 2003.

SARS Expert Committee. *SARS in Hong Kong: From Experience to Action*. Government of the Hong Kong Special Administrative Region, October 2, 2003. https://www.sars-expertcom.gov.hk/english/reports/reports/reports_fullrpt.html.

"SARS Fast Facts." CNN, September 2, 2013. https://www.cnn.com/2013/09/02/health/sars-fast-facts/index.html.

Schweitzer, Dahlia. *Going Viral: Zombies, Viruses, and the End of the World*. New Brunswick, NJ: Rutgers University Press, 2018.

Sedgwick, Eve Kosofsky. *Epistemology of the Closet*. Berkeley: University of California Press, 1990.

Sedgwick, Eve Kosofsky. *Touching Feeling: Affect, Pedagogy, Performativity*. Durham, NC: Duke University Press, 2003.

Seno, Alexandra A., and Alejandro Reyes. "Unmasking SARS: Voices from the Epicentre." In Loh and Civic Exchange, *At the Epicentre*, 1–15.

Shah, Nayan. *Contagious Divides: Epidemics and Race in San Francisco's Chinatown*. Berkeley: University of California Press, 2001.

Shah, Sonia. *Pandemic: Tracking Contagion, from Cholera to Ebola and Beyond*. New York: Sarah Crichton, 2016.

Sharpe, Jenny. *Ghosts of Slavery: A Literary Archaeology of Black Women's Lives*. Minneapolis: University of Minnesota Press, 2002.

Shih, Shu-mei. *Visuality and Identity: Sinophone Articulations across the Pacific*. Berkeley: University of California Press, 2007.

Shute, Nancy. "SARS Hit Home." *US News and World Report*, May 5, 2003.

The Silent Killer: SARS. Films Media Group, 2008.

"Singapore Woman Linked to 100 SARS Cases." Fox News, April 9, 2003. https://www.foxnews.com/story/singapore-woman-linked-to-100-sars-cases.

Siu, Helen, and Jane Chan. "Eulogy and Practice: Public Professionals and Private Lives." In *SARS: Reception and Interpretations in Three Chinese Cities*, edited by Deborah Davis and Helen Siu, 75–102. New York: Routledge, 2007.

"Solid Response to SARS—Almost." *Nature Medicine* 9, no. 5 (2003): 479.

Stein, Ruthe. "Joan Chen's Ode to Jews in Shanghai." *SFGate*, July 18, 2013. https://www.sfgate.com/movies/article/Joan-Chen-s-ode-to-Jews-in-Shanghai-4673712.php.

Tam, Arthur. "The Death of Cantonese?" *Time Out*, May 8, 2016.

Tan, Teri. "Booking Their Space." *Publishers Weekly*, October 3, 2005.

Tang, Xiaobing. *Visual Culture in Contemporary China: Paradigms and Shifts*. Cambridge: Cambridge University Press, 2015.

Tao Dongfeng. "Making Fun of the Canon in Contemporary China: Literature and Cynicism in a Post-Totalitarian Society." Translated by Yang Ling. *Cultural Politics* 3, no. 2 (2007): 203–22.

Teo, Stephen. "The 1970s: Movement and Transition." In Poshek and Desser, *Cinema of Hong Kong*, 90–110.

Teo, Stephen. *Hong Kong Cinema: The Extra Dimensions*. New York: Palgrave Macmillan, 1997.

Teo, Stephen. "*Promise* and *Perhaps Love*: Pan-Asian Production and the Hong Kong–China Interrelationship." *Inter-Asia Cultural Studies* 9, no. 3 (2008): 341–58.

Thornber, Karen Laura. *Global Healing: Literature, Advocacy, Care*. Leiden: Brill, 2020.

To, Johnnie Kei-fung, and Wai Kar-fai, dirs. "Kong soeng kuk"/"Kuangxiangqu" [Rhapsody]. In *Project 1:99*. Panorama, 2003.

Tsing, Anna Lowenhaupt. *The Mushroom at the End of the World: On the Possibility of Life in Capitalist Ruin*. Princeton, NJ: Princeton University Press, 2015.

Tsui Hark, dir. "Seon bat seon jau nei"/"Xin bu xin you ni" [Believe it or not]. In *Project 1:99*. Panorama, 2003.

Veg, Sebastian. *Minjian: The Rise of China's Grassroots Intellectuals*. New York: Columbia University Press, 2019.

Veloo, Ravi. "Lee, Russell (1964–)." In *Encyclopedia of Post-Colonial Literatures in English*, 2nd ed., edited by Eugene Benson and L. W. Conolly, 834. New York: Routledge, 2005.

Voigt, Kevin. "Outbreak Bad Luck for One Hong Kong Business." CNN, May 4, 2009. https://www.cnn.com/2009/BUSINESS/05/04/hk.metropark.luck/.

Wagner, Tamara S. "Singapore's New Thrillers: Boldly Going beyond the Ethnographic Map." *ARIEL* 37, nos. 2–3 (2006): 69–89.

Wald, Priscilla. *Contagious: Cultures, Carriers, and the Outbreak Narrative*. Durham, NC: Duke University Press, 2008.

Wang, Qi. "Young Feminist Activists in Present-Day China: A New Feminist Generation?" *China Perspectives* 3, no. 114 (2018): 59–68.

Wei Yi. "Xianggang feidian xungen" [Getting to the roots of Hong Kong and SARS]. Sina, May 30, 2003. http://finance.sina.com.cn/roll/20030530/1748346946.shtml.

Whaley, Floyd. "The Hanoi-French Hospital: Dr. Urbani's Alert." In World Health Organization, *SARS*, 167–72.

Whaley, Floyd. "Solving the Metropole Hotel Mystery." In World Health Organization, *SARS*, 141–48.

Whaley, Floyd, and Osman David Mansoor. "SARS Chronology." In World Health Organization, *SARS*, 3–48.

"WHO Points at 'Super Spreaders' as Key to Stopping SARS." *Medical Letter on the CDC and FDA*, May 4, 2003, 37.

Whyte, Kyle. "Against Crisis Epistemology." In *Routledge Handbook of Critical Indigenous Studies*, edited by Brendan Hokowhitu, Aileen Moreton-Robinson, Linda Tuhiwai-Smith, Chris Andersen, and Steve Larkin, 52–64. New York: Routledge, 2021.

Wolfe, Nathan. *The Viral Storm: The Dawn of a New Pandemic Age*. New York: St. Martin's Griffin, 2012.

Wong, James Jum-sum [Wong Jim]. "Yueyu liuxing qu de fazhan yu xingshuai: Xianggang liuxing yinyue yanjiu (1949–1997)" [The rise and decline of Cantopop: A study of Hong Kong popular music (1949–1997)]. PhD diss., University of Hong Kong, 2003.

World Bank. "World Bank/IMF Spring Meetings 2021: Development Committee Communiqué." April 9, 2021. https://www.worldbank.org/en/news/press-release/2021/04/09/world-bank-imf-spring-meetings-2021-development-committee-communique.

World Health Organization (WHO). "Consensus Document on the Epidemiology of Severe Acute Respiratory Syndrome (SARS)." 2003. https://apps.who.int/iris/handle/10665/70863.

World Health Organization (WHO). "Coronavirus Disease 2019 (COVID-19) Situation Report—37." February 26, 2020. https://www.who.int/docs/default-source/coronaviruse/situation-reports/20200226-sitrep-37-covid-19.pdf?sfvrsn=6126c0a4_2.

World Health Organization (WHO). "If Dr. Carlo Urbani Were Alive Today." March 12, 2019. https://www.who.int/vietnam/news/detail/12-03-2019-if-dr-carlo-urbani-were-alive-today.

World Health Organization (WHO). "Impact of COVID-19 on People's Livelihoods, Their Health and Our Food Systems." October 13, 2020. https://www.who.int/news/item/13-10-2020-impact-of-covid-19-on-people's-livelihoods-their-health-and-our-food-systems.

World Health Organization (WHO). *International Health Regulations (2005)*. WHO Press, 2008.

World Health Organization (WHO). *SARS: How a Global Epidemic Was Stopped*. Geneva: World Health Organization Regional Office for the Western Pacific, 2006.

World Health Organization (WHO). "Severe Acute Respiratory Syndrome (SARS)—Multi-Country Outbreak—Update 30." April 15, 2003. https://www.who.int/csr/don/2003_04_15/en/.

World Health Organization (WHO). "Severe Acute Respiratory Syndrome—Singapore, 2003." *Weekly Epidemiological Record* 78, no. 19 (2003): 157–68.

World Health Organization (WHO). "Update 17—Travel Advice—Hong Kong Special Administrative Region of China, and Guangdong Province, China." April 2, 2003. https://www.who.int/csr/sars/archive/2003_04_02/en/.

Worobey, Michael, Joshua I. Levy, Lorena Malpica Serrano, et al. "The Huanan Seafood Wholesale Market in Wuhan Was the Early Epicenter of the COVID-19 Pandemic." *Science*, July 26, 2022.

Wu Xia and Li Nannan. "Bu xiang bei ren ji zhe de feidian shouli" [The SARS index case who does not want to be remembered]. *360doc*, February 1, 2013. http://www.360doc.com/content/13/0201/03/200041_263516716.shtml.

Xiao, Hui Faye. *Family Revolution: Marital Strife in Contemporary Chinese Literature and Visual Culture*. Seattle: University of Washington Press, 2014.

Xia Yang. "Feidian 'duwang' shi nian yingxingmaiming shi" [Ten incognito years of SARS's "poison king"]. *Sina Daily*, February 26, 2013. http://style.sina.com.cn/news/p/2013-02-26/0937116933.shtml.

Xiong, Yong, Hande Atay Alam, and Nectar Gan. "Wuhan Hospital Announces Death of Whistleblower Doctor Li Wenliang." CNN, February 7, 2020. https://www.cnn.com/2020/02/06/asia/li-wenliang-coronavirus-whistleblower-doctor-dies-intl/index.html.

Xu, Rui-Heng, Jian-Feng He, Meiron R. Evans, et al. "Epidemiologic Clues to SARS Origin in China." *Emerging Infectious Diseases* 10, no. 6 (2004): 1030–37. https://doi:10.3201/eid1006.030852.

Yang, Guobin. *The Wuhan Lockdown*. New York: Columbia University Press, 2022.

Yang, Jeff. *Once Upon a Time in China: A Guide to Hong Kong, Taiwanese, and Mainland Chinese Cinema*. New York: Atria, 2003.

Yang Lin. "Feidian shi nian: Shouli bingren Pang Zuoyao" [Ten years later after SARS: Index patient Pang Zuoyao]. Sina, November 15, 2012. https://blog.sina.com.cn/s/blog_5f0b84100102e6eo.html.

Yang Xi. *Huang Zhan* [Wong Jim]. Hong Kong: Chung Hwa, 2016.

Yan Lianke. *Dream of Ding Village*. Translated by Cindy Carter. New York: Grove Press, 2011.

Yapp, Hentyle. *Minor China: Method, Materialisms, and the Aesthetic*. Durham, NC: Duke University Press, 2021.

Yeoh Chee Yan. Foreword to *Wet Markets: Community Heritage Series II*, by Singapore Heritage Society, 1. Singapore: National Heritage Board, 2013.

Yeoh En-lai. "Singapore Woman Linked to 100 SARS Cases." UCLA Department of Epidemiology School of Public Health, April 9, 2003. https://www.ph.ucla.edu/epi/bioter/singaporewomanSARS.html.

Yip, Paul S. F., K. W. Fu, Kris C. T. Yang, Brian Y. T. Ip, Cecilia L. W. Chan, Eric Y. H. Chen, Dominic T. S. Lee, Frances Y. W. Law, and Keith Hawton. "The Effects of a Celebrity Suicide on Suicide Rates in Hong Kong." *Journal of Affective Disorders* 93, nos. 1–3 (2006): 245–52. https://doi:10.1016/j.jad.2006.03.015.

Young, Emma. "The New Plague." *New Scientist*, May 9, 2015.

Yu, Verna. "Can Cantonese Survive?" *America: The Jesuit Review*, June 5, 2018. https://www.americamagazine.org/politics-society/2018/06/05/can-cantonese-survive-230027.

Zeng Zifan. *Xianggang yueyu guanyongyu yanjiu* [Hong Kong Cantonese idioms]. Hong Kong: City University of Hong Kong Press, 2008.

Zhan, Mei. "Civet Cats, Fried Grasshoppers, and David Beckham's Pajamas: Unruly Bodies after SARS." *American Anthropologist* 107, no. 1 (2005): 31–42.

Zhang, Hong. "Making Light of the Dark Side: SARS Jokes and Humor in China." In Kleinman and Watson, *SARS in China*, 148–70.

Zhang, Hong. "SARS Humor for the Virtual Community: Between the Chinese Emerging Public Sphere and the Authoritarian State." In *SARS: Reception and Interpretations in Three Chinese Cities*, edited by Deborah Davis and Helen Siu, 119–45. New York: Routledge, 2007.

Zhang, Xudong. *Postsocialism and Cultural Politics: China in the Last Decade of the Twentieth Century*. Durham, NC: Duke University Press, 2008.

Zhang, Yunpeng, and Fang Xu. "Ignorance, Orientalism and Sinophobia in Knowledge Production on COVID-19." *Journal of Economic and Human Geography* 111, no. 3 (2020): 211–23.

Zhang Minzhou. Foreword to *Ji feng jing cao* [The storm that tests the grass], edited by Zhang Minzhou et al., 7–9. Guangzhou: Guangdong renmin, 2003.

Zhang Minzhou, et al., eds. *Ji feng jing cao: Zhongzheng jianhushi (ICU) ziji de gushi* [The storm that tests the grass: Personal stories from the ICU]. Guangzhou: Guangdong renmin, 2003.

Zheng Xiaoling, Wang Changchun, and Chen Gang. "Foshan Bitang xiang: Qijin faxian de Guangdong diyili de yixue diaocha" [Foshan Bitang village: A medical investigation into Guangdong's first known case]. Sina, May 18, 2003. http://finance.sina.com.cn/x/20030518/1555341755.shtml.

Zhong, N. S., B. J. Zheng, Y. M. Li, et al. "Epidemiology and Cause of Severe Acute Respiratory Syndrome (SARS) in Guangdong, People's Republic of China, in February, 2003." *Lancet* 362, no. 9393 (2003): 1353–58. https://doi: 0.1016/s0140-6736(03)14630-2.

Zhou Lixin, Tan Jiaju, Wu Min, Luo Hongtao, Yu Tieou, Kang Ping, Fang Bin, Li Yinan, Wen Weibiao, and Zou Yicheng. "Guangdong sheng Foshan shi yanzhong jixing huxi zonghezheng shouli baogao" [The first case of severe acute respiratory syndrome in Foshan]. *Zhonghua jiehe he huxi zazhi* [*Chinese Journal of Tuberculosis and Respiratory Diseases*] 26, no. 10 (2003): 598–601.

Zhu, Ping. "Introduction: The Study of Laughter in the Mao Era." In *Maoist Laughter*, edited by Ping Zhu, Zhuoyi Wang, and Jason McGrath, 1–16. Hong Kong: Hong Kong University Press, 2019.

INDEX

Abbas, Ackbar, 120, 124, 155

Abraham, Thomas, 192

Adams, Jerome, 16–17

affect ordinariness, 33–37

affects: affective sovereignty, 26, 35, 76; reshaping of, 26, 28, 34–35, 81; ugly feelings, 25–26, 35–36, 50–53, 75. *See also* emotion

affect theory, 18–20, 25

Africa: Ebola epidemic (2014–2016), 6, 11; georacialized as source of disease, 11, 12, 200

"Against Crisis Epistemology" (Whyte), 7–8, 26–27

Agamben, Giorgio, 8, 15, 24, 44, 243n50

agency: cultural, 96, 113, 127; epidemic, 16; of fans, 107; "heroic," 21, 23; non-Western forms of, 23, 25; sexual, 37–39; Western erasure of Chinese, 35. *See also* lateral agency/lateral politics; microagency

The Age of Irreverence (Rea), 77–78

Ahmed, Sara, 9, 26, 71–72; legitimate and illegitimate lives, 18, 35, 81, 214. *See also* emotion; pain, politics and sociality of

Ai Fen, 109–10

Almenoar, Maria, 224

Almost Complete Collection of True Singapore Ghost Stories (TSGS) (Lee), 32, 233–37

amnesia, 23, 45, 165–67, 172

And the Band Played On (Shilts), 198

anglophone archive, 28; conspiracy theories, 180–81, 203–4; English as language of, 238–39; erasure of first patients from, 191–92; inaccuracies and distortions in, 31, 180–83, 191–201, 217–18, 224–25, 238–41; non-otherizing, 216; "Poison King" misinformation, 194–95; and SARS origin stories, 180–83; "superspreader" concept in, 197–201; unjust memories within medical archives, 211–14; and writing of diasporic elites, 192–93. *See also* first patients/index patients

animals: blurred boundaries with human, 193–94; considered SARS carriers, 51–52; human-animal companionship, 52, 55–56. *See also* "wet markets"

anti-Asian violence, 2–7, 12, 16, 197

apocalypse, slow, 120

Appadurai, Arjun, 158

Applause Pictures, 145–46, 176

archiving projects, pandemic, 21–22, 25

Arendt, Hannah, 47, 54, 126
arrogance, postcolonial, 18
Asia, trope of as origin of pandemics, 12–13
Asian financial crisis (1997), 117, 152
Associated Press article, misinformation in, 217–18, 224, 225
Atkins, Paul, 6
avian flu, 12, 95, 203, 204

Bakhtin, Mikhail, 83
bare life, 44, 52
Barthes, Roland, 53
Beggar So (martial arts folk hero), 131
Berlant, Lauren, 11, 28; crisis ordinariness, 20–21, 34, 36, 55, 79; cruel optimism, 20, 190; slow death, 20, 55, 127, 190. *See also* lateral agency/lateral politics
Berry, Michael, 73
bio-orientalism, 10–13, 19, 29; China as totalizing terror state, 192; of ecophobia, 200; and first patients accounts, 31, 181–83, 192–97; historical repetition of, 12–13, 182–83; humor culture as alternative to, 81; "medicalized nativism," 196; religion as alternative to, 227; threats to survival in crisis discourse, 11–12, 111, 181–82; "wet markets" discourse, 181–82, 193–94. *See also* pandemic crisis discourse
biopolitical and biosecurity critiques, predictive failure of, 14–15, 19
biopolitics: communist history connected to SARS governance, 45, 48–51; isolation ward conflated with prison, 48–50; nonexceptional, 56; outsourced to Asia, 9–10
biosecurity, 13–16, 19, 196, 203
bioterrorism, 13, 95
Bitang (town, Foshan), 184–85
Bordwell, David, 116, 125
Breiman, Robert, 188, 199
Bren, Frank, 124
Britain, as "soft touch nation," 9
British Columbia CDC, 215
Busse, Kristina, 107

California, 13, 242n17
Canada, SARS outbreaks, 215–16
canon-mocking literature (*dahua wenxue*), 83, 104–5, 106, 108, 110
Cantonese, 3, 30, 122–23; in *Golden Chicken 2*, 158; local slang in SARS films, 128, 133, 135, 147–51, 153–54, 156
Cantophone, 30, 121–23; extinction consciousness of, 126, 146; local memory cues, 128; local slang and period references, 147–56; memory retrieval cues, 168–70; multimedial culture, 158–59, 172; as nontransportable, 156, 157; rise of, 126; self-resuscitation, 128–29; social comedy films, 130–31, 136, 137; subimperial status, 120, 123–24, 146, 150, 171; ur-genre for resilience in social comedy, 130–31. *See also* Hong Kong; SARS films (2003)
Cantopop, 123, 132–33, 136; "04 Bless You," 178; "Ask Me," 170–71; in *Golden Chickens* films, 168–74; "Gone with the Wind," 175; "Just Loving You," 172–73; "Keep Smiling," 178; "Keep Smiling with the God of Songs" concerts, 177–78; "Riding in the Same Boat," 178; "Silence Is Golden," 179; "What Does One Ask for in Life," 173–74. *See also* Hui, Sam; *Project 1:99* (film)
care, 5–6, 19, 25–28; and humor, 81, 93–94, 96, 100; and microagency, 110–11; self-care neglected by caregivers, 228; self-care practices, 55–56, 93–94, 96, 100, 187–88, 190
carnivalesque, 30, 83, 94, 104, 141
cartoons, 3, 106, 131
Catlin, Jonathan, 21, 112
CDC Office Public Health Preparedness and Response, 184
censorship: countercensorship practices, 109–10; crafting of disease information, 90; and Li Wenliang's death, 74; misattribution of, 192–93; portrayed in literary works, 41–42; restrictions on reporting SARS, 249n53; of *Such Is This World*, 40, 46–48, 80, 245–46n21

286 INDEX

Centers for Disease Control, 16

Central Intelligence Agency, 14

Chan, Danny Pak-keung, 172–73

Chan, Eason Yik-shun, 132

Chan, Gordon, 130, 131

Chan, Grace Lai-sze, 171

Chan, Jackie, 148

Chan, Jane, 119

Chan, Joseph Man, 252n45

Chan, Peter Ho-sun, 129–30, 143, 155, 158, 161; and Applause Pictures, 145–46, 176

Chang, Eileen, 33–36, 38, 75

Chen Baozhen, 29, 39, 59–73, 80, 100, 140. See also *SARS Bride* (Chen)

Chen Chunming, 3

Chen, Joan, 29, 37–39, 61, 245n15

Chen, Johnny, 213, 214

Chen, Kuan-Hsing, 14, 123. *See also* subempire.

Chen Wenqiao, 59–60

Cheng, Albert, 252n45

Cheng, Steve Wai-man, 136, 254n89

Cheung, Leslie Kwok-wing: death of, 115–17, 119, 122, 126, 138; and extinction consciousness, 115, 126; in "Gone with the Wind" serial, 175; private ceremonies for, 119; "Silence Is Golden" duet with Hui, 179

Cheung, Jacky Hok-yau, 169

Chey, Jocelyn, 86, 96

China: authoritarianism blamed for early handling of SARS crisis, 17; censorship regime as vague, 40; Cold War epistemologies of, 22, 192; continuity between Mao and post-Mao capitalist eras, 44, 87; criticism of during SARS, 48–50; Cultural Revolution, 47, 57, 87; democracy movement, 45; dialectic of lack and surplus, 189; food incidents, 69; fragmented authoritarianism of, 43, 67, 89; Great Famine (1958–61), 189; as "horizon of horizons," 19; Long March, 66; "major and proper" vs. "minor," 24; number of COVID-19 cases, 243n50; party-state bureaucracy, 43–44; post-Mao reform era, 43, 82; postsocialist rhetoric, 47–48;

public secrecy, 23–24; Qing court's smallpox management, 12–13; sense of terror in, 44–47; state media, 67–68; state secret laws, 90; Tiananmen massacre (1989), 29, 45–48, 54, 57, 149; Western anxieties about rise of, 10–12

China Central Television (CCTV), 67, 85

China Syndrome (Greenfeld), 201–3

Chinese Communist Party: applications to by medical personnel, 68; humor directed at, 82, 83

Chinese diaspora, 3, 59–60, 67, 123

Chinese people: affinity with the nonhuman attributed to, 10–11, 181–82, 184, 189, 193–94; deexceptionalizing humanity of, 35; legitimate and illegitimate lives in Western viewpoints, 18, 35, 81, 214; stereotype of as susceptible to disease, 12–13; Western erasure of agency, 35

Chiu, Samson Leung-chun, 155

Choi, Po-King, 122

Chor Yuen, 130

Chow, Stephen Sing-chi, 134–36, 139, 141, 177, 255n112

Christian spirituality after SARS, 226–33

Chua Beng Huat, 223, 230

Chua Mui Hoong, 223–26

City of SARS (film), 30, 73, 121, 136–42, 165; elevator as zone of heightened danger, 140, 200

Clark, A. E., 40, 245n21

closure, narratives of, 24

Cold War epistemologies, 22, 192

colonialism, 18, 25, 83–84, 120; epistemologies of crisis used to mask, 7–8, 11; Indigenous responses to, 26–27; Qing Empire, construction of, 182

Comaroff, Joshua, 236

communal politics and ethics, 39

communism: biopolitics of, 44–45; connected to SARS governance, 45, 48–51, 87; continuance of Cold War epistemologies, 22, 192; critique of in SARS literature, 41–43; erasure of pre-1949 comic cultures, 77; portrayed as disease, 13; symbols of used during SARS pandemic, 10

Confucian primers, 99

"Congee Cure Song," 100

conspiracy theories, 180–81, 203–4

consumer goods, 69, 72; panic buying, 90, 95, 100

Contagion (Soderbergh), 28, 142

containment narrative, 90–91

"CoronaGothic" fiction, 233

Cosy House Publisher, 59–60

COVID-19, 1–3, 239–40; anti-Asian violence during, 2–7, 12, 16, 197; as "China virus" or "Wuhan virus," 11, 200; digital prosociality and quarantine humor, 109–11; ghost sightings and paranormal activities during, 233–34; labeled as unprecedented, 8; origin stories, 180, 182; quarantine hotels, 212; Sam Hui's concerts, 178; small humor, 110; Wuhan lockdown, 14, 73–76, 110, 240

Covid Resilience Ranking (Bloomberg), 113

crisis: banalities of, 1–2; as fact of life, 20; genre of, 11; rhetoric of, 20; systemic, 20; used to mask power deployments, 7–8, 11

crisis epistemologies, 7–14, 28, 78, 112, 120; denaturalization of, 35; orientalist facets of, 10–11; overturning of, 156; presentism of, 7–8, 11; unprecedentedness and urgency, 7–8

crisis ordinariness, 20–21, 29, 34, 36, 51, 55; and humor, 79, 98

cruel optimism, 20, 190

Cruel Optimism (Berlant), 20

cruelty, trope of Chinese, 19

cultural commons, 96, 105

Cultural Revolution, 47, 57, 87

Curtain, Michael, 175–76

cycle of fortune/misfortune, 109, 134, 141–42

daa gung zai (working-class guy), 132

Davis, Benjamin, 21, 112

dead farmer narrative, 31, 183–84, 186, 193, 195, 204

decolonization, 23, 25, 35, 83–84, 120, 236

deexceptionalization, 19, 35, 39, 56, 165, 221–22

deextinction, 30–31; in biology, 113; extinction/deextinction dyad, 113–14, 119–29; as response to Cheung's suicide, 115–16; reversals in SARS films, 161–63; self-extinction farce in *City of SARS*, 136–42; self-resuscitation, 128–29; subimperial double consciousness, 120, 123–24, 146, 171; underdog comeback trope, 31, 124, 127, 128, 130, 135, 143–44, 150, 155–65. *See also* Cantophone; entertainment industry, Hong Kong; extinction; Hong Kong

A Defining Moment: How Singapore Beat SARS, 223–24, 234

deimperialization, 14

Deleuze, Gilles, 80

Deng Xiaoping, 149

digital archive, participatory, 21–22. *See also* internet, Chinese

Ding, Huiling, 78, 81, 89, 90, 95, 100, 226

disability justice movement, 27

disappearance, culture and politics of, 120, 124–25, 155

disease: Africa georacialized as source of, 11, 12, 200; communism portrayed as, 13; destigmatization of, 27; diseased other, 12–13; as naturally occurring, 50–51

disease phobia, 85

dissidence hypothesis, 22–26, 65, 74, 83, 192

"documentary impulse," 21–22, 109

domesticity, 29, 34, 81, 98, 108; alternative, 63; redomestication of women as response to socialist history, 56–57. *See also* everyday life; ordinariness

double consciousness, subimperial, 120, 123–24, 146, 171

"double take," 146

Dream of Ding Village (Yan), 246n36

Drunken Master (film), 148

Dugas, Gaétan, 198

Ebola epidemic (2014–16), 6, 11

ecogothic imagination, 181, 182, 196, 200

Economist, 10

ecophilia/ecophobia, 200

egao (wicked-making) culture, 83, 84

elevator trope, 140, 200–202

elites: film producers and crew as, 145; material excesses during capitalist era, 87; next generation or *guanerdai,* 51; "residual elitism," 57

"elitist historiography," 22, 120

emotion: cultural politics of, 18–19, 35, 81, 214; "just emotions," 26; patriarchal economy of, 36; quasi-animalizing framework, 35; Western attitudes toward Chinese, 35. *See also* affects

enigmatization, 146, 148, 152–53, 156

Enjoy Yourself Tonight (television variety show), 132

entertainment industry, Hong Kong, 114–16; art-house cinema, 121–22, 125; audience fatigue, 117; bipolar styles, 127–28; Canto-comedy genre, 130–31; cultural aesthetics from below, 135; decline of, 116–17; de/extinctionist aesthetics, 121, 131, 156, 159; funding structure, 124–25; gambling-themed movies, 133–34; and Mandarin language, 125, 127; multi-media stardom, 122; New Wave cinema, 124–25, 144; 1972 low point, 125, 130; post- SARS, 117, 175; real-life relationships and celebrity gossip, 161; sexism in, 144; as subsistence subempire, 124; visuality and sound in, 122. *See also* Cantopop; Hong Kong; Hong Kong Film Awards; SARS films (2003); television

epicenters, global pandemic, 14, 22, 113; postepidemic renewal at sites of, 191; as sites of crisis resilience, 236. *See also* Foshan; Hong Kong; Singapore

epistemologies of coordination, 26–27

epistemologies of pandemic microagency, sociality, and care, 19–28

Erni, John Nguyet, 146

Estok, Simon, 200

European travelers: distortion of Qing court's health management, 12–13

Evasdottir, Erika, 23

everyday life, 1–2; "contradictions and chaos" of, 80–81; crisis ordinariness, 20–21, 29, 34, 36, 51, 55, 79, 98; gendering of, 56–59; as nonexceptional, 39, 41, 56, 59, 134, 156; participatory digital archive, 21–22; survival practices, 25, 30–31, 49, 52, 55, 74, 80–81, 97. *See also* pandemic ordinariness

extinction, 12, 28; Cantophone consciousness of, 126, 146; doom, trope of, 10–11, 193, 205; extinction/deextinction dyad, 113–14; and local vernacular practice, 153; of local world, 115; pandemic ordinariness alongside, 39; species extinction discourse, 175–76. *See also* deextinction; entertainment industry, Hong Kong

face mask usage, 16–17

fake news, 114

familiar devices as shared comfort, 95–96, 137

fanfiction, 103, 106–9

Fang Fang, 42, 73–76, 110

"A Farewell to Secretary Shuyun at Xuanzhou's Xietiao Villa" (Li Bo), 101

Farquhar, Judith, 189

The Fate (television serial), 170

Faucher, Carole, 235–36

fear, 47; naturalization of, 44–45, 196; socialist rhetoric about, 92–93; and "superspreader" metaphor, 199–200

Fearnley, Lyle, 182

Fedtke, Jana, 75

feidian (atypical pneumonia), as term for SARS, 87, 187, 249–50n63

female feelings and relationships, 29, 54–55; "compulsory sympathy," 36; female-female camaraderie, 60–68; patriarchal and patriotic emotive norms, 35; professional female sociality, 61; sexual agency, 37–39; transfer of primary emotional attachment, 61; *yiqi* (spirit of loyalty between friends), 71. *See also* gender

feminist activists, 71–72

Ferrari, Git, 203

INDEX   **289**

Fidler, David, 9

film: China-oriented, 176; Mandarin productions, 125, 127, 158; pan-Asian, 146, 176. *See also* entertainment industry, Hong Kong; SARS films (2003); specific films

Films Media Group, 200

first patients/index patients, 8–9, 28, 180–237; anglophone misinformation about, 183–84; blame assigned to, 197–98, 201–3, 212, 232; contact history not available, 187; elected local official as, 184; epidemiological and medical archives, 31–32, 205–6, 211–14; and global pandemic crisis discourse, 183, 197; Huang Xingchu, 194–95, 197; humanity of eclipsed, 182; impact of misinformation on, 187–88, 195; media dodged by, 186–88, 195; mental health of, 187–89, 229–30; microagency of, 190–94, 233; as "non-valuable life," 196; outbreaks that never were, 214–16; "patient zero" discourse, 31, 197–98, 201–3, 212, 224; primary cases vs. index cases, 185–86; as racialized aliens, 198; resilience of, 190, 226–28, 233; and SARS origin stories, 180–83; shifts in reporting on, 220–23; survival of, 185, 188, 190–92, 194, 204–5, 210–11, 213, 216–17, 225–26; and unjust memories, 211–14; Vietnam, 212–13. *See also* anglophone archive; Liu Jianlun; Mok, Esther; Pang Zuoyao

First People's Hospital of Foshan, 183, 185

folk cultures: ghost tales, 32, 236; humorous, 24, 83; recipes, 99–100. *See also* humor

food incidents, China, 69

Foshan (Guangdong province), 184–85; First People's Hospital, 183, 185

Foshan outbreak (Guangdong province), 31, 89, 183–84; as intrafamilial cluster, 185, 192

"Four Major Classic Love Stories: The SARS Edition," 107–9

The Fourth-Generation Women (Hu), 56–57

fragmented authoritarianism, 43, 89

"From Super Scientist to Great Infector: Patient Zero of the Killer Virus" *(La Repubblica)*, 203

"From the Ashes" (Chang), 33–36

Games Gamblers Play (film), 130, 132, 135

Gan, Wendy, 97, 105

gender: gendering of everyday life, 56–59; redomestication of women as response to socialist history, 56–57; and "super-spreader" concept, 216–18. *See also* female feelings and relationships

ghost sightings and paranormal activities, 32, 233–37, 266n244; guerilla funerals, 236

Glick, Megan, 196

Global Healing (Thornber), 27

global health: exceptional biopolitics outsourced to Asia, 9–10; purpose of "patient zero" discourse, 197; Western failure of timely intervention, 17–18. *See also* World Health Organization (WHO)

Globe and Mail (Toronto), 192–93

Golden Chicken 1 (film), 30, 142–43, 146; localism and vernacular in, 147–56; making-of featurette, 154–55; phoenix allegory in, 154–55

Golden Chicken 2 (film), 30–31, 121, 136, 142–46, 154, 156–65, 212, 255n112; Cantopop songs in, 170–74; memory and amnesia in, 165–75; underclass assemblages in, 156–65, 171–72

Golden Chicken SSS, 176–77

"Gone with the Wind" (ATV serial), 175

"good-life fantasy," 20

grassroots (*minjian*) intellectuals, 58–60, 69

"grassroots wit," 83

Great Famine (1958–61), 189

Greenfeld, Karl Taro, 201–3

greetings, during SARS, 93–97

"ground zero" rhetoric, 11, 197–98, 200

Guangdong Health Administration, 89

Guangdong province: February 11 press conference, 89, 91, 206; WHO travel advisory against, 114. *See also* Bitang (town, Foshan); Foshan outbreak (Guangdong province)

Guangzhou, 61

Guangzhou Military General Hospital, 194

Guattari, Félix, 80

guerilla funerals, 236

guerilla media, 78, 81, 91; and panic-inducing rumors, 95; as survival device, 226

Guo, Shaohua, 24, 78

Hall, Stuart, 83–84

Han Han, 57

handover paradigm, 22, 120–22

Hanoi-French Hospital, 213

Happy Camp (television series), 79

Harrison, Victoria, 233

hate crimes, 2–4

Hayes, Steven, 6

Hayot, Eric, 19

healing, collective, 27

health care: advanced access to, 185; common people's lack of access to, 15–16

health humanities scholarship, 27

health practices, Asian, Western ridicule of, 17

Heinrich, Ari, 12

Heise, Ursula, 127

Hellekson, Karen, 107

Hero (film), 106

Heymann, David, 199

Heyuan outbreak, 194–95

Hilditch, Tom, 136

Hillenbrand, Margaret, 23

Ho, Patrick Chi-ping, 157

Hollywood films, 117

homelessness and mental illness, 4–5, 7

Hong Kong, 112–79; 1970s working class, 132; Amoy Gardens housing estate, 114, 141; autonomous status terminated in 2046, 167, 172; cultural studies of, 113; *daa hei* (lifting of spirit), 178; disappearance, culture and politics of, 120, 124–25, 155; "doing things for yourself," 130; "elitist historiography" of, 22, 120, 124; emigration from, 158; entertainment industry, 114–19; as epicenter of SARS pandemic, 113, 114; excolonial status, 28, 31, 116, 119–20; handover, 22, 24, 26, 116, 117, 120, 154–55, 174, 178, 252n45; handover reductionism in scholarship on, 22, 121–22; identity construction, 124–25, 128, 158, 171; imperial imagery of, 119; indigenous culture of, 122; under Japanese rule, 33–34; *kau chim* ritual, 157; loss of world, 126–27; luck practices, indigenous, 129, 131–34, 138, 143, 155–56; Metropole Hotel outbreak, 31, 196, 198, 200, 202; print and radio journalism, 252n45; prodemocracy protests (2019), 22; protectionist quotas on, 117; public eulogies as civic practices, 119; resilience, local ethos of, 30–31, 113, 117, 128–30, 133, 136, 144, 155, 166; self-reliance, aesthetic of, 128–29, 132; signature cultural artifacts, 128; Umbrella Movement (2014), 22; underclasses, postcolonial, 157–65; unemployment rate, 117; WHO travel advisory against, 114. *See also* Cantophone; deextinction; entertainment industry, Hong Kong

Hong Kong Film Awards, 114–19

Hong Kong Film Directors' Guild, 129

Hong Kong Legislative Council, 205, 210

Hong Kong Stock Exchange, 152

Hong Zhaoguan, 92–93

Ho Sau-sun, Ivan, 132

The House of 72 Tenants (film), 130, 132, 158

"How One Person Can Fuel an Epidemic" (*New York Times*), 199

huaji (quick wit of jesters and clowns), 96–97

Huang, Nicole, 34

Huang, Yanzhong, 89–91

Huang Xingchu, 194–95, 197

Hu Fayun, 29, 39–44, 73, 80, 140, 212, 239; critique of totalitarian resilience, 57; *The Fourth-Generation Women*, 56–57. *See also Such Is This World@sars.come* (Hu)

INDEX   **291**

Hui, Michael, 130–35, 136, 138, 143

Hui, Ryan, 178

Hui, Sam, 132–33, 135, 177–78; "04 Bless You," 178; "Keep Smiling," 178; "Keep Smiling with the God of Songs" concerts, 177–78; "Riding in the Same Boat," 178; "Riding in the Same Boat" miniconcert, 178–79; "Silence Is Golden," 179. *See also* Cantopop

humanism, 9–10, 19, 21, 31–32, 65, 86; infrahumanist ontologies, 196, 227

humor, 28, 77–111; affective economy of, 30, 81; amiable, 97; associated with wit and social savvy, 87, 88; bathos, 81, 99; from bioevolutionary standpoint, 94–95; canon-mocking literature (*dahua wenxue*), 83, 104–5, 106, 108, 110; care and self-care, 81, 93–94, 96, 100; carnivalesque, 30, 83, 94, 104, 141; Chinese-specific linguistic, 86–87; comic cultures of pre-1949 decades, 77; during COVID-19, 109–11; and crisis ordinariness, 79, 98; cultural studies theories of, 83; *egao* (wicked-making) culture, 83, 84; *feidian*, 87–88, 249–50n63; folk cultures of, 24, 83; forms of, 29–30; genre mashing, 103; homophones and double entendres, 86–87; *huaji* (quick wit of jesters and clowns), 96–97; laughing with, 30, 94; and microagency, 79, 93, 95–96, 105; *minyao* (folk rhymes), 83; 1920s Shanghai farce culture, 97; psychological models of, 80–81; rebellion/subservience binary, 83–84; and resilience, 80–81, 86; in *SARS Bride*, 72–73; in SARS films, 130; satire and parody, 30, 73, 81, 82, 84–85, 87, 91, 94; *shunkouliu* (slippery jingles), 83; small, 30, 73, 81, 93–97; socialist, 84–86, 92–93; spectrum of social expressions, 79, 80; subaltern, 96; subculture of SARS jokes, 78–79; subversive and satirical attributed to United States, 84; *youmo*, 86, 96–97. *See also* internet, Chinese; SARS jokes

Hungry Ghost Festival (Singapore), 236

Ibahrine, Mohammed, 75

ignorance, production of, 17–18

Indigenous peoples, 26–27

influenza pandemic (1918), 8, 237–35

infrahumanist ontologies, 196, 227

Institute of Policy Studies think tank (Singapore), 223–24

intellectuals: complicity with party-state, 45–49; grassroots (*minjian*), 58–60, 69; universal, 57

International Health Regulations, 9

internet, Chinese, 28–30, 240; bloggers, rise of, 57; digital archive, participatory, 21–22; micro digital practices, 30; Pang's story readily available on, 192; reception of *Such Is This World*, 56–57; regional websites, 79; rise of, 60, 109; SARS romances on, 40; as site of residual feelings, 52–53; as space for prosociality, 24, 74; use in 2003, 78; Western narratives of, 24, 74. *See also* humor; SARS jokes; *Wuhan Diary* (Fang)

internet, COVID-era, 2–3

isolation ward, political use of, 48–49, 51

Jenkins, Steven, 4–7

Jiang Yanyong, 90

Jiang Zuohao, 92

Jing Ke, 106

Jin Yong, 106, 133

Journal of Infectious Diseases, 198

Jumping Ash (film), 171

Jurassic Park, 117

"Keep Smiling with the God of Songs" (Hui), 177–78

Khalik, Salma, 221–22

Khan, Ali, 184

killer bees, racialized trope of, 200

knowledge production, 6, 17–18

Koetse, Manya, 110

Kraut, Alan, 196

Kwan, Sui-Chu, 216

Kwong Wah Hospital (Hong Kong), 207, 208

Lai, Linda, 146, 168

Lai, Gigi Chi, 131

Lai, Michael Siu-tin, 171

Lam, Dante, 131

Lam, Desmond, 133

language, 6; Chinese-specific linguistic humor, 86–87; in digital spaces, 24; of films, 125; ideological policing of, 87; Mandarin, 87. *See also* Cantonese; Cantophone

lateral agency / lateral politics, 20–23, 27, 70; within crisis ordinariness, 36, 55, 79; and humor, 95, 111. *See also* Berlant, Lauren; microagency

Lau, Andy Tak-wah, 132, 133, 161, 167–68

Lau, James Tai-kwan, 114–15

Lau, Jenny, 22, 120, 121, 125. *See also* handover paradigm

Lau, Sean Ching-wan, 133

Laughing at SARS (Petroleum Industry Press), 79, 88, 91–93; folk recipes in, 99–100; "Four Major Classic Love Stories: The SARS Edition," 107–9; mimic poems in, 102; small humor in, 79, 88, 91–93, 96

Laughlin, Charles, 23

laughter, from bioevolutionary standpoint, 94–95

Law Kar, 124

Lee, Bruce, 125, 158

Lee, Haiyan 35, 42, 52

Lee Hsien Loong, 223

Lee, Leo Ou-fan, 34

Lee, Russell, 32, 233–37, 266n244

Lee, Tom, 215–16

Lee, Vivian, 144, 145

Lee, Yoon Sun, 25

Legend of the Condor Heroes (Jin Yong), 106, 133

Legend of the White Snake (SARS fanfiction), 107–8

Leung, Gigi Wing-kei, 131

Leung Ping-kwan (Ye Si), 1, 32, 111

Leung Sing-bor, 136

Leung, Tony Ka-fai, 153, 160

Leung, Wing-Fai, 122

Leu Siew Ying, 186, 192

Li Bo, 101, 104

Li Cheuk-to, 120

Li Ka-shing, 152

Li Tzar-kai, Richard, 152

Li Wenliang, 73–75, 109–10

Lieberthal, Kenneth, 43

Lii, Ding-Tzann, 123

Lim Hng Kiang, 218, 220

Lin, Shiqi, 21–22, 109

Lin Yutang, 96

linguistics, 122–23

Link, Perry, 40, 56, 83

literary fiction, 28–29; continuity between Mao and post-Mao capitalist eras in, 44; conventional epidemic genres, 28; intellectual characters' complicity with party-state, 45–47; officials' banal decisions, 54–55; responsibility of Chinese writers to document corruption and abuse, 43; revolutionary rhetoric in, 64–66. *See also* SARS romances

Liu Jianlun, 31, 195, 196–216; as an already symptomatic body, 200, 201; avian allusion, 204; blame of for SARS outbreak, 197–98, 201–3, 212; brother-in-law's death from SARS, 210; Cantonese spoken by, 209; career as medical professional, 205–6; direct infections not attributable to, 207–9, 214–16; erasure of family in news reports, 204–5, 219; extended clan and family circle, 209–11; first symptoms and disease trajectory, 206–9; ground zero metaphor used for, 197–98; last days reconstituted, 205–11; narrative isolation of, 204–5; as "patient zero" and "superspreader," 197–205, 207–9; self-disclosure of SARS, 209; Urbani's media narratives compared to, 212–14; wife of, 31, 204–7, 210, 211, 213, 220

Liu Xiaobo, 83

lives, legitimate and illegitimate, 18, 35, 81, 214

Looking Back in Anger (television drama), 173

"Love Poem in the Time of SARS" (Leung Ping-kwan), 1, 32, 111 luck practices, indigenous, 129, 131–34, 138, 143, 155–56; divination readings, 156–57

Lynteris, Christos, 182, 207

Ma, Eric Kit-wai, 252n45

Macron, Emmanuel, 74

Mandarin film productions, 125, 127, 158

Mao era, humor during, 84

Maoist Laughter anthology, 84

Maoist revolutionary drama, 65

Mao Zedong, 10, 84

marriage, 61–62; "bourgeois conjugality" and revolutionary bride, 65

Marx, Karl, 84

McBurney, Eric, 5, 6, 7

McKay, Richard, 198

media, Chinese, 67–68; blackout on SARS new, 89–90; containment narrative, 90–91; guerilla media, 78, 81, 91, 95, 226; on Pang, 186–88; "risk communication vacuum," 91; sanitizing imperative of, 68; SARS downplayed in, 67–68; unauthorized reporting as treason, 90

media, Hong Kong, 113, 120

media, Western: aggressive SARS reporting, 90–91; sinophobic stereotypes portrayed in, 3, 10, 17–18, 111, 182, 218, 239

"medicalized nativism," 196

medical records and scientific writings, 28, 31–32, 205–6; extra-epidemiological human details, 205; on Liu, 205–12; on Mok, 218–19; on Pang, 184–85, 192; readily accessible on internet, 192. *See also* media, Chinese

medical workers: applications to Chinese Communist Party, 68; bravery of, 67; female, 35–36, 60–68; ghostly experiences of, 234–35; and guerilla media, 91; Hong Kong, 118–19; panic toward, 162–63, 221; spread of SARS to, 162, 183; Vietnam outbreak, 213; vulnerability of, 67–68. *See also* Liu Jianlun

Meinhof, Marius, 18

memory: and ghost tales, 235–36; retrieval failure, 168; retrospective and prospective, 168

mental health, 162–63; alternative support networks, 226; of first patients, 187–89, 229–30; of recovered SARS patients, 187–88, 229

Metropark (Wei Jing) hotel, 212

Metropole Hotel (Hong Kong): damp interior of building, 207–8; elevator area, 201–2, 206–7; renaming of, 211

Metropole Hotel outbreak (Hong Kong), 31, 196, 198, 204–8, 260n111; *China Syndrome* misinformation, 201–3; due to environmental contamination, 202; recreation of for books and film, 200–202; zero staff infected, 209, 214. *See also* Liu Jianlun; Mok, Esther

microagency, 20–22, 29, 34, 109, 120; and care, 110–11; and digital platforms, 78; of first patients, 190–94, 233; guerilla funerals, 236; guerilla media as, 78; and humor, 79, 93, 95–96, 105; in minor styles and minor genres, 25; private care work as activism, 27; recovery of, 34, 191; during Wuhan lockdown, 75. *See also* lateral agency/lateral politics

microepistemes, 29

Mid-Autumn Festival, 103

migrants, rural women, 69–71

mimic poems, 101–5

Ministry of Health (Beijing), 89

Mirsky, Jonathan, 40

Miss Hong Kong Pageant, 132

missing body, metaphor of, 45–50, 55

mnemonic schemes, 168

modernity, 13, 25, 34, 66, 97, 237

Mok, Esther, 31, 216–33, 240; Associated Press article, 217–18; delay in diagnosis of, 219; disease trajectory, 224–25, 228–29; family closeness, 225–26, 228, 229–30; family members infected, 220, 221, 225; Hong Kong visit, 217–19, 224, 228; as hyperinfectious Asian female body, 218; labeled as "super-infector," 218, 220–22, 226–27, 229;

medical records of, 218–19; multiple story arcs, 230–31; ordinariness of, 219, 222, 224, 227; and outbreaks that never happened, 219–20; Philippines experience, 231–32; public questioning of media, 220–21; shift in reporting on, 220–23; spirituality after SARS, 226–33; state biopoliticization of, 223; story of in own words, 223–26; *A Tale of Two Esthers* (film), 226–33

Mo Yan, 23

National Heritage Board (Singapore), 182
National Intelligence Council, 13
National People's Congress meeting (March 2003), 89, 90
natural disasters, as human disaster, 42–43
neoliberalism, 6, 11, 20, 55, 113, 116; and decline of Hong Kong entertainment industry, 116–17
New York Times, 9, 199–200
The Next Pandemic (Khan), 184
Ng, Sandra Kwan-yu, 143–44, 161, 121, 176–77. *See also Golden Chicken* films
Ngai, Sianne, 25–26, 36
Nixon, Rob, 127
No. 2 Affiliated Hospital of Zhongshan Medical University, 206
Nobel Prize in Literature, 23
"nonce taxonomies," 24, 120
nonexceptional, the, 39, 41, 56, 59, 134–35, 156; and desire for postprecarity, 190–91
nonhuman, affinity with attributed to Chinese, 10–11, 181–82, 184, 189, 193–94
Not SARS Just Sex (Ferrari), 203

"obedient autonomy," 23
Oksenberg, Michel, 43
Old Master Q (comic strip), 131
omertà, law of, 23
Ontario SARS Commission report, 216
ordinariness, 20–21, 29; ethics of, 60; and shame, 72. *See also* affect ordinariness; crisis ordinariness; pandemic ordinariness; ugly feelings

orientalism, 3, 10; "amiable" Anglo-American humor, 97, 105; "new," 18; self and other, partitioning of world into, 24–25; sinophobic racism, 18; techno-orientalism, 28. *See also* bio-orientalism
origin stories, SARS, 10–11, 180–83; human, 182; zoonotic, 10–11, 180–82, 189–90
otherness: China as totalitarian other of West, 192; diseased other, 12–13; "wet markets" as emblems of, 182
outbreak narrative, 28, 30, 198

Pacific Century CyberWorks (PCCW), 152
pain, politics and sociality of, 18, 81
Pak Ho, 4
"Pandemic as Method" (Kong), 13
pandemic crisis discourse, 183, 197; georacial sinicization of, 199–200; outbreaks that never happened, 214–16; secularized, 233. *See also* bio-orientalism; media, Western
pandemic ordinariness, 29, 38–43, 59; affect ordinariness, 33–36; alongside crisis narrative, 39; alternative paradigm of, 35, 44–45, 55–56, 64; and totalitarian history, 40. *See also* everyday life; SARS romances
Pang Zuoyao, 183–94, 204, 219; advanced health care treatment for, 185; anglophone misinformation about, 31, 184, 191–94, 204, 239; dead farmer narrative of, 31, 183–84, 186, 193, 195, 204; as deputy chief of Bitang Village, 184–85, 187, 192; erasure from anglophone archive, 191–92; impact of disease experience on, 186–89, 239–40; initial experience with SARS, 185; local eco-activism by, 189–90; media interactions with, 186–87; reconstructing life of, 184–90; self-care practices, 187–88, 190; stigmatization of, 188
panic, 118–19
panic buying, 90, 95, 100
"paranoid reading," 24, 26

INDEX 295

"patient zero," discourse of, 31, 195, 196, 197–201

People's Action Party (PAP) (Singapore), 223

People's Daily, 85

"people's war" rhetoric, 65, 90

Petroleum Industry Press, 79

photo-forms, 23

photography, SARS-era, 182

Piepzna-Samarasinha, Leah Lakshmi, 27

places, attachment to, 236

poetry, mimicry of, 101–5

popular music, Chinese, 105. *See also* Cantopop

postepidemic renewal, 191

postsocialist era, 55; humor of, 80; redomestication of women, 56–57; rise in gender crimes, 71

power, 6; crises used to mask deployments of, 7–8, 11; layered histories of, 13; state of exception, 8, 15, 44, 50–52, 134

precarity: colonial, 120; in comic suicide films, 139; of housing project residents, 141; human and animal, 44, 52; as life without the promise of stability, 190; social, 20

"Prelude to Water Melody" (Su Shi), 102–4

presentism, 7–8, 11

Project 1:99 (film), 30, 121, 129–36, 165, 239; "Believe It or Not," 131; deextinctionist themes in, 129–32; "Hong Kong Will Sure Win," 134–35; "Memories of Spring 2003," 146; "The Private Eyes," 132–33; "Rhapsody," 132–33; "Waiting for Luck," 131–32; "Who's Miss Hong Kong?" 132

Prosocial (Arkins, Wilson, and Hayes), 6

prosociality, 1–7, 25, 30, 80–81; community building performed by SARS jokes, 88; COVID-19 and humor, 109–11; public eulogies as civic practices, 119; transnational and translingual, 5–6; Xie Xiao Zhen incident, 2–7. *See also* care; humor; small humor; sociality

Provine, Robert, 94–95

pseudomedical ditties, 99–100

public citizenship, 81

public health: bio-orientalism in, 12–13; draconian measures, 9, 85; foreign-born linked to to disease and contamination, 196; medical surveillance phone calls, 211; neoliberal co-optation of resilience, 113; and state deployments of power, 8; uneven knowledge among officials and ministries, 89–90

public secrecy, 23–24

publishing industry, 59–60

Qing Empire, 12–13, 182

Qin Shi Huang, 106

Qin Yingyun, 99

Qi Wang, 71

Quammen, David, 192

Quek, Tracy, 221

"Quiet Night Thoughts" (Li Bo), 101

racism: anti-Asian violence, 2–7, 12, 16, 197; flaunted during pandemics, 10; georacial chauvinism, 16, 81; grief, politics of, 18–19; historical patterns, repetition of, 7, 12–13, 182; pathological, 13

Ratanapakdee, Vicha, 4

Rea, Christopher, 77–78, 84, 97

reparation, 26–27

La Repubblica, 203

resilience, 28, 239; alternative, 112–14; of authoritarian state, 86; in COVID era, 112–13; of first patients, 190, 226–28, 233; and humor, 80–81, 86; local ethos of in Hong Kong, 30–31, 113, 117, 128–30, 133, 136, 144, 155, 166; on more-than-ordinary scales, 227–28; neoliberal co-optation of, 113; and peopleness, 113, 240; in *Such Is The World*, 52–53, 57, 64; of systemic racism, 7; technologies of, 226; ur-genre for in Cantonese social comedy, 130–31. *See also* Hong Kong

retrieval failure, 168

revolution, narratives of, 24, 64–66

rhizome, 80

rumors, 78, 91, 92, 95, 103, 114

Said, Edward, 24–25

SARS (severe acute respiratory syndrome), 1–2; array of scenes, 28–32; attributed to "wet markets," 31, 111, 181–82, 193; Beijing outbreak coverup, 90; Canada outbreaks, 215–16; as "Chinese virus," 200; elevator as zone of heightened epidemic danger, 140, 200–202, 206–7; as epidemic of "firsts," 9; expansion of biopower justified by, 8; *feidian* (atypical pneumonia) as term for, 87, 187, 249–50n63; female medical workers, 35–36, 60–68; first known case, 89; Foshan outbreak, 31, 89, 183–85, 192; governance of connected to communist history, 45, 48–51, 87; Heyuan outbreak, 194–95; hunger and destitution as greater threat, 163; infectious period, 207; internationalization of, 199; internet technologies during, 78; labeled as unprecedented, 8–9; in longer timeline, 38; mental health impacts of, 188; names for, 249–50n63; no fatalities in United States, 13; noncrisis epistemologies of, 25; nosocomial clusters, 218–19; origin stories, 180–83; pets considered viral carriers, 51–52; quotidian effects of, 72–73; timeline of information, 88–89; travel advisories, 9, 114; Vietnam outbreak, 213; and yellow peril ideologies, 196–97, 203–4; zoonotic origin theories, 10–11, 180–82, 189–90. *See also* first patients/index patients; Metropole Hotel outbreak (Hong Kong); Singapore

SARS Bride (Chen), 29, 39, 59–73, 100, 212, 239; ceremonious gestures in, 64; deviations from party line in, 67–68; endemic social issues in, 68–73; female-female camaraderie in, 60–68; humor in, 72–73; limited print run, 60, 80; preface to, 67; publication of, 59–60; revolutionary rhetoric in, 64–66; sex trafficking and exploitation of rural women in, 69–71

SARS: Down But Still a Threat (National Intelligence Council), 13

SARS films (2003), 28; amnesia motif, 164–65; audiences interpellated as accomplices, 144; bad body fluid humor, 141; bankruptcy motif, 158–59; de-extinctionist themes in, 129–32, 138, 142, 146, 154, 156, 168; enigmatization in, 146, 148, 152–53, 156; gambling themes, 133–34; little-guy protagonist, 132, 135, 138, 141–44; localism and vernacular in, 147–56; media clips in, 152–53, 163; mental illness motif, 164–65; minor roles for disease and sickness, 128; pedagogical ideals in, 155, 166; satire of disaster capitalism, 137; stylistic polarities in, 127–28; suicide motif, 138–41, 160–62. *See also* Cantophone; City of SARS (film); Golden Chicken 2 (film); Project 1:99 (film)

SARS jokes, 79–80, 236–37, 240; background to, 88–91; capaciousness and flexibility of, 88; Chinese New Year text greetings, 91; community building performed by, 88; death-by-SARS, 85; as elusive and replicable, 80; epidemic chatter function of, 86, 88, 89, 91; fanfiction, 106–9; feminist queer subtext, 108; folk recipes (parodic pseudomedical ditties), 99–100; government promotion of, 84–85; greetings, 93–97; mimic poems, 101–5; new subgenres, 87, 92, 93, 97, 99, 106; nonpartisan, 80, 86–92; parodic pseudomedical ditties, 99–100; political, and politics of, 82–86; state appropriation of, 85–86; sweet-talk messages, 97–98; taxonomy of, 82; timeline of, 91; trivial and hackneyed, 88; as type of mass culture, 80; as uncommoditized ephemera, 80; as "weapons of the weak," 81; "What the Party Has Failed to Do, SARS Has Succeeded," 82; *wo feidian* and *feidian* (atypical pneumonia), 87–88, 249–50n63. *See also* humor; Laughing at SARS (Petroleum Industry Press)

"SARS Prevention Song," 99

SARS romances, 33–76, 245n5; affect ordinariness in, 33–36, 33–37; criticism of communist regime in, 41–43; and gender politics, 41, 56–59; postcrisis optimism in, 39; sexual agency of women in, 37–39; ugly feelings in, 35–36, 50–53, 75. *See also* literary fiction; SARS Bride (Chen); *Shanghai Strangers* (Chen); *Wuhan Diary* (Fang)

Science, 181

Sedgwick, Eve, 24, 26, 120. *See also* "nonce taxonomies"; "paranoid reading"

sex trafficking, 69–71

sexual agency, 37–39

sex work, 144–45; airport conceit, 150–51; *bak gu* (northern mainland women), 149–50; eras of, 147–49; nightclub dance girls, 147–48; one-woman operations, 154

Shanghai: 1920s farce culture, 97; during SARS, 37–38

Shanghai Strangers (Chen), 29, 37–39, 62

Shaw Brothers productions, 158

Shi, Nansum, 131

Shih, Shu-mei, 122–23. *See also* Sinophone

Shilts, Randy, 198

Shiwan People's Hospital, 185

Shi Yan Wu Tian, 245–46n21

Shum, John Kin-fun, 129

Shum, Lydia Din-ha (Fei-Fei), 132

The Silent Killer: SARS (film), 200

Sina (news portal), 40, 78

Singapore, 28, 31; indigenous traditions, 235–36; influenza outbreak (1918), 235, 237; Ministry of Information, Communications and the Arts, 223–24; open-air food markets, 182; popular literature of, 235; SARS outbreak, 216–33; *True Singapore Ghost Stories*, 233–37; urban demolition and redevelopment policy, 236; World War II memories, 235. *See also* Mok, Esther

Sino-British Joint Declaration, 124–25

sinophobia, 3, 10, 17–18; during COVID-19, 200; parading of during pandemic

crises, 10; "wet markets," focus on, 31, 111, 182

Sinophone, 122–23

sinophone media, 3, 16, 24

Siu, Helen, 119

slow death, 20, 55, 127, 190

slow violence, 127

small humor, 30, 73, 81, 93–97; and COVID-19, 110; familiar literary devices as shared comfort, 95–96; as good-humored, 94; socius, concern with, 30, 94

smallpox management, 12–13

Snow.Wolf.Lake (musical), 169

sociality: lateral, 23; maximal, 25; microsociality, 78; professional female, 61; toward epistemologies of, 19–28; tyranny of politics without, 76. *See also* humor; prosociality; SARS jokes

social justice thought, 19, 26–27

social problems, endemic, 68–73

socius: affable community, imagined, 94, 105; and local films, 121; small humor's concern with, 30, 94

Soderbergh, Steven, 142

sonic cultures, 28, 128, 172. *See also* Cantophone; Cantopop

sousveillance, 75–76

South China Morning Post, 186, 192

sovereignty, affective, 26, 35, 76

species barrier, 12

species extinction discourse, 175–76

Spielberg, Steven, 117

Spillover (Quammen), 192

Spring Festival (2003), 78

state: appropriation of SARS jokes, 85–86, 91–93; co-optation of Mok's experience, 223; co-optation of traditional Chinese medicine, 100; culture of secrecy and surveillance, 204; deployments of power, 8; "logic of a total surveillance," 223; necropolitics of, 49; and timeline of SARS information, 88–89

stateless peoples, 126

state of exception, 8, 15, 134; alternatives to, 55, 64; biomedical, 44–45, 50–52

298 INDEX

Stop AAPI Hate, 4

The Storm That Tests the Grass (Guangdong People's Publishing House), 68

Straits Times (Singapore), 220–24

subempire, 31, 123–24, 128, 145. *See also* Chen, Kuan-Hsing

Such Is This World@sars.come (Hu), 29, 39–59, 62–63, 190, 212, 239; animal and the internet as themes in, 51; censored Beijing edition, 40, 46–48, 80, 245–46n21; Chinese versus Western reviewers, 56–57; English translation, 40, 245n21; female bonding in, 54–55; gendered reception of, 56–59; intellectual complicity with party-state in, 45–49; isolation ward conflated with prison, 48–51; missing body, metaphor of, 43–50, 55; online versions, 40, 245–46n21; redomestication of women in, 56–57, 62–63; resilience in, 52–53, 57, 64; romance and domesticity in, 51–56; sense of terror in, 43–51; ugly feelings in, 50–53; uneventful ending, 55

suicide: of celebrities, 115–16, 117, 126, 172; in comic films, 136–42, 160–62; economic, 139, 162; in humorous poems, 101; ideation and survivors' guilt, 229

"superinfector" label, 220–22, 226–27, 229

"superspreader" concept: in anglophone writing, 197–201; as discursive construct, 198–200, 208; flaws in, 207–8; and gender, 216–18; "hyperinfectious" theory, 199, 201, 207–8, 218; outbreaks that never were, 214–16, 218–19; public dissension around, 221–22; Typhoid Mary comparisons, 217, 218; in WHO official language, 218. *See also* Liu Jianlun; Mok, Esther

survival, 1, 34; attitude required for, 101; in capitalist terms, 46; collaborative, 191; and disability activism, 232–33; everyday practices of, 25, 49, 52, 55, 74, 80–81, 97; of first patients, 185, 188, 190–92, 194, 204–5; and guilt, 229; of Hong Kong cinema industry, 177; Hong Kong spirit of, 30, 113, 120, 124, 127–30, 133, 135, 146, 152, 154, 158, 163; and humor, 101, 104, 110; as process of corporeal maintenance, 190; reinvention of new idioms of the political, 21, 55, 80; scarcity economy of, 95; and sex work, 149; subaltern, and endemic violence, 68–73; techno-orientalism as technology of, 28, 217; threats to in bio-orientalist crisis discourse, 11–12; translated into healing service, 232–33. *See also* microagency

Su Shi, 102–5

sweet-talk messages, 97–98

Taishanese people, 3

Taiwan, 123, 125

A Tale of Two Esthers (film), 226–33

talk radio, 252n45

Tan Tock Seng Hospital (Singapore), 218–2220, 225–26

Tang, Xiaobing, 22, 65, 74, 83, 120, 192. *See also* dissidence hypothesis

Tao Dongfeng, 83, 104

Tea Cup in a Storm (Cheng), 252n45

techno-orientalism, 28, 217

television, 67, 129; ATV, 175; Cantopop songs in, 168–69; film actors and themes drawn from, 136–37, 158; TVB, 125–26, 136, 158, 174; variety shows, 79, 132

Television and Entertainment Licensing Authority (Hong Kong), 129

Teng, Teresa, 105

Ten Years (film), 122

terror, 44–51, 69, 192; sense of, 44–47

Thatcher, Margaret, 124

"Theses for Theory in a Time of Crisis" (Davis and Catlin), 21, 112

Thornber, Karen, 27

Thousand Character Classic (Confucian primer), 99

Three Character Classic (Confucian primer), 99

Tiananmen massacre (1989), 29, 45–48, 54, 57, 149

Time, 10, 12

Tin, Kristal Yui-nei, 161

To, Chapman Man-chat, 142–43, 161
To, Johnnie Kei-fung, 132, 133
Toronto, SARS outbreak, 215–16
totalitarianism, 40, 44–49; biopolitical model of, 44–45; isolation ward conflated with prison, 48–49; lack of artistic tradition, 47–48; persistence of, 42, 44; terror as key instrument of, 47
toxins, metaphorical, 161
travel restrictions, 9, 114
trickster, 104–5
True Singapore Ghost Stories (TSGS) (Lee), 32, 233–37
Trump, Donald, 200
"Try a Little Kindness" editorial (Quek), 221
Tsang, Eric Chi-wai, 117–19, 121, 137, 160
Tse, Chi-Kwan, 216
Tsing, Anna, 190, 191
Tsui Hark, 129, 130, 131
Twenty-First Century Plague (Abraham), 192
2046 (film), 166–67
Typhoid Mary comparisons, 217, 218

ugly feelings, 25–26, 35–36, 50–51, 75; over internet, 52–53
underclasses, postcolonial, 157–65
underdog comeback trope, 31, 124, 127, 128, 130, 135, 143–44, 150, 155–65; "golden chicken spirit," 155–56; local lineage of, 136, 144
United States: conspiracy theories about origin of COVID-19, 180; as COVID epicenter, 14; demonization of Chinese by health officials, 13; no SARS fatalities in, 13; passivity toward COVID, 18; racial contours of COVID outbreak, 15; subversive and satirical humor attributed to, 84
unprecedentedness and urgency, 7–9, 11; focus on China, 50–51; and Hong Kong Cantophone, 30; toughness, emphasis on, 9
Urbani, Carlo, 212–14
US Army Medical Research Institute of Infectious Diseases (Fort Detrick), 181

Vancouver, SARS outbreak, 215–16
Veg, Sebastian, 57
Vietnam, 213
violence, slow, 127
visual culture, 23–24, 122, 164, 168, 172. *See also* entertainment industry, Hong Kong

Wai Kar-fai, 132
Wald, Priscilla, 11–12, 28, 198
Wang, Yuting, 75
We Pictures, 176
Wen Jiabao, 90
West: and "amiable" humor, 97; China as totalitarian other of, 192; "softness" attributed to, 9–10
"wet markets," 31, 111, 181–82, 193, 204. *See also* animals
Whyte, Kyle, 7–8, 10, 14, 20, 26–27, 50, 112, 120
Wilson, David Sloan, 6
Wong Chak (Alfonso Wong), 131
Wong, Dayo Tze-wah, 131
Wong, Faye, 105
Wong, Felix, 173
Wong, Jan, 192–93
Wong Jim, 136, 171
Wong Kar-wai, 129, 166–67
World Health Assembly, 9, 16
World Health Organization (WHO), 9, 91, 114, 163; access to Guangdong, 199; "superspreader" terminology used by, 218; and Urbani, 212–13; visit to Pang, 188
Wu Fung, Bowie, 132
Wuhan, China, 42; Li Wenliang honored by, 74–75; lockdown, 14, 73–76, 110, 240
Wuhan Central Hospital, 73–74, 109–10
Wuhan Diary (Fang), 42, 73–76; as performance of sousveillance, 75–76
Wuhan Institute of Virology, 180
Wuhan lab leak conspiracy, 181, 204
The Wuhan Lockdown (Yang), 240

Xiao, Hui Faye, 56–57, 65
Xie Xiao Zhen, 2–7, 29

Xiu Xiu: The Sent Down Girl (Chen), 245n15

Xu, Fang, 17–18, 182

Yamamoto, Rick, 227

Yan, Geling, 245n15

Yan Lianke, 246n36

Yang, Guobin, 109, 240

Yang, Jeff, 127

Yapp, Hentyle, 24

yellow peril ideologies, 13, 196–97, 203–4

yewei (wild animals), consumption of, 189

youmo (humor), 86, 96–97

Yuen, James Sai-sang, 142–43

Zeng Bihua, 59–60

Zhan, Mei, 10–11, 181, 184

Zhang, Hong, 65, 78–79, 81, 82–83, 85, 87, 91

Zhang, Xudong, 80–81

Zhang, Yunpeng, 17–18, 182

Zhang Yimou, 106

Zhong Nanshan, 187

Zhou, Kate, 83

Zhu, Ping, 84, 92